PHONOLOGY: DEVELOPMENT AND DISORDERS

PHONOLOGY: DEVELOPMENT AND DISORDERS

Mehmet Yavaş, Ph.D.
Florida International University
Miami, Florida

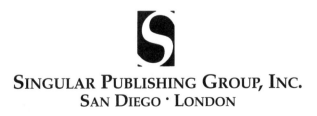

SINGULAR PUBLISHING GROUP, INC.
SAN DIEGO · LONDON

Singular Publishing Group, Inc.
401 West "A" Street, Suite 325
San Diego, California 92101-7904

Singular Publishing Ltd.
19 Compton Terrace
London, N1 2UN, UK

Singular Publishing Group, Inc., publishes textbooks, clinical manuals, clinical reference books, journals, videos, and multimedia materials on speech-language pathology, audiology, otorhinolaryngology, special education, early childhood, aging, occupational therapy, physical therapy, rehabilitation, counseling, mental health, and voice. For your convenience, our entire catalog can be accessed on our website at **http//www.singpub.com**. Our mission to provide you with materials to meet the daily challenges of the everchanging health care/educational environment will remain on course if we are in touch with you. In that spirit, we welcome your feedback on our products. Please telephone (**1-800-521-8545**), fax (**1-800-774-8398**), or e-mail (**singpub@mail.cerfnet.com**) your comments and requests to us.

Typeset in 10/12 Palatino Light by So Cal Graphics
Printed in the United States of America by Bang Printing

Library of Congress Cataloging-in-Publication Data

Yavas, Mehmet S.
    Phonology: development and disorders / Mehmet Yavas
        p. cm.
    ISBN 1–56593–702–3 (pbk. : alk. paper)
    1. Articulation disorders.   2. Phonetics.
    [DNLM: 1. Phonetics.   2. Phonation.   3. Speech Disorders.   P 217
Y35i 1998}
RC424.7.,Y38   1998
616.85'5—dc21
DNLM/DLC   97–42817
for Library of Congress   CIP

CONTENTS

PREFACE

This book is an attempt to respond to the need for an introductory book on phonology for speech-language pathology students and people who are interested in applied phonology. A delicate balance should be reached between material coming from a technical field and its use in applied fields. On the one hand, one wants to be faithful to the principles and methods of analysis of the technical field with no distortions and, on the other hand, one would like to make the material comprehensible and useful to people in applied fields without making the presentation impossible to follow. I have had the opportunity to work with students from diverse fields during my teaching career. To linguistics students, I have always tried to emphasize the relevance and use of different models of phonology in the real world. I have used real-world situations such as phonological development, disorders, bilingualism, and second-language acquisition in evaluating competing models and descriptions. To students coming from programs such as TESOL (ESL) and/or speech-language pathology, my goal has always been to show the importance of linguistic knowledge (in this particular case phonology) for their fields of study or practice. My repeated message to them has been that remediation that is related to sound systems cannot be achieved without a good grasp of phonology. This might require more detailed and technical knowledge about language than they wished for, but results cannot be obtained in remediation without it.

Dealing with students with these diverse interests and backgrounds has taught me to look at matters from varying angles, and this book has benefitted from these interactions. I hope the end product meets the goals of addressing the concerns and the interests of the individuals who come from different but related fields.

I would like to thank my students who have helped me by asking questions and making comments that made me think and rethink about the field of phonology and its relevance to remediation. Special thanks go to Cynthia Core whose enthusiastic and tireless efforts in reading and commenting on the manuscript have resulted in significant improvement of the text. Finally, I am indebted to the two reviewers from Singular Publishing Group for their comments on the earlier draft of this text. Their constructive comments are deeply appreciated. Needless to say, all imperfections that remain are solely my responsibility.

NOTE TO
THE INSTRUCTOR

Anyone who writes a text on phonology has the hard task of deciding on the organization of the material. This concerns the question of whether the material should be ordered chronologically or presented on the basis of topic unity. In this book, the former principle is followed. The basic reason is that each model is built on the previous one and it is easier to follow the text given the background of preceding chapters. This way, phonemics was followed by generative phonology, which in turn was followed by natural phonology. The topics discussed in Chapters 9 and 10 (syllables, feet, feature geometry, and underspecification) are the products of the last two decades and thus come later in the book. I have no doubts that some instructors might prefer to follow the topic unity principle rather than chronological ordering in their teaching. This should not create any problems, as some minor adjustments will yield the desired result. For example, combining Chapter 4 and Chapter 10 gives the opportunity to deal with features as a single topic, if desired. Another reorganizational matter that might be thought of concerns the material in Chapter 7. Certain sections of this chapter may be deemed very complex and can be omitted for students of speech and language pathology. Also, the first and second sections may be added to Chapter 2, and the instructor might want to incorporate the fourth section of Chapter 7 into Chapter 9, and the fifth section into Chapter 6. These are a few points that come to mind in attempts to reorganize the material and make the text more profitable. These points give the instructor flexibility while not disturbing the effectiveness of the text.

As for many of the exercises, there is no rigid requirement to work only in relation to the model presented in the chapter that contains them. In particular, the solutions using data-based material can and should be attempted with different models. After all, the same data would lend itself to different interpretation by different methods of analysis.

Chapter 1

INTRODUCTION

Phonology is an area of linguistics that is concerned with the sounds of language. Naturally, once we start talking about sounds, another area of study, phonetics, comes to mind as well.

Then, the reasonable question to ask is: What is the difference between these two areas? Although the dividing line between the two areas is not clearly defined, we can attempt the following formulation: The human vocal apparatus can produce a wide variety of sounds, and this is the concern of phonetics. On the other hand, a small number of these sounds are used in any given language to construct its words and sentences. It is generally stated that phonetics is the study of sounds as phenomena in the physical world and the physiological, anatomical properties of human beings who make these sounds, whereas phonology is concerned with the function, behavior, and organization of them. Thus, in studying phonology, linguists look at the way speech sounds form systems and patterns in human language.

PHONOLOGICAL KNOWLEDGE

One of the major goals of phonologists is to discover universals or universal tendencies of sound systems of languages. This is attempted by studying the commonly occurring patterns in phonological inventories, phonological acquisition, and phonological changes. In a phonological description of a language, we try to account for the phonological knowledge of a native speaker of that language. In other words, what does a speaker know about the phonology of his or her language?

Phonological knowledge allows a speaker to do a variety of things. To start with, it gives one the ability to judge whether a given form is a possible word in his or her language. For example, in English, we can start a word with one, two, or three consonants. This is exemplified in *ray, tray,* and *stray.* However, there are regularities and restrictions concerning this sequencing, and not every consonant or consonants are allowed to appear in this position. For example, we cannot start a word with the consonant sound that appears at the end of the word *sing* (phonetically /ŋ/). For two-consonant words, the possibilities are more limited. Although combinations such as *pl, tr,* and *fl* are allowed (e.g., *play, train, flu*), we cannot start a word with clusters like *ts, pf,* or *mb.* The restriction on three-consonant clusters are even greater. In such sequences, the first consonant must be an *s,* the second *p, t,* or *k,* and the third is chosen from among *r, l, w, y* (e.g., *splash, script*). These regularities allow us to judge whether a given form can be a possible English word. Thus, although we do not, at present, have words such as *plerg* or *strun* in English, we judge these as possible combinations. The judgment, however, will be entirely different if we are asked to evaluate forms such as *dzol* or *fmit.* These restrictions are not possible due to the impossibility of pronouncing these strings. In fact, many combinations that are not allowed in English are part of other language systems.

Phonological knowledge also allows us to create accurate morphological forms in adding appropriate endings. For example, in plural formation we have different sounds used for the ending. While *cat* becomes *cats* (with a final sound phonetically [s]), the plural of *dog* is realized with a different sound, [z]. To test whether this behavior is a memorized reaction to forms like *cat* and *dog* or an internalized phonological reality, we can attempt to pluralize some nonoccurring forms. For example, if we are asked to pluralize a new form such as *glak,* we quickly respond with *glaks* (with an [s] sound). If, on the other hand, the form given is *glar,* then the response will be a [z], similar to the ending we give to *dog*[z]. Note that this behavior is totally unrehearsed and no memorization is involved. This particular example demonstrates another thing that taps into the knowledge of the speaker. The fact that we make the plural of *glar* as *glar*[z] should not suggest that, in English, the sound combination *rs* cannot occur at the end of a word, as we have words such as *course, horse, source,* and so on. The combination is allowed as long as *s* does not have an independent meaning. When the plurality is marked, *r* must be followed by [z]. Thus, although a native speaker of English will not reject new words such as *smurs,* or *flars* where the final *s* does not denote plurality, she or he will reject a plural like *glar*[s].

Another situation in which native speakers' phonological knowledge is manifested is the area of speech errors such as spoonerisms. This can be illustrated by moving the initial consonant of the first word of *scotch tape* to the beginning of the second word. This results in a combination that will be pronounced [kʰ ʌtʃ step]. Although meaningless, this sequence is phonologically perfect, and it shows the instant adjustments made. In English, *p, t, k* sounds (as in the initial position of *pill, till,* and *kill*) are produced with an extra puff of air that is called aspiration (shown by a raised h [pʰ] in phonetic transcription). However, this is restricted to the beginning position of a stressed syllable, and in other positions these sounds are unaspirated. In the above example, the target *scotch tape* (phonetically [skʌtʃtʰep] has an unaspirated [k] in the first word, because it is not in the syllable-initial position, and an aspirated [tʰ] in the second, because it is in the syllable-initial position). When the speech error is committed and the first consonant of the first word is moved to the initial position of the second word, the first word begins with a [kʰ], as it is in the syllable-initial position. The moving of *s* from its original position to the beginning of the second word removes the *t* from its original position and thus eliminates the aspiration. The unconscious knowledge of the speaker is responsible for these instant adjustments. The end product is semantically empty but phonologically perfect.

The phonological knowledge of his or her own language enables the speaker to differentiate between an acceptable and an unacceptable variation. This relates to a situation in which the pronunciation of a heard word is different from that of the speaker. For example, a word such as *rental* can be pronounced differently by speakers of American English. The variations include the change in the vowel of the first syllable (it could be [ɛ] as in *bet*, or [ɪ] as in *bit*), and the elimination of *t* at the beginning of the second syllable. Thus, we can have [rɛntl̩], [rɪntl̩], [rɛnl̩] or [rɪnl̩]. All of these forms will be acceptable, as the variations are within native limits. The variation concerning the two different vowels in the first syllable of *rental* that is judged acceptable cannot be transferred to other words freely. While it is possible to find the same variation in the first vowels of *sense* and *generally*, replacing [ɛ] with [ɪ] will not be acceptable in *pet, fresh,* or *bare*. In short, the listener knows that the vowel variation in question can occur only before nasal consonants like [n].

Similarly, the deletion of *t* in *rental* [rɛnl̩] will be judged normally acceptable in many other words such as *dental, winter, enter,* and so on, but will immediately be judged as nonnative in a word such as *contain*. This shows that a speaker of American English has the phonological knowledge that allows him or her to accept the deletion of *t* after an *n* in an unstressed syllable. Because the deletion of *t* in *contain* occurs in a stressed syllable and thus violates the regularity, it will not be judged as an acceptable variation.

The reality of the native language phonology is also well reflected in foreign language learning. Many pronunciation errors made in the attempt to speak a foreign language reveal a person's native phonological patterns. For example, the expected (and indeed observed) erroneous productions of the final consonant of the word *Bill* will be different by speakers of Spanish and Portuguese. Although these two languages are very closely related, the different phonological patterns would render the target English final *l* in *Bill* differently mispronounced. Spanish speaker's off-target pronunciation is due to the different quality of the *l* sound in Spanish. In American English, this sound is produced with the tip of the tongue touching the area behind the upper teeth (alveolar ridge) while the back of the tongue is raised towards the back part of the upper surface of the mouth (soft palate). The Spanish *l* does not have any raising of the back of the tongue and results in a very different quality. The Portuguese situation is somewhat different. Although the *l* in the beginning position is similar to that of English, in the syllable-final position it is pronounced as [w]. As a result, whereas a word like *lake* is not problematic for a speaker of Portuguese, *Bill* is pronounced as [bɪw].

APPLIED PHONOLOGY

Besides revealing information about the universal properties of sound systems and accounting for the phonological knowledge of the speaker of a language, phonological description has many practical applications. It should be obvious from the discussion of foreign accents that the field of foreign language teaching makes good use of phonological analysis. Learners' errors, whether they are caused by the conflicts of the patterns of their native language and those of the languages they are learning or are the result of some universally determined factors, reveal systematicness. Phonological analysis helps greatly in determining the regularities of error patterns. This determination is indispensable in the preparation of remedial material.

Another field in which phonological analysis is vital is speech-language pathology. Here, speech patterns of individuals with disabilities are compared to and contrasted with those who have developed normally. Thus, we need a good description of normal acquisition to make any judgments on the patterns exhibited by the subjects with disabilities.

In addition to these two areas, applications of phonology are also found in the training of actors and spies and in forensic work by the police.

PHONOLOGY IN REMEDIATION

Three groups of people especially draw our attention when we deal with applied phonology: children acquiring their native language, foreign language learners, and individuals with speech-language disorders. What these three groups share is their deviance in production when compared to the ambient language (the norm). Although the productions we hear from the members of these groups are, to varying degrees, in disagreement with the target norm they attempt, the renditions are not haphazard. This is the starting point of the phonologist. In other words, one takes the view that, in all of these populations, productions have underlying systematicity. The motto is: "There is order in disorder." In fact, this is the only path for the investigator to follow, because the contrary assumption (i.e., considering the productions to be chaotic with no systematicity) results in attributing to an individual with a disability or disadvantage a rather superhuman characteristic: the capacity to be able to store a vast amount of information that has no systematicity. Once we recognize that such a view is untenable, the only alternative is to think that the productions of these groups are different from the ambient language, but nevertheless are systematic. Thus, the task of the investigator is to discover this systematicity.

If our purpose is to apply phonological principles to intervention, normally developing children can be singled out and excluded from the rest, as they do not require any remediation. Their productions agree with the ambient language when the time comes in their developmental timetable. This leaves us with the individuals in the other two groups, whose productions cannot be expected to agree with the ambient language without remediation. Obviously, the characteristics of the two groups, foreign language learners and individuals with phonological disorders, are not identical. The members of the former group have problems in their productions of a foreign language, whereas the individuals in the latter group have difficulties in productions of their native language. Although the difference between these two groups is obvious, one also can find a commonality between them: Both groups require remediation.

Speech-language pathologists and teachers of foreign language who work with these populations have recognized that any attempt at remediation requires a detailed phonological profile of the client. The importance of an accurate phonological profile for remediation of an individual has long been recognized in the field of second language phonology. Starting in the 1940s, using the structuralist framework, linguists worked with comparisons between the two languages of the learner to predict the difficulties and prepare material for remedial teaching. Lado's (1957) *Linguistics Across Cultures* and Fries' (1945) *Teaching and Learning English as a Foreign Language* are the two landmarks of this movement. Linguistically based activity of the same magnitude in the field of speech-pathology had to wait until the publication of Ingram's (1976) classic, *Phonological Disability in Children*. This book, which set the stage for the application of phonological principles to clinical populations, was a precursor to an explosion of phonologically based studies of disordered sound systems over the last 30 years. A field called **Clinical Phonology**, which is concerned with the application of phonological investigation to speech-language pathology, has emerged. Assessment, diagnosis, and treatment, which are three aspects of clinical work, rely crucially on phonological analysis.

Individuals who require remediation may belong to one of three categories: (a) those whose deviance from the norm may be phonetic, (b) those whose deviance from the norm may be both phonetic and phonological, and (c) those whose deviance from the norm may be phonological. To exemplify (a), we can think of a situation in which the individual's productions are not different from the target functionally, but the sounds are not exactly the same. For example, in English the production of the first sound of the word *take* involves the touching of the tip of the tongue to the alveolar ridge, and the sound is classified as alveolar. In Romance languages, on the other hand, the sound that is represented by the same orthographic letter *t* is produced somewhat differently by touching the tip of the tongue to the back of the upper teeth. Thus, in languages such as Spanish and Portuguese, this sound is described as dental. Therefore, a speaker of one of these languages may have a phonetic problem in which the target alveolar is pronounced as dental when she or he attempts English. Although this example is from foreign language learning, it should be mentioned that it also could easily occur in an individual with a disability in his or her own native language.

The situation given in (b) involves errors in articulation as well as the differences in the sound system of the client. For example, we may have a case in which English targets demanded for underlined portions of <u>th</u>in, e<u>th</u>er, and too<u>th</u> are realized with a dental *t* sound which is a more forward articulation than the regular English *t* sound. In this case, we have a situation in which the individual misses the target for *th* phonologically (because *th* and *t* contrast in English) by replacing it with a *t*, while at the same time he or she does not articulate the *t* exactly like the ambient language.

Finally, (c) refers to a situation, for example, in which the *th* targets (e.g., t<u>h</u>in) are realized as *t*, and *s* targets (e.g., <u>s</u>ick) are produced as *th*. If an individual makes the substitutions *thin* → *tin*, *sick* → *thick*, while correctly pronouncing *miss* and *tall*, we would have the following correspondences:

Target   Realization

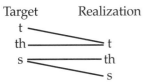

In such a case, the mismatches are not phonetic in that the sounds in question are not misarticulated; the individual can pronounce the two targets *th* and *s*. The errors are due to faulty organization of the phonology. The use of phonological principles and methods will be needed for diagnosis and remediation planning for individuals who belong to groups (b) and (c).

Once we establish the fact that the deviance is phonological, the exact nature and details have important implications for intervention. Successful remediation requires relevant treatment/teaching planning, and this, in turn, requires accurate diagnosis of the problem. To arrive at an accurate diagnosis, we need a detailed phonological description of the system of the client; this is the client's phonological profile. To discover the regularities in the data, the professional or clinician needs a good grasp of phonology. Phonological descriptions used in establishing the profile of the client are based on different phonological models. Manuals prepared for phonological analyses use elements that are provided by phonological models. Articles and books written on phonological remediation also use the same elements. Thus, it is not hard to envision that, in order to be able to understand and apply phonological principles to remediation, a practitioner needs to be familiar with the concepts and models of phonology.

The need for phonological knowledge for professionals dealing with remediation has been made very clear during the last three decades. This is beautifully reflected in the following quote by Crystal (1984):

> Times have changed, with new training courses. A new generation of therapists has emerged who do not have to be convinced of the desirability or efficacy of clinical linguistic techniques. (p. 25)

Today, the issue debated seems to be just how comprehensive the phonological analysis of a client should be. The answer we would like to give is "as detailed as needed." This might encounter objection because many therapists contend that they have little time to allocate to evaluation before starting treatment. To this, Crystal (1984) has the most succinct answer: "If you want understanding, insight and remedial confidence, time must be spent. Such prizes are not glibly won" (p. 23). Crystal also states the trade-off elegantly:

> The question of time has to be seen in the long term, and weighed against the criteria of success . . . . A day devoted to linguistic analysis early on in a case may seem trivial by comparison with the overall amount of time devoted to a patient in subsequent months. And how much time might not be saved by a better distribution of time and resources in the early stages of assessment? (p. 24)

The field of phonology has witnessed significant changes during the last three decades. Different models of phonological analysis have different degrees of success and impact in the area of phonological remediation. A certain model may be more popular than others due to its notational simplicity and its greater use of data from developmental phonology. This, however, does not mean that it answers all the questions. Thus, to be able to evaluate alternative views and suggestions with respect to remediation, professionals should be equipped with knowledge of several models. It is with this belief that this book aims to present the essentials of both older and more recent models and their implications for remediation.

Chapter 2

PHONETICS

Phonology is the study of sound systems; however, this cannot be done without the raw material, **phonetics**, which is the study of speech sounds. The dependence of phonology on phonetics is such that the reliability of the phonological analysis is entirely dependent on the accuracy of the phonetic data. As a corollary, students and professionals who deal with individuals with phonological disability and remedial teaching (i.e., those who have to have a phonological profile of the subject they are dealing with) cannot go very far without some knowledge of phonetics.

During the transmission of a message by sound, a whole range of events takes place, and these events are the concern of the field of phonetics. The speaker encodes meaning into sounds using the articulatory organs; the study of how the sounds are produced is the subject matter of **articulatory phonetics**. The hearer perceives the message through auditory processes; the physical effects of the speech on the human ear is the study of **auditory phonetics**. Finally, the acoustic properties of the sound waves in the message are the concern of **acoustic phonetics**. Among the three, articulatory phonetics, which focuses on the human vocal apparatus and describes sounds in terms of their articulation in the vocal tract, has been by far the most studied. The main reasons for the preference of articulatory phonetics over the others are as follows: First, very little information is available about the workings of the ear and the brain in terms of speech perception, and this creates difficulties for the study of auditory phonetics. Second, the highly technical and, consequently, the not-so-accessible nature of acoustic phonetics makes this subject a very specialized study. These factors make articulatory phonetics the only candidate for introductory texts.

PHONETIC TRANSCRIPTION

Before we examine the details of how sounds are produced by speakers and how they can be classified according to their properties, we would like to make clear the need for a special alphabet for the description of sounds. As everyday users of language, we are accustomed to seeing language written down by regular orthography, the writing system of a language. In many instances the number of letters we see representing a word is indicative of the number of sounds there are in that particular word. For example, speakers of English can judge that the word *water* has five sounds as well as five letters; similarly, *dark* has four of each, and *cat* has three. However, this one-to-one correspondence of sound-to-letter relationship is not found in a great many words. For example, both *freight*, and *knife* have four sounds but seven and five letters, respectively; *fish* and *phone* have three sounds each, but more than three letters. This is only one example to show that orthography is not a reliable tool to represent the sounds of the language.

There are additional inadequacies of orthography in its ability to represent the spoken language. One of these refers to the situation in which the same sound is spelled using different letters, as in the following words: grease, key, week, scene, believe, icy, seize. The opposite is also true; we frequently find the same letter for different sounds, as in electric, electricity, electrician, or sick, resume, measure, or chip, character, Chicago. There are still other anomalies such as a single sound being represented by a combination of letters as in they, tough, appear, or cases in which a single letter represents more than one sound as in example, or union.

The above examples clearly show that an ideal one-to-one relationship between sound and letter in an alphabetic system does not exist. This situation is not unique to English, although languages do vary as to the degree of discrepancy they display between their orthographies and the sounds of the spoken language. To eliminate the consequences of using orthography to represent spoken language, professionals dealing with language (phoneticians, speech-language pathologists, language teachers, linguists) use a special set of symbols in their phonetic transcription in which one sound is represented by one symbol, and each symbol represents a single sound. Although the effort to devise a universal system for transcribing the sounds of speech goes back as far as the 16th century, the most well-known system was developed by the **International Phonetic Association (IPA)** in 1888 and was revised in 1989. Most books written by American linguists use a modified version of the IPA. The symbols used in this book, going along with the tradition of clinical phonology, are those from the revised version of the IPA alphabet unless otherwise noted.

We will start our examination of speech sounds with those of English and add sounds from other languages as they become relevant to the discussion. Tables 2–1 and 2–2 provide a listing of English speech sounds.

THE VOCAL TRACT

Each speech sound is produced differently because of the different combinations of articulators and places of articulation that are utilized. In describing how speech sounds are made, we start with the air that comes from the lungs, passes through the larynx where the vocal cords are situated, and then arrives at the vocal tract (the air passages above the larynx) where it is shaped into specific sounds. In the production of sounds, we generally move the articulators from the lower surface of the vocal tract toward those that form the upper surface. Figure 2–1 illustrates the vocal tract. Starting from the outer extreme, we see the familiar lips and teeth. Going to the upper surface, we find the alveolar ridge, which is the small bumpy area right behind the upper teeth. After this, we get to a larger bony area in the upper surface, the hard palate, behind which is a softer area at the back of the mouth, the soft palate, or velum. The soft palate is a movable organ, which opens or closes the passage that links or unlinks the pharynx to the nasal cavity by being raised or lowered, respectively. Finally, at the very back of the soft palate we see a small appendage that is called the uvula.

In the lower part of the mouth, behind the lower lip and teeth, we describe the different parts of the tongue which participate in the production of many different sounds. After the tip and the blade, we have the center, back, and root, which are situated opposite the hard palate, soft palate, and the back wall of the pharynx, respectively. Finally, we have the epiglottis, which is attached to the lower part of the root of the tongue.

Table 2–1. English consonants (non-IPA American usage is shown in parentheses).

Phonetic Symbol	Initial	Medial	Final
p	*p*ick	a*pp*ear	ca*p*
b	*b*ook	ro*b*in	ca*b*
t	*t*ake	a*t*tempt	ca*t*
d	*d*ay	cra*d*le	pa*d*
k	*c*at	so*c*ket	ca*k*e
g	*g*et	a*g*o	do*g*
f	*f*ish	ele*ph*ant	cou*gh*
v	*v*ase	ri*v*er	ca*v*e
θ	*th*ink	au*th*or	fif*th*
ð	*th*at	fa*th*er	tee*the*
s	*s*it	Ja*s*on	pa*ss*
z	*z*oo	pu*zz*le	buse*s*
ʃ (š)	*sh*oe	wa*sh*ing	ru*sh*
ʒ (ž)	_____	mea*s*ure	gara*ge*
h	*h*ome	a*h*ead	_____
tʃ (č)	*ch*ip	na*t*ure	tea*ch*
dʒ (ǰ)	*j*ail	bu*dg*et	fu*dge*
m	*m*oon	cru*m*ble	sa*m*e
n	*n*o	bo*n*y	ru*n*
ŋ	_____	fi*n*ger	ri*ng*
j (y)	*y*es	be*y*ond	bo*y*
w	*w*eek	a*w*ake	co*w*
ɹ (r)	*r*ed	Mo*rr*is	ca*r*
l	*l*ake	a*l*arm	pa*l*e

Table 2–2. English vowels and diphthongs.[1]

Phonetic Symbol	Initial	Medial	Final
i	*e*at	b*ee*t	k*ey*
ɪ	*i*t	b*i*t	_____
e	*a*te	b*ai*t	b*ay*
ɛ	*e*gg	b*e*t	_____
æ	*a*pple	b*a*t	_____
ʌ	*o*ven	b*u*t	_____
ə	*a*mong	alph*a*bet	sof*a*
a	*a*rch	c*a*r	sp*a*
ɔ	*au*to	wr*o*ng	j*aw*
o	*o*cean	b*oa*t	g*o*
ʊ	_____	f*oo*t	_____
u	*oo*ze	b*oo*t	sh*oe*
aj (ay)	*I*	b*i*te	p*ie*
ɔj (ɔy)	*oi*l	b*oi*l	t*oy*
aw	*ow*l	l*ou*d	c*ow*

DESCRIPTION AND ARTICULATION OF SOUNDS

Voicing

When speech sounds are produced, air is set in motion. The supply of air comes from the lungs, but the sound source is in the larynx where we have the vocal cords. As the air is pushed from the lungs up the trachea, it passes through the space between the vocal cords, the **glottis**. The vocal cords can be positioned in a number of ways, and the different configurations of the vocal cords are responsible for different types of sounds.

When the vocal cords are apart, as in normal breathing, the air passes freely through the glottis. Sounds produced with this configuration of the vocal cords are called **voiceless**. However, when the vocal cords are brought close together, the air passing through them creates vibration. Sounds produced with this configuration are called **voiced**. It is important to stress that the vocal cord vibration is not a consciously controlled muscular movement; rather, the vocal cords are positioned fairly close-

1. Lips
2. Teeth
3. Alveolar ridge
4. Hard palate
5. Soft palate (velum)
6. Uvula
7. Pharnyx
8. Epiglottis
9. Glottis
10. Tip of tongue
11. Blade of tongue
12. Back of tongue
13. Root of tongue

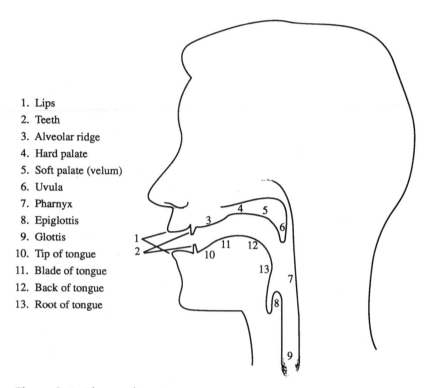

Figure 2–1. The vocal tract.

ly together and the passing airstream from the lungs creates a suction effect and pulls the cords together. This is called the Bernoulli effect. As soon as the cords are together, the suction is no longer there and they come apart. As soon as the cords are apart, the Bernoulli effect is reinitiated and pulls them together again. This quick cycle of opening and closing of the cords is the vibration in voiced sounds.

To observe the difference between voiced and voiceless sounds, try the following: Say the word *sue* and then say the word *zoo* and concentrate on the first sounds of these words; in the second but not the first word you should hear initial vibration at the beginning of the word. If you cannot feel the difference in the vocal cord activity, place your index finger on your Adam's apple while saying the first sounds of these two words alternately (*sss zzzzzz sssssss zzzzzz*). You will notice a buzz while you are saying the first sound of the word *zoo* which is absent from the first sound of the word *sue*. This is the effect of the vocal cord vibration in the voiced sound. The same can be felt by placing both index fingers in both ears while alternating between [s] and [z].

The two configurations of the vocal cords are relevant in the description of sounds in all languages. However, there are two additional states of the glottis that are important in the description of other languages.

The first of these is called **creaky voice** (sometimes called laryngealized), in which the arytenoid cartilages at the front of the glottis are tightly together, and the vocal cords vibrate at the other end, creating a low-pitched sound. Many Chadic languages (e.g., Hausa of Nigeria and Southern Niger) use laryngealization to make a change in meaning when used in opposition to a regularly voiced sound.

The other state of the glottis is responsible for the sounds that are called **murmur** (also called breathy voice) in which the vocal cords are apart at the back, while they vibrate at the front portions. Hindi and many other languages spoken in India have murmured stops.

Consonant Articulation

In the formation of consonants, the airflow through the vocal tract is obstructed by the placement of the tongue or by lip configurations. Consonants are classified according to the place and manner of this obstruction. Figure 2–2 shows the vocal tract with the different places of articulation.

Places of Articulation

Bilabial: Sounds that are made with the two lips such as the English [p, b, m] in pick, boy, and moon are called bilabials. In addition to the stops and nasals that are exhibited by the English examples languages may have voiceless and voiced bilabial fricatives ([ɸ, β] of Ewe of West Africa). The affricate [pf] that is found in German (*pferd*) "horse" is a bilabial stop released into a labiodental fricative.

Labiodental: Sounds that are made with the lower lip and upper teeth as in the English fricatives [f, v] in feel, and veal are called labiodentals. Bilabials and labiodentals are together called **labials**.

Dental: Sounds that are made with the tip or blade of the tongue and upper front teeth, as in the English [θ, ð] thin, and that are dentals. For many speakers, these sounds are articulated by placing the tongue in be-

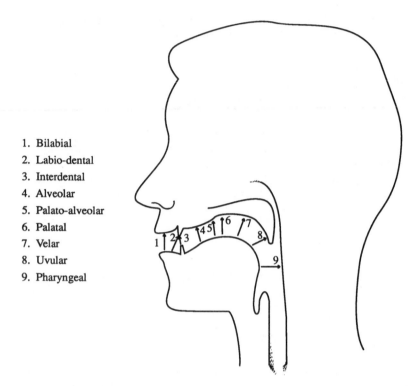

Figure 2–2. Places of articulation.

tween the upper and lower teeth and, thus, are known as **interdentals**. Dental stops in which the tongue tip touches the teeth are found in many languages including Spanish (*dia*, "day") and Portuguese (*dar*, "to give").

Alveolar: Sounds that are made with the tip or the blade of the tongue and the alveolar ridge as exemplified by the English stops, fricatives, nasals, and laterals [t, d, s, z, n, l] as in take, day, sake, zoo no, and lake are called alveolars. All of these sounds are very common in many languages.

Palato-alveolar: Sounds that are made with the blade of the tongue and the back of the alveolar ridge, as in the English fricatives and affricates [ʃ, ʒ, tʃ, dʒ] in shoe, measure, cheap, and jam, are referred to as palato-alveolars.

Retroflex: Sounds that are made by curling the tip of the tongue up and back toward the back part of the alveolar ridge, as in the English [ɹ] in rain are called retroflex sounds. Retroflex stops [t̪, d̪], nasal [n̪], and fricatives [ṣ, ẓ] are found in many languages spoken in India including Tamil and Malayalam.[2]

Because the constriction for both palato-alveolars and retroflexes is made at the back of the alveolar ridge, Ladefoged (1993) suggested that the differentiation between these two groups of sounds can also be made by using the terms **apical** (with the tip of the tongue) and **laminal** (with the blade of the tongue). Looked at this way, retroflexes are considered apical postalveolar, whereas palato-alveolars are laminal postalveolars.

Palatal: Sounds that are made with the front of the tongue articulating against the hard palate, as in the English [j] in yes are called palatals. Palatal stops [c, ɟ] , although not very common, are found in different languages (e.g., Hungarian, Basque, Turkish), whereas the nasal [ñ] is quite common (e.g., French, Spanish, Portuguese, Vietnamese). Also found are palatal fricatives, which can be voiceless [ç] (Irish, Bengali, Norwegian) or, less frequently, voiced [ʝ], (Greenlandic, Margi).

Velar: Sounds that are made with the back of the tongue articulating against the soft palate (velum), as exemplified by the English stops [k, and g], and the nasal [ŋ] in keep, go, and sing are velars. Velar fricatives (voiceless [x], and voiced [ɣ]) are found in several languages including Greek, Spanish, Irish, and Vietnamese.

Uvular: Sounds that are made with the back of the tongue articulating against the uvula are called uvulars. Uvular sounds do not occur in English, but are found in the French word rouge [ʁuʒ] (voiced uvular fricative or approximant). Uvular stops [q, G], and nasals [N] are found in many Amerindian languages.

Pharyngeal: Sounds that are made by pulling the epiglottis back toward the pharynx wall are pharyngeals. English does not have any pharyngeal sounds; pharyngeal fricatives [h, ʕ] are found in Arabic.

Glottal: Sounds that are made at the glottis, as in the English [h] in home, and [ʔ] in Batman are glottals.

Manners of Articulation

Nasals: A basic distinction in manner of articulation separates oral and nasal sounds. Compare the words *beat, bead,* and *bean,* which differ in their final sounds. The sounds of the first two words are different because of voicing. For [t], the glottis is open, whereas for [d], the vocal cords are vibrating. However, if we compare the second and the third words, we do not find any difference in terms of voicing, as [n], like [d], involves vocal cord vibration. Yet, we clearly feel that these two sounds are different, and the difference lies in the oral/nasal dimension. In the production of [d], the soft palate, or velum, is raised and the passage that links the pharynx with the nasal cavity (velopharyngeal opening) is closed. Consequently, [d] is produced with air going out through the mouth. Sounds that are articulated with such velopharyngeal configurations are called **oral** sounds. On the other hand, when we produce [n], the velopharyngeal passage is open, and the air goes out through the nasal cavity as well as through the mouth. Sounds that are articulated in this manner are called **nasal** sounds. English has three nasal consonants: [m, n, and ŋ] as in <u>m</u>oon, <u>n</u>ame, and si<u>ng</u>. All other consonants in English are oral.

Stops: Stops are made with complete closure of the articulators so that the airflow through the oral cavity is blocked before the release. In English [p, t, k, b, d, and g] are stop sounds. In addition to these, the nasal sounds [m, n, ŋ] are sometimes considered stops because they, too, have blockage of the air flow through the oral cavity. This last group, however, is classified separately as **nasals**, as indicated above, and will not be considered as stops here as air is escaping through the nose.

Fricatives: Sounds that are made with a close approximation of the articulators which creates a partial obstruction of the airflow while allowing it to escape with audible friction are called fricatives. In English [f, v, θ, ð, s, z, ʃ, ʒ, h] are fricative sounds.[3] Fricatives are further classified according to their characteristics of pitch and intensity. The sounds [s, z, ʃ, ʒ] are called sibilants. Sibilants are high-pitched and intense and have greater amounts of acoustic energy at higher frequencies than those that are less noisy.

Affricates: The release of a stop sound is quick and abrupt; however, if a stop is released gradually, creating friction, the resulting sound is an affricate. In other words, phonetically speaking, an affricate is a combination of a stop and a fricative. This is evident from the phonetic symbols assigned to affricates. English has two of the most frequent affricates [tʃ and dʒ]. In some other systems a single symbol [č, or ǰ] is used, relating to their phonological status of behaving like a single sound unit in the language. Like fricatives, some affricates are sibilants and some are not. The sibilance of an affricate is determined by its fricative component. If the fricative component is sibilant, as in [tʃ] or [dʒ], then the affricate is a sibilant. If, on the other hand, the fricative component is nonsibilant, as in [pf] of German (*pferd* "horse"), then the affricate is a nonsibilant. Both of the English affricates are sibilants.

Approximants: These are sounds that are made in such a way that one articulator is close to another without narrowing the vocal tract to create the friction necessary to be a fricative. These sounds may be thought of as "frictionless fricatives"; that is, further narrowing in the vocal tract would create a fricative. The criteria for differentially classifying a segment as an approximant or as a fricative include acoustic/auditory and aerodynamic considerations as well as articulatory factors. Typical cross-sectional areas of the maximum constriction in a fricative range from about 3 to 20 mm². If this measurement is greater than 20 mm², then the segment is an approximant (Catford, 1977). In English, the category of approximants includes [l, ɹ , j, w] of lake, rake, yes, and week. The American English *r* is a retroflex approximant made either by curling the tip of the tongue back, or by bunching the tongue upward and back in the mouth, often with some lip rounding. Different dialects and even different speakers within the same dialect produce r-sounds differently; therefore, it is difficult to provide a single description for this sound. The approximant [l] is a lateral sound in which the tongue is articulated against the roof of the mouth, but air is allowed to escape around the sides of the tongue. Languages of the world exhibit numerous variants of laterals and r-sounds which form the class called **liquids**.

English [w] is a labio-velar approximant because it involves two places of constriction: rounding of the lips and the raising of the back of the tongue toward the velum. Finally, [j] is a palatal approximant for which the tongue is humped up toward the hard palate. These two approximants are called **glides** or **semivowels**. The term semivowels is used because they are vowel-like sounds that occupy the spaces of consonants in words. Phonetically, the production of [j] is quite similar to the vowel [i]. The same can be said about the labio-velar glide [w] and the vowel [u]. However, the phonological sequencing in the structure of the language determines whether a given occurrence will be interpreted as a vowel or a consonant. Glides, for example, do not occupy the place of the nucleus, or center, of the syllable that is normally taken by vowels, and thus they behave as consonants. The deciding factor, then, is the function of the segment, rather than its phonetic characteristics.

Trills, taps, and flaps: In languages, r-sounds present a variety of articulations. Apart from the approximant *r*-sounds of English (retroflex in American and alveolar in British English), taps, flaps, and trills dominate the picture.

Both taps and flaps involve a momentary contact between articulators. In a **tap**, one articulator is thrown at the other, makes a momentary contact, and immediately is withdrawn to its point of origin. The American English *t* or *d* between vowels (*latter* or *ladder*), or the single *r* of Spanish (*caro* "expensive," *pero* "but") are the most well-known tongue-tip (apical) taps, where there is a flicking movement of the tip of the tongue against the upper articulator.

Although sometimes equated with a tap, a flap typically is different in that the active articulator starts in one position, strikes the place of articulation in passing and finishes the movement in a position different from that in which it began. In other words, the momentary contact does not occur with a flicking motion as is the case for a tap. A typical example is the retroflex flap of Hausa ([baɽa] "servant"), in which the tip of the tongue is curled up and back, then shoots forward, momentarily striking the upper surface of the mouth, and then flaps down with the tip forward in the mouth.

Trills, on the other hand, are made by the repeated tapping of one flexible articulator against another. A common trill is the dental/alveolar trill in which the tip of the tongue multiply taps against the alveolar ridge; Spanish [r] as in *carro* ([karo] "cart") and *perro* ([pero] "dog") is of this kind. Another well-known trill is the uvular trill, [R], which is found in German and in some varieties of French. It is made by raising the back of the tongue so that the airstream causes the uvula to vibrate against it. It is important to note that trills are not made via conscious control of tongue movements. Instead, the multiple vibrations are produced by aerodynamic forces, similar to those described earlier for vocal cord vibration. Once the tongue is placed in its appropriate position with the right tension and the air is blown through the space between the articulators, the Bernoulli effect pulls the articulators together. Once they are together, the airstream from the lungs pushes them apart again. The cycle repeats itself quickly several times, creating the trill.

Sonorant vs. Obstruent: The above groupings classify consonants in terms of their manner of articulation. There is, however, a further binary grouping that categorizes these sounds according to the vocal tract obstruction necessary for their production. The term **obstruent** refers to sounds that are produced with a considerable amount of obstruction of the air in the vocal tract. Accordingly, stops, fricatives, and affricates are obstruents. The opposing group, **sonorants**, which is composed of liquids, glides, and nasals, requires only a negligible amount of obstruction in the vocal tract.

Although this binary grouping is justified by the sound systems of languages, it is not problem-free. This is essentially due to liquids. Although liquids are in the sonorant group, some r-sounds in certain languages are fricatives. Also, laterals are like stops in that they often involve closure (see Chapters 4 and 7 for more on this topic). Figure 2–3 summarizes the consonants discussed in this section.

Airstream Mechanisms

Plosives, implosives, ejectives, and clicks: The great majority of speech sounds in languages are made by the use of an airstream flowing out from the lungs. Sounds produced in this way are said to use a **pulmonic egressive airstream mechanism.** However, this is not the only airstream mechanism used in languages of the world.

In some languages, stops are produced by the movement of different bodies of air. The glottalic airstream mechanism uses the larynx as the initiator, and thus employs the air above the larynx. If the closed larynx is raised, together with a closure somewhere in the mouth and a raised velum, the air pressure within this chamber is increased. Upon release of the closure in the vocal tract, the air rushes out. Stops that are produced this way are called ejectives. Because the glottis of the raised larynx is closed, ejectives typically are voiceless. These sounds are common in many Amerindian languages (Nez Perce, Klamath, Nootka, Dakota), Circassian languages (Kabardian, Georgian), and African languages (Zulu, Hausa).

		Labial										
		Bilabial	Lab.dental	Interdental	Alveolar	Retroflex	Pal-alveolar	Palatal	Velar	Uvular	Pharyngeal	Glottal
OBSTRUENT	Stop	p b			t d	ṭ ḍ		c ɟ	k g	q G		ʔ
	Fricative	Φ β	f v	θ	s z	ṣ ẓ	ʃ	ç ʝ	x ɣ	X ʁ	ħ ʕ	
	Affricate	pf					tʃ d					
SONORANT Approx.	Nasal	m			n	ṇ		ɲ	ŋ	N		
	Liquid				l r	ɭ						
	Glide	w						j	w			

Figure 2–3. Consonant chart.

The opposite of an ejective is the stop sound called implosive, which is made by the glottalic ingressive airstream mechanism. Implosives involve a downward-moving larynx, which sucks the air inward. In general, the downward movement of the larynx cannot be accomplished with a closed glottis and, thus, there is a leak of air from the lungs which causes vibration of the cords, producing a voiced sound. Implosives can be found in many African languages (Zulu, Hausa, Swahili). Implosives and ejectives are often referred to as "glottalized" or "laryngealized" consonants.

The third airstream mechanism is the velaric airstream mechanism. Stops produced using this airstream mechanism ingressively are called clicks. In the production of a click, the back of the tongue is drawn against the velum and forms a closure at the back of the oral cavity, while another closure is formed forward (lips, alveolar ridge, or palate), trapping this mouth air in a chamber as in the click sound frequently used to call a horse, or the one that expresses the "tsk" of disapproval in English. Then, the body of the tongue is pulled down and drawn backward, which rarefies the air. When the front closure is released, the air rushes in, creating a clicking sound. As ordinary consonants, clicks are found only in languages of southern Africa.

Voice Onset Time

Before we finish our discussion of manners of articulation, we will deal with one other aspect of stop consonants that is related to their production and the timing of vocal cord vibration. This is relevant in the separation of the stop sounds regarding their voicing and/or aspiration. For example, the initial sounds of the words *paper* and *papel* in English and Spanish, respectively, are very different. The first is a voiceless aspirated stop that is produced with a perceptible puff of air, whereas the second is a voiceless unaspirated stop that lacks this puff of air. The quality of the Spanish [p] is similar to the second sound of the English words *speak*, and *sport* in which these English [p] sounds are unaspirated.

Voice onset time (VOT) is the time between the release of a stop closure and the onset of glottal vibration (voicing). Stop release is the reference point in time (0 msec) and VOT is measured relative to that point. Voice onset that occurs before stop release is assigned a negative VOT value and is referred to as **voice lead**. Voice onset that occurs after the stop release is assigned a positive VOT and is called **voice lag**.

Although VOT is a continuum, our perception of it is categorical. If the timing relationship is one in which the onset of voicing falls within + or

−20 msec of the release of the stop, it will be perceived as simultaneous onset and will be classified as a voiceless unaspirated stop. In order to be perceived as aspirated (voice lag), the delay in the onset of voicing must occur more than 25 msec after the release of the stop. Similarly, for a stop to be perceived as voiced (voice lead), the beginning of voicing typically precedes the release of closure by more than 25 msec. There are different degrees of voiced and aspirated stops within these categories in different languages. Figure 2–4 illustrates the differences in VOT continuum.

In Figure 2–4, the first of the two vertical lines indicates the moment of closure for the stop and the second represents the moment of release for this stop closure. Between these two vertical lines (i.e., during the closure period for the stop), the dotted line indicates voicelessness and the zigzag line indicates vocal cord vibration (voicing). While French [p] is unaspirated (voicing is simultaneous with the moment of release), English and

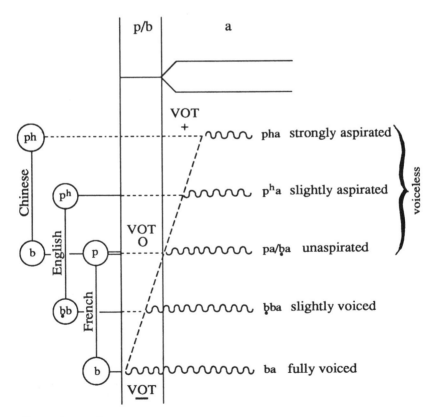

Figure 2–4. The VOT continuum.

Chinese [pʰ] are aspirated. The fact that Chinese starts the voicing of the vowel later than English creates the difference between slightly aspirated and strongly aspirated. In strongly aspirated Chinese stops there is a greater delay of the voicing of the following vowel. In comparing the voiced stops, we see that English [b, d, g] are slightly voiced, as opposed to French, Spanish, or Portuguese fully voiced stops. This means that, in these Romance languages, vocal cord vibration starts from the beginning of the closure, as opposed to the partial devoicing that occurs in English sounds.

Certain segment internal factors are influential regarding the amount of VOT of the stops within the same language. One of the most well-known is the place of articulation of the stop; /k/, in general, has a longer VOT than /t/, and /t/, in turn, has a longer VOT than /p/. In other words, as we move the place of articulation from the lips (bilabial) farther back, the VOT is increasingly longer. This is evident in the following VOT values (in milliseconds) (Lisker & Abramson, 1964).

English (voiceless aspirated stops)	:	[p] 58	[t] 70	[k] 80
Dutch (voiceless unaspirated stops)	:	[p] 10	[t] 15	[k] 25
Thai (voiceless unaspirated stops)	:	[p] 3	[t] 15	[k] 30
Thai (voiceless aspirated stops)	:	[p] 78	[t] 59	[k] 98
Cantonese (voiceless unaspirated stops):		[p] 9	[t] 14	[k] 34
Cantonese (voiceless aspirated stops)	:	[p] 77	[t] 75	[k] 87
Hindi (voiceless unaspirated stops)	:	[p] 13	[t] 15	[k] 19
Hindi (voiceless aspirated stops)	:	[p] 70	[t] 67	[k] 92

The difference between the velar [k] and the others is unequivocal. However, the differential effect between the dental/alveolar [t] and the bilabial [p] appears much less clear, although the general tendency of [t] to have a longer VOT than [p] is observed.

The length of VOT of the segment also appears to be related to the quality of the following voiced segment. For example, the aspiration of the initial [p] of *pack* [pæk], *pick* [pɪk], and *play* [ple] increasingly rises as we move from the first to the second and then to the third word. What seems to be affecting this is the nature of the second segment in question. In the first word, [p] is followed by a vowel that is produced with a low tongue position; in the second word, it is followed by a vowel that is produced with a raised tongue position; and in the third, it is occupied by a lateral liquid. In other words, there is an increasing narrowing in the articulation of the second segment. Thus, we can say that the VOT of a segment is longer if the following segment is articulatorily more close.

In addition to these segment internal effects, VOT can be influenced by other factors such as the tempo of speech, the number of syllables in the word, and the sentence length. As expected, faster speech, words with more syllables, and longer sentences have the effect of reducing VOT.

Secondary Articulations

In the production of some consonant sounds in languages, we observe addition of a secondary, lesser constriction to the primary articulation. The distinct sound that is superimposed on the original creates the secondary articulation. Four types of secondary articulation are common: labialization, palatalization, velarization, and pharyngealization.

Labialization: This term refers to the addition of lip rounding, resulting in the rounded vowel quality of the type seen in *boot*. An example of a labialized consonant is found in the initial sound of the word *quick*. The common symbol for labialization is a raised [ʷ] as in [kʷɪk]. Labialized consonants contrast with nonlabialized consonants in some African languages.

Palatalization: This is the raising of the blade of the tongue toward the hard palate without touching the roof of the mouth. It can be considered as the addition of [j] to the primary articulation, and the symbol for palatalized consonants is a raised [ʲ]. Russian and other Slavic languages have palatalized consonants contrasting with the regular consonants ([brat] "brother" vs. [bratʲ] "to take").

Velarization: This term refers to the raising of the back of the tongue toward, but not touching, the velum, as for the vowel [u] without the lip rounding. The symbol for velarization is [~]. Scots Gaelic contrasts velarized and nonvelarized consonants ([balə] "town" vs. [baɫə] "ball/wall").

Pharyngealization: This term refers to the lowering of the back of the tongue and a retraction of the root toward the pharynx wall, resulting in a narrowing of the pharynx. The same symbol that is used for velarization is commonly used for pharyngealization, as no language makes a contrast between these consonant types.

Of the four secondary articulation types, labialization is the only one that involves lip rounding and can be combined with any of the remaining three which involve movements of the tongue.

Vowels

Although varying degrees of obstruction of airflow characterize consonants, vowels can be described as sounds with the least constriction in
which the air escapes most freely. This distinction, however, is not definitive and is blurred in cases like the glide/vowel separation discussed
earlier.

Consonants are described by place and manner of articulation. Vowels,
on the other hand, are characterized by the height and the front-
ness/backness of the tongue, and by the position of the lips.

High, Mid, Low

If you say the words *beat, bit, bait, bet,* and *bat* in the order given, you will
notice that you progressively open your mouth more and the body of the
tongue is lowered. A similar tongue movement along the back vertical
axis can also be observed in words like *pot, hall, boat, put,* and *boot,* although this time the direction is from lower to higher. Traditionally, three
degrees of vowel height are recognized: **high, mid,** and **low.** Vowels in
beat, bit, put, and *boot* [i, ɪ, ʊ, u] respectively, are called high vowels, because the body of the tongue is raised in their production. Conversely, the
vowels in *bat* and *pot* [æ, a] are low vowels, because they involve the lowering of the body of the tongue from its neutral position. The vowels of
bait, bet, bought, and *boat* [e, ɛ, ɔ, o], respectively, are produced with an intermediate tongue height and are called mid vowels. We should mention
that in many American dialects the two vowels [ɔ, o] are not distinguished in many words. For example, these speakers pronounce *cot* and
caught identically, with a more [a]-like vowel. However, the difference between these two vowels is not overlooked in words like *course,* and *hall,*
and the vowel [ɔ] appears in both of these words. The vowels [ʊ] as in
pull and [u] as in *pool* also vary. Many speakers employ a rather unrounded vowel in *book* and a rounded but central vowel in <u>poor</u>.

The two remaining vowels of English, [ə] of <u>above</u>, and [ʌ] of <u>but</u>, are
considered mid and low, respectively. However, in some books, one does
encounter the classification of mid for both.

Front/Central/Back

If the movement of the tongue along the vertical axis is relevant for high,
mid, and low vowels, the movement along the horizontal axis defines the

front, central, and back vowels. If, in the production of a vowel, the tongue is pushed forward, then we have a front vowel [i, ɪ, e, ɛ, æ]. If the tongue is retracted, or pulled back, then we have a back vowel [a, ɔ, o, ʊ, u]. For central vowels [ə, ʌ], the body of the tongue remains neutral and is centrally located.[4]

Rounded/Unrounded

Another dimension of vowel quality is related to lip position. In the production of some vowels, [ɔ, o, ʊ, u], the lips are rounded. Therefore, these vowels are called round vowels. All other vowels are unrounded. In English, all front vowels are unrounded and all nonlow back vowels are rounded. However, vowels that counter these tendencies are found in other languages. For example, the high front round vowel [y] is commonly found in languages such as German, French, Danish, Finnish, Turkish, Mandarin Chinese, and Hungarian. German, Danish, Norwegian, French, and Hungarian also have the higher mid front round vowel [ø] (the round counterpart of [e]). The lower mid front round (round counterpart of [ɛ]) vowel [œ] is found in German, Norwegian, Danish, French and Turkish. Although not as common as these front rounded vowels, high back unrounded vowel [ɯ](unrounded counterpart of [u]) is found in Turkish, Korean, Japanese, and several Amerindian languages.

Tense/Lax

In addition to the parameters describing vowel quality, tongue height, backness, and lip rounding, another dimension is needed to distinguish between certain vowels. If we look at the vowels [i] and [ɪ] as in *beat* and *bit*, we immediately realize that both are classified as high, front, and unrounded; in other words, the three dimensions we have dealt with are not enough to distinguish these two vowels. A similar problem arises when we compare the vowels [u] and [ʊ], which are both high, back, and round. To remedy this situation, another distinction is made in terms of a tense/lax parameter. Tense vowels are those that require more muscular effort to produce, are longer in duration, and have a higher tongue position than their lax counterparts. Looked at in this way, the pairs of vowels [i — ɪ], [u — ʊ], [e — ɛ], and [o — ɔ] can be distinguished on the basis of this new dimension; in all of these pairs, the first member is tense and the second is lax. In summary, tense/lax grouping helps distinguish the vowels in these four pairs that are not distinguishable via tongue height, frontness, and lip rounding. This can be seen in Figure 2–5 in which the vowels of English are displayed.

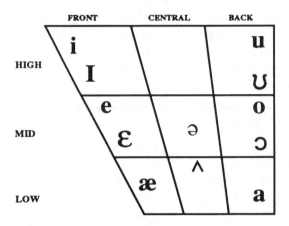

Figure 2–5. Vowels of English.

Although this phonetically defined tense/lax grouping is quite well established, it is not free of controversy. Some books suggest classification of tense/lax on the basis of the occurrence of these vowels in different types of syllables. Defined in this way, tense vowels occur in open syllables (syllables that end in a vowel) (e.g., bee, bay) and syllables closed by [ɹ] (e.g., beer, bare), whereas lax vowels occur in syllables closed by [ŋ](e.g., sing, length), and syllables closed by [ʃ] (e.g., wish, fresh) (Ladefoged, 1993). This way of classifying the vowels in tense/lax groups creates problems, and due to the number of exceptions required for this explanation, it will not be pursued here.

Cardinal Vowels

Although we frequently see labels such as high front unrounded and mid back rounded used for the vowels in different languages, the exact quality of these vowels may not be, and in most situations is not, identical from one language to another. For example, the high front unrounded vowel of language X may not be the same as the high front unrounded vowel of language Y. To resolve this problem, phoneticians usually refer to the Cardinal vowel system to describe the vowels in various languages. The Cardinal vowel system serves as a precise reference tool by arbitrarily picking certain vowels as basic, and describing the vowels of languages in terms of their relationship to these cardinal vowels. Figure 2–6 illustrates the primary and secondary cardinal vowels.

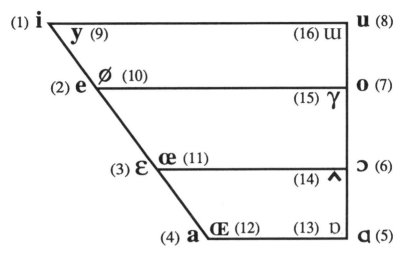

Figure 2–6. Primary and secondary cardinal vowels.

The vowels 1[i], and 5[ɑ] define two extreme corners of the vowel continuum. The first represents a vowel that is the highest and most front possible (a higher and more front articulation would result in a palatal consonant) and the second represents the lowest and most back vowel possible (a more back and lower articulation would result in a pharyngeal consonant). The other corners, 4 [a] and 8 [u], also represent the extremes in high back and low front. The situation repeats itself with the secondary cardinal vowels 9 [y], 12 [œ], 13 [ɒ], and 16 [ɯ], this time with opposite lip rounding. The vowels 1–4 (front) and 5–8 (back) are equidistant from one another and the same is true for vowels 9–12 and 13–16. As we mentioned earlier, these vowels are arbitrary reference points and do not represent any particular language, although certain vowels of one language may be very similar, or even identical, to some of the Cardinal vowels.

Once we have these reference points, we can describe any vowel in any language. For example, English [æ] is a little higher and a little farther back than Cardinal vowel 4. Danish [œ] is a little higher and a little farther back than 11.

Nasalization

All of vowels described until this point have been oral, that is, they are produced with the velum raised, cutting off the nasal cavity. However, any of these vowels can be nasalized. This is done by pronouncing the vowels while passing the air through the nasal cavity as well as through the mouth. The symbol for a nasal vowel or nasality is a tilde [˜] above the vowel symbol. Some languages have nasal vowels that parallel the oral vowels. Portuguese has a contrast between *vi* [vi] "I saw" and *vim* [ṽi] "I came." A similar nasal-oral contrast can be seen in French *lin* [lɛ̃] "flax" versus *lait* [lɛ] "milk."

Diphthongs

The syllable nucleus of the words such as *night*, *sound*, and *boy* are not simple vowels, but consist of two parts: a vowel and a glide, [aj], [aw], and [oj], which are called diphthongs. Some books use two vowels to represent the diphthongs, for example, [ai], [au], and [oi]. In [aj], the tongue starts out in the low position with [a] and moves higher toward the position for the palatal glide [j]. For [aw], the starting point is the same but the movement is toward the labio-velar glide [w]. Finally, [oj] starts with [o] (or [ɔ] for some speakers) and moves to the palatal glide. Figure 2–7 illustrates these movements.

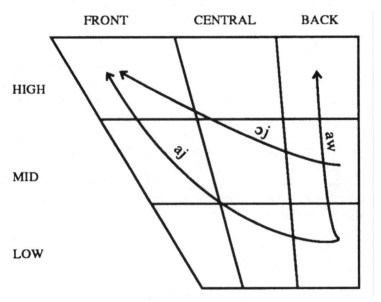

Figure 2–7. English diphthongs.

There is considerable variation in diphthongs [aj] and [aw]. For many speakers, [aj] as in *bite* and *sign* does not have a movement to higher than a mid front vowel and results in a production which sounds like [baɛt]. The other diphthong, [aw], as in cow, may start with a more front quality in the low vowel, and may go as far front as [æ] for some speakers. In most Canadian dialects and some American dialects, [aj] and [ʌj], and [aw] and [ʌw] are positional variants of each other. Diphthongs starting with [ʌ] occur before a voiceless consonant as in *ice* [ʌjs] or *out* [ʌwt]. In other word positions, diphthongs starting with [a] are found (e.g., *eyes* [ajz] or *loud* [lawd]).

Suprasegmentals

Vowels and consonants are normally considered as segments in a linear sequence of the speech stream. There are other characteristics of speech that are used simultaneously with the segmental vowels and consonants, and with syllables, which are units greater than segments. These aspects of speech, known as suprasegmentals, include pitch, stress, and length.

Pitch

The **pitch** of the voice refers to the frequency of the vocal cord vibration and is affected by the tension of the cords and the amount of air that passes through the cords. Several different kinds of information are discernible from the pitch of the speaker. Among these are the gender, possibly the age, and the emotional state of the speaker. Linguistically, two kinds of controlled pitch seem to be significant and define the difference between tone and intonation. Speakers of all languages reveal changes in pitch while they talk. However, depending on the unit to which it applies, the variation in pitch makes a significant difference. In English, when we utter the sequence "His brother is leaving tomorrow" with a falling pitch, it will be taken as a simple statement. However, if the same sequence is produced with a rise in pitch at the end of the last word, the hearer will interpret this as a question. Such falls and rises, sometimes called the melody of a phrase or a sentence, are known as intonation.

In other languages, however, differences in word meaning are signalled by pitch differences. In these languages, known as tone languages, even a monosyllabic word uttered with different pitches results in different meanings. For example, in Mandarin Chinese the sequence [ma] can mean "mother," "hemp," "horse," or "scold" depending on whether it is uttered by a high level, high rising, falling rising, or a low falling tone, respectively. In some tone languages, the pitch of each tone is level; in others there is a gliding movement from high to low or from low to high. Tones that have gliding movements are called **contour tones** and tones that do not glide, but can be described in terms of points within a pitch range, are called **register tones**.

The lexical change that is accomplished in a tone language cannot be repeated in an intonation language like English. For example, no matter what kind of pitch variation we use in uttering the word *book*, the meaning of this item cannot be altered.

Lexical change accomplished by pitch variations is a characteristic of all tone languages. In some tone languages, however, the tone shift is used for changes in grammatical meaning as well. Examples include tone shifts used to show tense shift (Bini of Nigeria), to separate the main clause and the relative clause (Shona of Zimbabwe), or to indicate possession (Igbo of Nigeria).

Stress

An important suprasegmental feature that applies to syllables is stress. Stressed syllables are pronounced with a greater amount of energy than unstressed syllables. In general, three characteristics separate a stressed syllable from an unstressed syllable. The first is the loudness or intensity. Because more air is pushed out of the lungs, stressed syllables are louder than unstressed syllables. The second characteristic relates to duration: The length of a stressed syllable is greater than an unstressed syllable. Finally, a stressed syllable is higher in pitch than an unstressed syllable. Studies dealing with the perceptual cues of lexical stress in English (Fry, 1955, 1958, 1965) show that higher pitch was the most influential cue in separating the stressed syllable from the unstressed. The second most influential cue was length and the third was intensity. Although all languages and dialects (varieties) distinguish stressed syllables from unstressed by causing the former to be perceived as prominent, the phonetic realizations of the three factors (loudness, length, and pitch) can differ widely.

Apart from its use for special emphasis, stress functions to distinguish noun/verb pairs with identical sounds in English. For example, *import* and *insult* are nouns if the stress is on the first syllable; in their verb forms, however, the stress falls on the second syllable. The majority of the seemingly comparable pairs, however, are not distinguished in their noun versus verb form only by a shift in stress, but also by a change in the quality of the reduced vowel (Householder, 1971). Words such as *object* and *permit* change their first vowels to [ə] when the stress shifts to the second syllable in the verb forms. The position of stress in English and other Germanic languages is rather variable. However, in many languages lexical stress is predominantly fixed in a given word position. Hyman (1977) investigated 306 languages with fixed stress and found a strong tendency for the trailing edge of words to be stressed (174 languages, 57%). The preferences for final (31.7%, e.g., French), and penultimate (25.2%, e.g., Polish, Welsh, Swahili), syllable stress is attributed to the demarcative function of stress to indicate where the word boundary is for the listener. This explanation gains further support by 114 languages (37.3%) in which the fixed stress is predominantly on the first syllable (e.g., Czech, Finnish), making the other edge of the word clearly marked.

Variations in the use of stress result in different rhythms in different languages. Accordingly, it is customary in the literature to see languages divided into two categories according to their different rhythms. The typical definition of a **stress-timed language** revolves around the tendency for stresses to recur in regular intervals. A **syllable-timed language** is defined as one in which syllables, rather than stressed syllables, recur at regular intervals. English, German, Russian, Arabic, and Brazilian Portuguese are examples of the former, and French, Italian, Greek, Spanish, Turkish, and Hindi are said to belong to the latter group.

The above binary split has been challenged (Dauer, 1983; Giegerich, 1992), and the situation may better be shown as a continuum. Apart from the rejection of the dichotomous grouping, the differences of rhythms between languages are suggested to lie not in the durations of interstress intervals, but rather in the differences of length between the stressed and unstressed syllables, the greater variety of syllable structures, and vowel reductions. According to this characterization, in stress-timed languages, the difference of stressed versus unstressed syllable duration is greater; these languages also maximize this difference via vowel reduction of the unstressed vowels. Finally, stress-timed languages typically have a greater variety of syllable structures.

Length

Another suprasegmental feature in which languages may vary is length of vowels or consonants. In English, vowel length is predictable. For example, the vowel in *back* [bæk] is shorter than the vowel in *bag* [bæg], as the former is followed by a voiceless consonant and the latter by a voiced consonant. However, in many languages (Swedish, Danish, Finnish, Arabic, Japanese), long and short vowels occur in exactly the same context and change the meaning of the word.

Although not as common as in vowels, long and short consonants also can be utilized to change the meaning of the word. The long consonants, which are sometimes called **geminates**, are found in several languages such as Italian, Finnish, and Turkish.

Syllable

Although we have made several references to the syllable up to this point, we have not yet defined this unit. This may be precisely the point where we have a problem, as there is no agreed phonetic characterization of the notion syllable. We will not, however, go into the discussion of different phonetic definitions, as our concern is from a phonological point of view. Syllables are of considerable importance for the phonological organization of language and we will devote an entire chapter to the syllable later in this book. In the meantime, let it suffice to state that a syllable is a small unit of speech, and can conveniently be described as having the components of **onset**, **nucleus**, and **coda**. The last two together are referred as the **rhyme**. The onset is the initial consonant or consonant cluster of the syllable. For example, the onset of the monosyllabic word *strap* is /str/, the onset of *trap* is /tr/, and the onset of *rap* is /r/. The onset is not obligatory in English in that a well-formed syllable may not have one (e.g., *at*, *in*, *out*). The rhyme is the remaining part of the syllable after the onset; in the above examples /æp/ is the rhyme of all three words *rap*, *trap*, *strap*. A rhyme may have a short or diphthongized vowel and a consonant or consonant cluster (e.g., *sit*, *seat*, *tent*, *taint*) or a long or diphthongized vowel without anything following it (e.g., *bee*). Within the internal structure of the rhyme, the vowel or the diphthong is the nucleus, or peak, and the consonant or consonants following are the coda.[5] Like the onset, a coda is not an obligatory in English. Syllables that have a coda are called **closed syllables** (e.g., *beet*). Those that lack a coda are called **open syllables** (e.g., *bee*).

NOTES

1. In comparison to consonants, there is even greater diversity for vowel symbols among various sources. The following list shows the differences in some of the most commonly referred to publications.

Key Word	LF	Ladefoged	E & G	K & K	P & R	F & R	Webster's
beat	i	i	i	iy	iy	i	e
bit	ɪ	ɪ	ɪ	ɪ	ɪ	ɪ	i
bait	e	eɪ	e	e	ey	e	a
bet	ɛ	ɛ	ɛ	ɛ	ɛ	ɛ	e
bat	æ	æ	æ	æ	æ	æ	a
car	a	ɑ	ɑ	ɑ	a	a	a
cut	ʌ	ʌ	ʌ	ʌ	ə	ʌ	ə
wrong	ɔ	ɔ	ɔ	ɔ	ɔ	ɔ	o
boat	o	oʊ	o	o	ow	o	o
foot	ʊ	ʊ	ʊ	ʊ	ʊ	ʊ	u
boot	u	u	u	u	uw	u	u
bite	ay	aɪ	aɪ	aɪ	ay	aj	ɪ
boil	oy	ɔɪ	ɔɪ	ɔɪ	ɔy	ɔj	oi
loud	aw	aʊ	aʊ	aʊ	aw	aw	au

LF = *Language files* (6th ed.) (1996). Columbus: Ohio State University Press.

Ladefoged = Ladefoged, P. (1993). *A course in phonetics* (3rd ed.). Orlando, FL: Harcourt Brace Jovanovich.

E & G = Edwards, H.T., & Gregg, A. (1997). *Applied phonetics workbook* (2nd ed.). San Diego: Singular Publishing Group.

K & K = Kenyon, J.S., & Knott, T.A. (1953). *A pronouncing dictionary of American English.* Springfield, MA: C. Merriam.

P & R = Prator, C., & Robinett, B.(1985). *A manual of American English pronunciation* (4th Ed.). New York: Holt Rinehart and Winston.

F & R = Fromkin, V., & Rodman, R. (1993) *An introduction to language* (5th ed.) Orlando, FL: Harcourt Brace Jovanovich.

Webster's = *Webster's new international dictionary* (3rd ed). (1961). Springfield, MA: C. Merriam.

2. One difference from the IPA symbols for consonants has to be noted. In this book, retroflex consonants are transcribed with a diacritic, a subscript dot ([Ç]). The reason for this divergence is twofold. First, more phoneticians adhere to this practice and second, students find this much more straightforward and less confusing.

3. Some books, adhering strictly to the requirement of turbulent airstream, do not consider [h] as a fricative. Some linguists prefer to put h-sounds, together with [ʔ], into the class of laryngeals (Schane, 1973), others emphasize its quality of being a voiceless counterpart of an abutting vowel.

4. We must mention that the height and the backness of a vowel is better characterized acoustically. Accordingly, the frequency of the first formant is inversely related to the height of the vowel; the difference between the frequencies of formant two and formant one characterizes its backness. The details of these are not within the scope of an introductory book of this kind, and the reader is referred to Ladefoged (1993) for more information.

5. In some languages, English included, liquids and nasals may form a syllable of their own. These syllabic consonants are represented by a diacritic C̩. In English, nasals may become syllabic in final position after an obstruent (e.g., *sudden* [sʌdn̩], *madam* [mædm̩]), and liquids may become syllabic in final position following any consonant (e.g., *channel* [tʃænl̩], *razor* [rezr̩].

EXERCISES

1. Circle the correct alternative:
   a. Consonants produced without vocal cord vibration are known as nasal/voiced/voiceless consonants.
   b. To produce a stop/fricative/affricate, the outgoing breath stream is completely stopped behind a closure somewhere in the vocal tract, then released abruptly.
   c. Glides share articulatory characteristics of vowels/ consonants, and the functional characteristics of vowels/consonants.
   d. To produce a fricative/liquid/glide, the outgoing breath stream is forced through a very narrow passage.
   e. English affricates are produced when the tongue tip/ blade/root touches the back of the alveolar ridge.
   f. Sonorants/obstruents are normally voiced, whereas sonorants/obstruents can be voiced or voiceless.
   g. The soft palate is lowered and the velopharyngeal passage is open during the production of oral/ nasal/ voiceless sounds.

h. The obstruent category includes fricatives/affricates/ liquids/and nasals.

i. In a voiceless aspirated stop voice onset occurs before/ after the stop release.

j. The secondary articulation that is accomplished by the raising of the blade of the tongue toward the hard palate is called labialization/palatalization/ velarization.

k. A stressed syllable has higher/lower pitch than an unstressed syllable.

2. Circle the words that have
   a. Bilabial sounds
      mother, cheap, grass, zero, shoe
   b. Alveolar sounds
      cheap, fickle, safe, rag, chess
   c. Approximants
      roses, mouth, laugh, hang, cloth
   d. Fricatives
      matched, laugh, copper, pudding, taxi
   e. Palato-alveolar sounds
      sip, ticket, nation, wish, judge
   f. Diphthongs
      night, conclude, prepare, report, sound
   g. High vowels
      door, bazooka, set, bathe, realize
   h. Back vowels
      anger, nation, rotten, Asia, ruler

3. Identify the phonetic symbol represented by the following descriptions.

Voiced bilabial fricative   [   ]

Bilabial nasal   [   ]

Voiced labio-dental fricative   [   ]

Velar nasal   [   ]

Voiced inter-dental fricative   [   ]

Voiced velar stop   [   ]

Voiceless palato-alveolar fricative [   ]

Palatal glide   [   ]

Voiceless bilabial stop   [   ]

Low back vowel   [   ]

Mid front tense vowel   [   ]

Low front vowel   [   ]

High back lax vowel   [   ]

4. Give the phonetic descriptions for the following sounds:

[z] _____

[f] _____

[k] _____

[ɛ] _____

[ʒ] _____

[n] _____

[b] _____

[i] _____

[w] _____

[u] _____

5. State the shared phonetic characteristic in each of the following groups of sounds.

Example: p t g b   stops

j   z   b   dʒ   m   l   _____

v   z   ʃ   s   f   h   _____

s   d   n   t   z   l   _____

i   æ   ɛ   ɪ   e   _____

e   ɔ   ɛ   o   ə   _____

6. The underlined sounds in the following pairs of words share some phonetic properties and are different in other respects. Give the phonetic symbol for each underlined sound and state the shared feature(s) and differences.

   Example: [k] boo<u>k</u> - be<u>s</u>t [s] Both [k] and [s] are voiceless.

   [k] is a velar stop

   [s] is an alveolar fricative

   [ ] a<u>dd</u>er-fa<u>th</u>er [ ] _____

   _____

   _____

   [ ] e<u>th</u>er-ho<u>pp</u>er [ ] _____

   _____

   _____

   [ ] su<u>nn</u>y-lo<u>dg</u>er [ ] _____

   _____

   _____

   [ ] m<u>ai</u>d-c<u>a</u>p [ ] _____

   _____

   _____

[ ] plea<u>s</u>ure-<u>ch</u>op [ ] _____

_____

_____

17. Match the sounds under column A with one or more phonetic properties given in column B.

Example: [ʃ]   4,   7

A   B

[j] _____   11. voiced

[z] _____   12. round

[u] _____   13. alveolar

[m] _____   14. palatal/palato-alveolar

[d] _____   15. velar

[ð] _____   16. nasal

[g] _____   17. fricative

[l] _____   18. liquid

                 19. stop

                 10. labial

                 11. back

                 12. high

Chapter 3

PHONEMICS

If you ask a native speaker of English if any sound is shared by the words *pet* and *speak*, the answer will invariably be yes, and the sound identified will be *p*. However, if we examine the two sounds that are identified as the same further, we realize that they are actually different; the initial sound of the word *peak* is a voiceless aspirated stop [pʰ], whereas the sound in *speak* is a voiceless unaspirated stop [p]. The important thing is that the initial reaction of the native speaker is very clear and unambigious, and tells us that the phonetic distinction between these sounds is totally overlooked. If, however, we ask the same question of a speaker of Hindi or Korean, she or he will not be able to find any sounds shared by these two words. The phonetic distinction between [pʰ] and [p] will not be overlooked, and these sounds will be identified as different.

A similar test case comes from comparing Spanish and English. If we ask a native speaker of Spanish if there is any consonant sound repeated in the words *danza* [danza] "dance" and *casado* [kasaðo] "married," the answer would be yes, and the consonant identified would be *d*. It is clear, however, that the first consonant of the first word is a stop, [d], whereas the so-called same sound, which appears as the third consonant of the second word, is a fricative [ð]. It is also clear that the Spanish speaker can hear the difference between these two sounds after it is pointed out. Again, however, what is important is the spontaneous re-action of the native speaker, and this clearly shows that the phonetic difference between these sounds is not functionally relevant. Therefore, [d] and [ð] are treated as one sound by native Spanish speakers. If, on the

41

other hand, the same question were posed to a native speaker of English, the answer would be entirely different, and the two sounds would be identified as different.

The underlying message gained from these facts is that the same phonetic reality is treated differently by speakers of different languages. Now, the question arises as to why this is the case. The reason that English speakers disregard the differences between the aspirated [pʰ] and unaspirated [p] is that these two sounds are functionally the same in the language; they are allophones of the same unit, the phoneme. However, in Hindi and Korean, the same two sounds are functionally different and belong to separate units; they are members of separate phonemes. Consequently, the speakers of Hindi and Korean would be attuned to the difference between [pʰ] and [p].

A similar situation is observed for the pair [d] and [ð] with speakers of Spanish and English. Although the difference between these two sounds is very important for English (the two sounds belong to two separate phonemes), the same phonetic distinction is treated as irrelevant by Spanish speakers because the sounds are functionally the same in Spanish (the two sounds are allophones of the same phoneme).

Although we have described the different cases by these labels, we have not really explained what is meant by allophones or phonemes yet. To understand these concepts, we must examine the ways sounds are distributed in languages.

DISTRIBUTION OF SOUNDS

Complementary/Overlapping Distribution

Sounds in any language are in one of two possible types of distribution: complementary or overlapping. When we say that two sounds are in overlapping distribution, we mean that these sounds are capable of occurring in the same environment. For example, the words *cap* [kʰæp] and *gap* [gæp] provide an instance of an overlapping distribution for the sounds [k] and [g] in word-initial position, and the words *back* [bæk] and *bag* [bæg] provide examples for the same pair of sounds in word-final position. The environments for distribution may be defined in terms of word or syllable position, neighboring sounds (preceding and/or following sounds), or suprasegmentals. When two sounds are in overlapping distribution, they are said to be in a nonpredictable distribution in that, wherever X might occur, so can Y, and vice versa.

In a great number of cases, overlapping distribution of two sounds in two words such as the above pairs results in different meanings. The change in the sound results in a change in meaning and, in such a case, we say that the two sounds are in contrastive distribution and belong to separate phonemes. The contrast we see between the two sounds of English in the above examples comes from pairs of words in which everything is identical with the exception of the sounds in question, [k] and [g]. Such pairs provide contrasts in identical environments and are called **minimal pairs**. Here are some other examples of minimal pairs:

lake - rake	[l] [r] contrast in initial position
ether - either	[θ] [ð] contrast in medial position
sin - sing	[n] [ŋ] contrast in final position

Sometimes, it is not possible to find minimal pairs to establish the contrasts between two different sounds. In these situations, the investigator may make use of near minimal pairs that provide contrasts in analogous environments. A near minimal pair is a pair of words in which the two sounds in question appear in environments surrounded by the same neighboring sounds, although the more distant sounds may be different. For example, to establish the contrast between [p] and [b] in a language, we may use the hypothetical word pair [sepit] and [tebim]. Because the sounds [p] and [b] are surrounded by the same sounds, this will be sufficient to conclude that the two sounds contrast and belong to two separate phonemes. In summary, we can say that, if two sounds can occur in the same environment, and if the substitution of one sound for the other changes the meaning of the word, then the sounds are contrastive and they belong to two separate phonemes in the language.

We can now go back and examine the case of [d] and [ð] in English. Because these two sounds are in overlapping distribution (they can occur in the same environment), and the substitution of one for the other creates a meaning change (as in *day* [de] versus *they* [ðe]), they are functionally different and belong to two separate phonemes. The fact that they are functionally different makes the native speaker of English very sensitive to the difference in sound.

Sometimes, it is not possible to find even a near minimal pair because the sounds do not occur in the same environment of any sort. This may be due to structural aspects of the language. The distribution of [d] and [ð] in Spanish is a case in point. We do not find these two sounds in overlapping distribution (they never occur in the same environment); [ð] appears only between two vowels and [d] is found in other environments but never between two vowels. This is a situation in which the two sounds are in **complementary distribution**, and prediction of which sound will occur in a given environment is possible. In such a case, the sounds [d] and [ð] are said to be allophones of the same phoneme. This is the reason that Spanish speakers consider the two sounds to be the same despite the fact that they are phonetically different.

A similar situation arises when we look at the voiceless aspirated and the voiceless unaspirated stops, [pʰ] and [p], in English. Because these two phonetically different sounds never occur in the same environment (identical or analogous), they are in complementary distribution. A prediction regarding the occurrences of each is possible: [pʰ] occurs in syllable initial position followed by a stressed vowel, [p] occurs in other environments; these two sounds are, therefore, allophones of the same phoneme. This is why English speakers treat these two sounds as the same.

Complementary distribution is a necessary, but not sufficient, condition for two or more sounds to be allophones of the same phoneme. The case of English [h] and [ŋ] illustrates this point well. The distribution of these two sounds in English gives us the following picture: [h] occurs only in syllable-initial position and never in syllable-final position. [ŋ], on the other hand, has exactly the opposite distribution, occurring only in syllable-final position and never in syllable-initial position. In other words, we have a perfect case of a complementary distribution. Despite this, no one has suggested that these two sounds should be considered as allophones of the same phoneme. This is because they do not fulfill the other requirement of allophonic relationship, **phonetic similarity**. Sounds that are allophones of the same phoneme, in addition to being in complementary distribution, must have phonetic similarity. That is, they must share phonetic properties such as place or manner of articulation or voicing. If we examine these two sounds, we see that they have no similarities in their phonetic make up; [h] is a voiceless, glottal fricative, and [ŋ] is a velar nasal. There is no agreement in any of the dimensions (voicing, place of articulation, manner of articulation, or nasality) that are relevant for consonants. Thus, we can conclude that allophones of the same phoneme must be phonetically similar and be in complementary distribution.

Free Variation

There are two situations in which the above mentioned principles and practices are violated. In the first, we see cases in which allophones of the same phoneme may occur in the same environment without changing the meaning of the word. Note that this violates what we said earlier about the allophones of the same phoneme being in complementary distribution. By occurring in the same environment, we have a case of an overlapping distribution. For example, the final stops of American English are unreleased and unaspirated in the pronunciation *tap* [tæp], and *back* [bæk]. However, for certain speakers, it may be possible to release and aspirate these stops. Although these alternate pronunciations are possible, the words do not change meaning with the variation in pronunciation. Although the two sounds (aspirated and unaspirated) in these examples are in overlapping distribution, they are not in contrast. In these cases, they are said to be in **free variation**.

Although free variation commonly is mentioned in relation to allophones of the same phoneme, there is another type of case in which it can occur with allophones of separate phonemes. We can exemplify this situation by the following: The sounds [i] and [ɛ] are in contrast in English and belong to separate phonemes, as seen in the minimal pair *beat* [bit]—*bet* [bɛt]. The substitution of one vowel for the other is responsible for a change in meaning. However, for certain items in the language, this substitution does not result in a change in meaning. For example the word *economics* can be pronounced either as [ikənamɪks] or [ɛkənamɪks] with the same meaning. What we have here is a situation in which a normally contrastive pair of vowels that belong to separate phonemes do not perform this contrastive function in that particular item. A similar case is cited between [aj] and [i]. These sounds are in contrast in English and belong to separate phonemes, as shown in the pair *bite* [bajt]—*beat* [bit]. However, the words *either* and *neither* can be pronounced either as [iðər] or [ajðər], or [niðər] or [najðər], respectively, without any change in meaning. Here, again, we have a case of phonemic free variation.

PHONEMIC ANALYSIS

Although we have talked about the principles underlying the assignment of sounds to phonemes, we have not given a detailed account of how to do a phonemic analysis, which is an indispensible tool for linguists, language teachers, and speech-language pathologists. In the following, we will look at a step-by-step procedure of how to do a phonemic analysis.

The first task is to collect and transcribe the data phonetically. This is one of the most important steps in phonemic analysis, because the accuracy of the phonemic status of the sounds in the data correlates with the accuracy of the phonetic transcription. Greater care should be given to the fluctuations observed between phonetically similar sounds. Once that is determined, the next step is to establish the phonetic inventory of the sounds. This means placing the sounds in the right places in the phonetic chart according to their phonetic characteristics. Let us do this with the following data from Korean:

1. [us]	"upper"		13. [ʃinho]	"signal"
2. [sɛk]	"color"		14. [ʃigan]	"time"
3. [maʃi]	"delicious"		15. [ʃiktaŋ]	"dining room"
4. [inza]	"greetings"		16. [tadara]	"close it"
5. [tal]	"moon"		17. [paŋzək]	"cushion"
6. [talda]	"sweet"		18. [sul]	"wine"
7. [saram]	"person"		19. [tere]	"some"
8. [tʰaːl]	"mask"		20. [ʃilsu]	"mistake"
9. [pabi]	"cooked rice"		21. [son]	"hand"
10. [pʰado]	"wave"		22. [irure]	"reaches"
11. [kirim]	"picture"		23. [ʃipsam]	"thirteen"
12. [kʰigi]	"size"		24. [kamgak]	"sense"

Phonetic chart of Korean consonants

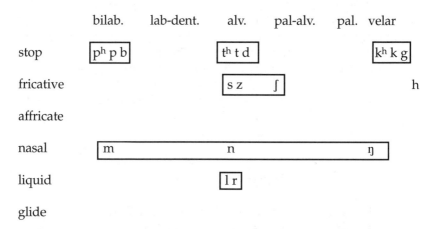

	bilab.	lab-dent.	alv.	pal-alv.	pal.	velar
stop	pʰ p b		tʰ t d			kʰ k g
fricative			s z	ʃ		h
affricate						
nasal	m		n			ŋ
liquid			l r			
glide						

Having placed all of the sounds in the phonetic chart, we are now ready to extract the suspicious pairs and groups. A suspicious pair or group of sounds is formed by the sounds that are phonetically similar and, therefore, are considered as potential allophones of the same phoneme. Our task is to determine whether these sounds are allophones of the same phoneme or if they belong to separate phonemes.

From the above chart, the relationships indicated by the broken lines will be examined for this purpose. As we can see clearly, in every one of these pairs (or groups), sounds share certain phonetic properties, that is, they are phonetically similar. Specifically, [p, t, k] share place, manner, and voicing characteristics with [pʰ, tʰ, kʰ] pairwise, but each pair differs in aspiration. The same group, however, share place, manner, and aspiration with [b, d, g], but differ in voicing. Another group of three sounds that will be considered suspicious are [s, z, ʃ]. Here, [s] shares the place and the manner of articulation with [z], and the two sounds differ only in voicing. As for the difference between [s] and [ʃ], we look at place of articulation, because the other characteristics (manner and voicing) are shared. Nasals always form a suspicious group, but it is generally the case that [n] and [ŋ] may form an allophonic relationship, and [m] remains as a separate phoneme. Finally, we look at the pair [l] and [r]; these two liquids are always suspicious because of their shared characteristics of manner and voicing. To summarize then, we have identified the suspicious sets of sounds that are phonetically similar. Next, we will determine whether the relationship between the pairs and the groups are distinctive (contrastive) or allophonic (predictable).

Looking at the set [p, t, k] in relation to [pʰ, tʰ, kʰ], we begin searching for minimal pairs for each place of articulation. For [pʰ - p] we cannot find a minimal pair, but we can use number 10 and number 17 to show that these two sounds occur in analogous environments (i.e., both sounds are in word-initial position and followed by the same vowel) and, thus, are in contrast. For [tʰ - t], the situation is a little easier as numbers 5 and 8 show these two sounds in the same environment and, thus, in contrast, also. Having spotted the bilabials and the alveolars contrasting between the aspirated and unaspirated stops, we have certain expectations for the remaining pair of velars. Symmetrical patterns regarding sets of sounds are common in languages. Thus, we also expect the velars to contrast. This, however, must be verified with the data. Although we cannot find an exact minimal pair, numbers 11 and 12 are sufficient to confirm this hypothesis. The two sounds in question, [kʰ - k], occur in an analogous environment and are in contrast. Thus, we can conclude that the aspirated and unaspirated voiceless stops of Korean belong to separate phonemes, and aspiration is a distinctive property of Korean phonology.

The next suspicious relationship occurs in the set [p, t, k] with the voiced version [b, d, g]. Again, we start the pairwise examination of distribution. The data do not reveal any cases of minimal pairs, nor do we find a near-minimal pair for an analogous environment for the suspicious pairs [p - b], [t - d], and [k - g]. In this case, the most fruitful strategy is to list the environments for each sound:

p	b	t	d	k	g
#__a(9)	a__i(9)	#__a(5,6)	l__a(6)	#__i(11)	i__i(12)
i__s(23)		#__e(19)	a__a(16)	#__a(24)	i__a(14)
			a__o(10)	a__#(24)	m__a(24

Here, the environments are given in terms of the immediately preceding and immediately following environments. The symbol # stands for the word boundary and indicates either the word-initial position (before the space bar), or word-final position (after the space bar). For example, the first occurrence of [p] is in word-initial position and is followed by [a]. This is described as #__a. The numbers in parentheses next to each environment indicate the number of the word in the data in which this particular environment occurs.

After we carefully screen the data and register the environments for each sound, we compare the environments for each pair in terms of a phonetic characteristic that could be of importance. Here, the most important point is the phonetic feature that distinguishes one sound from the other in the pair. Each of these three pairs, [p - b], [t - d] and [k - g], is separated by voicing. Consequently, we should examine the immediately preceding and immediately following environments in terms of this feature. This is because neighboring sounds may influence each other and may be responsible for the change (in this case, voicing). If we look at the environments that are listed, we find the voiced [b], [d], and [g] always in between two voiced sounds. This never happens with the voiceless [p], [t], and [k]. In other words, when we look at the surrounding environments, we do not find the voiced and voiceless sounds in the same environment with respect to voicing. This reveals a perfect case of a complementary distribution. Therefore, we can conclude that the sounds [p, b], [t, d], and [k, g], pairwise, are allophones of the same phonemes. Because the relationship is the same for bilabials, alveolars, and velars, it is obvious that the place of articulation is irrelevant and there is only one process that describes the situation: voiceless stops become voiced between voiced sounds.

Before we continue our phonemic analysis, we can stop for a moment and compare the situation of the stops of Korean with the stops of English. Phonetically, both languages make use of the nine sounds given in three sets, [p, t, k] [pʰ, tʰ, kʰ], and [b, d, g]. In Korean, these nine sounds are reduced to six in terms of phonemes, because the aspirated stops are in contrast with the unaspirated ones, whereas the voiced [b, d, g] are allophones of the voiceless /p, t, k/. Thus we have the following:

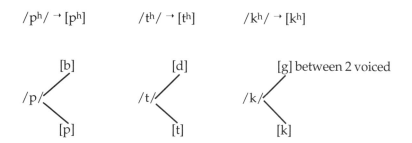

In English, however, the relationship among the same sounds is different. The set [p, t, k] contrasts with [b, d, g], but is in complementary distribution with the set [pʰ, tʰ, kʰ]. Thus, although there are also the same nine phonetically different sounds that are reduced to six, phonemically, the relationship assumes the following shape:

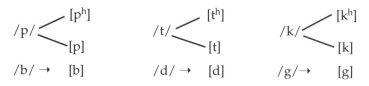

The rather different phonemic segmentation of the same phonetic reality certainly has many practical consequences. For example, a Korean speaker who is learning English (or an English speaker who is learning Korean) will need to adjust the relationships in his or her attempts in the target language. For example, we can predict that a Korean speaker would have a problem with an English item like *paper* [pʰepər] with regard to the second consonant [p]. Because it is not possible to have a [p] between two voiced sounds in his or her language (only [b] is allowed), the speaker might produce the target as [pʰebər]. Note that the first consonant in the same word will not be affected, because Korean allows [pʰ] in initial position. To consider the situation from the other perspective, we can talk about the attempt for the Korean item number 5, [tal] "moon" by a speaker of English. Because the word starts with a voiceless unaspirated stop, it would create difficulty for the speaker of English, as his or her language allows only the aspirated stop in this position. The rendition we would expect for this item is [tʰal], that is, with [tʰ]. This prediction happens to be a very accurate one when we look at the speakers of English in their attempts to speak Korean. Similar situations would be observed with regard to numbers 6, 9, 11, 16, 17, 19, and 24, for which initial unaspirated voiceless stops are demanded in Korean.

Such conflicting situations are not restricted to foreign language learners. Similarly, a child with a phonological disorder growing up in a Korean-

English bilingual home or a Korean-English bilingual person with aphasia will need to deal with these differences in their phonologies. We will have more to say about these cases later, but it is important to alert the reader to the importance of such differences, which cannot be overstated.

Let us now go back to our data and examine the other suspicious pairs/groups. The next subgroup on our list is the group [s - z - ʃ]. In this group, the phonetic similarity will be pairwise between [s - z] and [s - ʃ]. The first pair shares place and manner of articulation and differs in terms of voicing, and the second pair shares manner of articulation and voicing, but differs in place of articulation. We have no reason to consider [ʃ - z] because these two sounds differ in more characteristics (place of articulation and voicing) than they share (manner of articulation).

The examination of the pair [s - ʃ] does not reveal any minimal pairs, nor does it show any near-minimal pair. Note that the environments that are examined here should relate to place of articulation because the pair of sounds in question differs in that dimension. When we list the environments for each sound we find the following:

s	ʃ
u__# (1)	a__i (3)
#__ɛ (2)	#__i (13,14,15,20,23)
#__a (7)	
#__u (18)	
l __u (20)	
#__o (21)	
p__a (23)	

The distribution of these two sounds reveals that they do not occur in the same environment; we always find [ʃ] before [i], and this is the significant environment. The preceding environment cannot be a factor, as both of these sounds can occur in word-initial position. In addition, the vowel [i] is known to cause alveolar sounds to change in place of articulation to palatal sounds in many languages. This is phonetically motivated because the place where we raise the tip of the tongue to produce the vowel [i] corresponds to the palatal place of articulation. The fact that we find [ʃ] only before [i], and we never find [s] in the same environment, tells us that these two phonetically similar sounds are in complementary distribution and, thus, are the allophones of the same phoneme.

As for the situation between [s - z], the data do not provide minimal or near-minimal pairs. Here, again, we rely on a list of the environments.

Because we already have the distribution of [s] from the above case, all we need is the distribution of [z]:

z
n__a (4)
ŋ__ə (17)

If we compare the environments of [s] and [z], we see that the environment following the sound is irrelevant, as both sounds can be followed by the same sounds. However, the preceding environment seems to reveal a complemetary distribution because we find [z] only after nasals, and we never find [s] in this environment. The conclusion is that [s] and [z] are allophones of the same phoneme. Because we said the same thing for [s] and [ʃ] earlier, the complete picture is that all three sounds are in complementary distribution and belong to the same phoneme. To decide which sound to choose to represent the phoneme, we should choose the sound that is the least restricted in occurrence. Because [ʃ] occurs only before [i] and [z] occurs only after nasals, [s] is clearly the least restricted allophone and will represent the phoneme. We present the situation in the following manner:

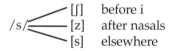

	[ʃ]	before i
/s/	[z]	after nasals
	[s]	elsewhere

As seen in this presentation, we write the more restricted, thus, more easily predictable, allophone(s) first, so that we can say "elsewhere" for the main (the least restricted) allophone of the phoneme.

The allophonic relationship of [s, z, ʃ] in Korean is very different from what we find in English for the same sounds. English provides examples of minimal pairs for the sounds in question: *sip, ship,* and *zip* are sufficient to conclude that [s, z, and ʃ] contrast and belong to separate phonemes /s/, /z/ and /ʃ/. This is illustrated in the following chart:

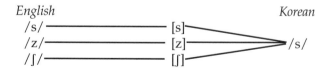

The practical consequences of such an uneven situation between Korean and English puts the Korean speaker at a disadvantage in learning English. The predicted, and often attested, case in which *sea shells*

[si ʃɛlz] is pronounced as [ʃi sɛls] tells the whole story. Note that the Korean speaker's difficulty regarding this example does not reside in learning to pronounce new, foreign sounds. The English sequence has three sounds which all are also available in Korean but, alas, all of them are at "wrong" places in Korean phonology. The speaker must learn to categorize them as different (contrastive) units rather than to treat them as distributionally related members of one unit, as they normally function in Korean. To start with, the word *sea* has [s] followed by [i] which, according to the Korean sound system, should be [ʃ], thus the rendition [ʃi]. The second word, *shells*, creates two problems that are related to the first and the last sounds. The first sound is [ʃ] in English, but this does not match the Korean system. Because the sound is followed by a vowel other than [i], Korean would not allow the [ʃ], and would replace it with [s], which would occur in that environment in the Korean system. Finally, the last sound in the English word *shells* is a [z]. Although Korean has [z], it appears only after a nasal and, because, in this word, [z] does not occur after a nasal, the Korean rendition would be [s]. This completes the picture for the rendition as [ʃi sɛls] for [si ʃɛlz].

Next, we will consider the nasal consonants of Korean, [m], [n], and [ŋ], which differ only in place of articulation. As usual, we begin the analysis with a search for minimal or near-minimal pairs. Without much difficulty, we can spot items 7, 14, and 15, in which we locate the three nasals in near-minimal pairs. All three sounds are found in word-final position after [a], and this is sufficient to conclude that they are in contrast and belong to separate phonemes /m/, /n/, and /ŋ/. The system of Korean nasals corresponds to the system of the English nasals:

English					*Korean*
/m/———————	[m]	———————	/m/
/n/———————	[n]	———————	/n/
/ŋ/———————	[ŋ]	———————	/ŋ/

Given this parallelism, we would not predict any difficulties for learners.

Finally, we look at the suspicious pair of liquids [l, r] in Korean. Because we cannot find any minimal or near-minimal pairs for the sounds in question, we list the environments for each:

r	l
a__a (7)	a__# (5)
i__i (11)	a__d (6)
e__e (19)	a:__# (8)
u__e (22)	u__# (18)
	i__s (20)

A close examination of the environments reveals that the occurrence of [r] is always in an intervocalic environment (between two vowels) and [l] never occurs in that environment. Thus, this is a case of complementary distribution, and these two sounds are allophones of the same phoneme. Because the distribution of [l] is the least restricted one (it occurs word finally as well as medially), [l] will be chosen to represent the phoneme and describe the distribution of [r] first:

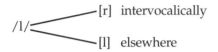

/l/ ⟨ [r] intervocalically
        [l] elsewhere

This situation is different from English, in which [r] and [l] contrast (*lay - ray*):

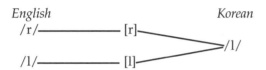

English   Korean
/r/——————— [r]
                                              /l/
/l/——————— [l]

Needless to say, this mismatch is responsible for commonly occurring errors such as [ærɪsən] for *Allison*, or [ærɪmɔni] for *alimony*.

Now, we are in a position to show the relationship of all the sounds shared by the two languages in question:

English phonomes   Korean phonemes

                            [pʰ] ———————/pʰ/
/p/ ⟨   [p] ———————/p/
/b/ ——————— [b]
                            [tʰ] ———————/tʰ/
/t/ ——————— [t] ———————/t/
/d/ ——————— [d]
                            [kʰ] ———————/kʰ/
/k/ ——————— [k] ———————/k/
/g/ ——————— [g]
/ʃ/ ——————— [ʃ]
/s/ ——————— [s] ———————/s/
/z/ ——————— [z]
/m/ ——————— [m] ———————/m/
/n/ ——————— [n] ———————/n/
/ŋ/ ——————— [ŋ] ———————/ŋ/
/r/ ——————— [r]
/l/ ——————— [l] ———————/l/

Going back to our data, now we can write the Korean words phonemically with the assumption that vowels belong to separate phonemes. To write words phonemically, only phonemes—the representations between slashes—are used. Here, only phonemic contrasts are recorded and phonetic details that are shown in bracketed phonetic representations are ignored. For example, number 3 is /masi/ phonemically, which then will be converted into the phonetic [maʃi] by the predictable distribution of /s/ → [ʃ] before [i]. Number 10 would be /pʰato/ and is converted into its phonetic representation [pʰado] by the rule that states that /t/ becomes a [d] between two voiced sounds. Finally, number 22 will start out as /ilule/ phonemically, and end in [irure] phonetically; the discrepancy between the two representations will be explained by the rule that states that the /l/ phoneme is phonetically realized as [r] whenever it occurs intervocalically.

PHONEMICS AND WRITING SYSTEMS

Although phonemics as an independent area of study is not very old, its practice is quite old. The discovery of alphabetic writing systems in the ancient Middle East reveals an understanding of the phonemic structure of language, which is a prerequisite for writing.

The intimate relationship between the phonemic structure of a language and the alphabetic writing system was made very clear by the title of K. L. Pike's (1947) book *Phonemics: A Technique for Reducing Language to Writing*. What seems to be the underlying principle of the alphabetic writing system is that each phoneme is assigned a letter, and the orthographic representation is phonemic. Having said this, we can see why, in English orthography, we do not need two different letters for two phonetically different but phonemically same p-sounds [pʰ - p]. The same is true for Spanish orthography, in which the letter *d* stands for the two phonetically different sounds [d] and [ð]. Because these two sounds are allophones of the same phoneme, /d/, and their distribution is predictable, an orthography that used only one letter would not have any problems. However, if we think about the same sounds in English, we realize that the use of one orthographic symbol for these two distinctive sounds would create problems, and English requires two separate symbols.

Although alphabetic writing systems *ideally* are phonemic, due to historical changes, there are many discrepancies today between the phonemic structure of languages and their orthographies. To cite some cases, let us consider the letter *k* in initial position before nasals in English in words such as *know*, *knee*, and *knife*,which are pronounced as [no], [ni], and [nayf]. Kindergartners are quick to realize the discrepancy between the pronunciation and the orthography, and the teachers' explanation of this letter being a "magical *k*" may satisfy the curiosity of some of this baffled audience. We know, of course, from old documents that there was a [k] sound at the beginning of these words and, at some point in the history of English, [k] sounds in initial position before nasals were dropped. The current orthographical shape represents this old pronunciation. Although we are not in a position to give the reader the actual date of the disappearance of this "magical *k*," we are certain about its historical origin.

Another historically caused mismatch can be seen in the orthographic combination *th* in English. If we do not know how to pronounce a word in English, there is no way that we can predict whether it would have a [θ] or a [ð] in its pronunciation by looking at the letters *th* in a given word. The reason for this is that the distribution of these two sounds is not predictable and the sounds belong to two separate phonemes, /θ/ and /ð/. However, the records show that, early in the history of English, there was only the voiceless interdental fricative /θ/ phonemically. The voiced allophone [ð] occurred between voiced sounds. During the Middle English period, due to the disappearance of certain inflections, the voiced allophone [ð] appeared word-finally, creating contrasts and, over time, achieving the present phonemic status. Because these two phonemes in present-day English are represented by the same combination, *th*, the orthography deviates from the basic principle of the alphabetic writing system, namely, that a phonemically accurate system would require two separate symbols for two different phonemes, /θ/ and /ð/.

Sometimes, one does hear remarks such as "the writing system of language X is excellent; it is phonetic." Such comments have to be taken very cautiously, because they are simply careless remarks about that language. There is no language with a fully precise phonetic writing system, as this would be an extremely cumbersome way of representing the sound patterns of the language. Because the occurrences of the different allophones of the same phoneme are predictable, the native speaker does not need to be shown every allophone in every environment. When a Spanish speaker sees the word *dedo*, she or he automatically uses a stop, [d], for the first consonant, but changes it to a fricative, [ð], for the second consonant, despite the fact that the orthography treats the two identically. One may ask "how a nonnative learner of Spanish would know this." The answer is, she or he would not, and cannot, know. The fact is, though, that writing systems are designed for the native speakers of that language.

CLINICAL RELEVANCE

Phonological Development

The importance of phonemic analysis between two languages also is relevant for other areas of practical application. One such situation is the case of phonological disorders, in which the client's sound structure would guide the type of remediation. The following examples from monolingual situations show how the sound system of a person may be very different from the ambient language phonemically. In other words, the deviance is structural rather than (or, as in most cases, as well as) phonetic. We will illustrate this point with the following examples (Bleile, 1991, p. 32):

	Target	*Child's realizations*
a.	key	[ti]
b.	go	[doʊ]
c.	big	[bɪk]
d.	stick	[tɪk]
e.	guy	[daɪ]
f.	coat	[toʊt]
g.	broken	[bwoʊdɪn]
h.	digger	[dɪdər]
i.	egg	[eɪk]
j.	Mike	[maɪk]

In addition to the obvious problems of the consonant clusters and the voicing of the stops, this child's system reveals that velar stops become alveolars in syllable-initial position.

Now, observe the following data from another child (Bleile, 1991, p. 37):

	Target	*Child's realization*
a.	ball	[bɔʊ]
b.	mama	[mama]
c.	pad	[bæ]
d.	big	[dɪʔ]
e.	boo	[bu]
f.	milk	[nɪʔ]
g.	bʌbʌbi	[babadi]
h.	me	[ni]
i.	pa	[pa]
j.	"B"	[dɪʔ]

Here, what we observe is that bilabial consonants become alveolars before a high front vowel. In other words, we can describe a situation in which bilabial and alveolar realizations are allophonically related as in /b/ → [d] before /i/.

Another interesting case was described by Camarata and Gandour (1984):

bee	[bi]	tea	[di]	kite	[gæ]
bath	[bæ]	key	[di]	tie	[gæ]
bus	[bʌ]	kick	[di]	clown	[gæn]
boot	[bu]	two	[du]	train	[gæn]
book	[bu]	cook	[du]	cup	[gʌ]
boat	[bo]			duck	[gʌ]
ball	[ba]			goat	[go]
pan	[bæn]			toe	[go]
				car	[ga]
				dog	[ga]

These data from a 3-year-old child with a phonological disorder reveal the productions of voiced stops [b], [d], and [g]. We can see that /b/ and /d/ contrast (*bee* [bi] versus *tea* [di]). On the other hand, [d] and [g] do not show any contrast. What we have here is a complementary distribution between these two sounds; [d] appears before high vowels (second column), and [g] appears before low or mid vowels (third column). This is another case in which the child has the voiced stops phonetically in a restricted set of phoneme classes.

Finally, let us examine the following data taken from another child (Bleile, 1991, p. 40):

	Target	*Child's realization*
a.	big	[bigŋ]
b.	egg	[ɛgŋ]
c.	read	[widn]
d.	drop	[dap]
e.	stub	[dabm]
f.	eat	[it]
g.	word	[wʊdn]
h.	talk	[dɔk]
i.	lightbulb	[jaɪtbabm]
j.	fit	[vɪt]

This time, the major pattern revealed concerns the voiced stops adding a homorganic nasal in final position. Thus, we can give the following account:

/b/ ⟨ [bm] / [b]   /d/ ⟨ [dn] / [d]   /g/ ⟨ [gŋ] final position / [g] elsewhere

In summary, the child's system involves using both sounds noncontrastively, the sounds are in allophonic variation. In all of these cases, the child has the ability to pronounce different allophones. Thus, what is needed is a restructuring of the system rather than simple articulation therapy.

Not all cases of disability would reveal situations like those presented above and, in some cases, articulation therapy would be required. For example, the individual may have one or the other phoneme missing entirely. For example, when all target /k/ phonemes are replaced by the alveolar /t/, the resulting situation would have the homophonous realizations [tæp] for the words *cap* and *tap*. In this case, she or he will need articulation therapy together with activities that will ensure the contrastive function of the new phoneme in the system.

Phonemic Awareness and Literacy Skills

Developing an ambient like phonemic system is necessary not only for spoken language skills, but has implications in acquiring literacy skills as well. Phonological awareness, which is the ability to reflect on and manipulate the structure (e.g., syllable, sounds), is a prerequisite for the acquisition of written code. Children who are learning a language like English that utilizes an alphabetic script must develop the awareness that a phoneme-grapheme link exists. Doing this requires the ability to segment words into phonemes. This phonemic awareness is dependent on a phonemic system that is intact. Any problems with the child's system may disrupt the development of this awareness. Research over the last two decades has shown that there is a strong relationship between spoken language impairment and the development of phonological awareness in that children with phonological disorders do not perform well in many tasks related to awareness (Bird & Bishop, 1992; Bird, Bishop, & Freeman, 1995; Marion, Sussman, & Marquardt, 1993; Webster &

Plante, 1992). If phonemic awareness is a strong predictor of literacy development, children with phonological disorders are at greater risk for deficiencies in their development of literacy skills.

There are different tasks to test phonemic awareness. Among them are phoneme identification, phoneme segmentation, and rhyming. In phoneme identification tasks, children are asked whether a target vowel or consonant is included in a number of words. The target sound appears in initial, medial, and final positions of the words. Phoneme segmentation tasks require children to indicate the number of phonemes in words that are varied in length and number of syllables. In rhyming exercises, children may be asked to produce spontaneous rhymes. Another task that is utilized is rhyme-detection. For example, children are shown three pictures that are named during conversation and the children's task is to indicate the two rhyming words among the three. Among these tasks for measuring phonemic awareness, phoneme segmentation and identification skills have been found to be more powerful predictors of literacy outcome than rhyming. The explanation for this may come from the fact that rhyming requires only partial segmentation of a syllable or word, whereas the other two tasks demand complete segmentation.

Because phonemic awareness is such a powerful predictor for literacy skills, and because children with phonological disorders in general are less successful than their normally developing counterparts in developing this awareness, to prevent later literacy problems, intervention programs to promote phonological awareness should be greatly emphasized.

SUMMARY

In this chapter, we have seen how sounds of a language system are distributed. Sounds may be organized in one of two ways: complementary distribution or overlapping distribution. To find out which sounds the language uses distinctively, it is necessary to conduct a phonemic analysis of the language. The process of identifying the phonemes and their allophones in a language may be useful in situations of language learning, language contact, teaching reading and writing, and remediation of disordered speech. Assessing the phonemic system of a subject with disordered phonological patterns may be useful to identify structural differences between their system and the target system. If the subject's system is different from the target system, it may be necessary to restructure the system, not just train specific sounds.

EXERCISES

1. Circle the correct alternative:

   a. If a difference between two speech sounds is phonemic/allophonic, they will contrast in the same environment.

   b. In words such as *pit* and *bit* or *tap* and *tab*, /p/ and /b/ are in complementary/contrastive distribution.

   c. When the difference between two sounds is functional, we say that it is phonetic/phonemic.

   d. Because, in English, we have no minimal pair [pʰɪn] - [pɪn], and because we do have minimal pairs like [pʰɪn] - [bɪn], we conclude that aspiration/voicing is a phonetic difference, whereas aspiration/voicing is a phonemic difference.

   e. Sounds in complementary distribution occur/do not occur in the same environment.

   f. Phonemic systems are never/sometimes/often the same for any two languages.

   g. Allophones of the same phoneme are sometimes/ often/always phonetically similar.

   h. Phonetics/phonemics deals with the production of speech sounds; phonetics/phonemics deals with the function of speech sounds.

   i. Portuguese has neither /θ/ nor /ð/. Voicing, however, is phonemic in Portuguese and the language contains both /t/ and /d/. If the speaker of Portuguese substitutes /t/ for /θ/ in English, she or he would be likely to substitute [t / d /p /b] for /ð/, as in the word *then*.

2. Match the following:

1. A pair of words differing by only one phoneme.

2. If the substitution of one sound for another in the same environment results in a change of meaning, we say that the two sounds _____.

3. A list of all of the perceptibly different speech sounds in a language.

4. Two phonetically different sounds can be interchanged in the same environment without causing a change of meaning.

5. A list of all of the functionally different speech sounds of a language.

a. phonetic inventory

b. minimal pair

c. phonemic inventory

d. contrast

e nonphonemic difference

3. For each of the following pairs of sounds give a minimal pair showing their occurrence in initial, medial, and final position.(Note that the spelling of the words is irrelevant in this exercise):

e.g.: [l] [r] *lake - rake, cold - cord, fall - far*

	Initial	Medial	Final
[i] [ɪ]			
[p] [b]			
[tʃ] [dʒ]			
[s] [ʃ]			
[s] [z]			
[p] [f]			
[m] [n]			
[k] [g]			

4. What sounds are contrasted in the following minimal pairs?

bib - babe	[-]		*west - vest*	[-]	
plea - play	[-]		*rope - robe*	[-]	
creased - crest	[-]		*rifle - rival*	[-]	
hill - hell	[-]		*deaf - death*	[-]	
bond - boned	[-]		*vowel - bowel*	[-]	
defend - descend	[-]		*lard - lord*	[-]	
shot - shout	[-]		*ether - eater*	[-]	
look - luke	[-]		*they - day*	[-]	

5. In the following data, [θ] and [f] are substitutes for the targets /f/, /s/, /ʃ/, and / θ/, and their occurrences are predictable. Give the generalization.

feather	[θɛdə]
soup	[fup]
fall	[fɔl]
thin	[θɪn]
fish	[fɪs]

sick	[θɪk]
ship	[fɪp]
shoe	[fu]
thought	[fɔt]

6. Examine the distribution of [s] and [ʃ] in the speech of T (4 years, 3 months), a child with phonological disorder, and determine whether the two sounds are in contrast or in complementary distribution.

Irish	[aɪrɪs]	*leash*	[lis]
fasten	[fæsən]	*fashion*	[fæʃən]
show	[ʃo]	*short*	[ʃɔrt]
shell	[ʃɛl]	*clash*	[kæs]
sip	[ʃɪp]	*shoe*	[ʃu]

7. Examine the following data from B (4 years, 1 month), a child with phonological disorder, and determine whether the realizations of /r/ targets are predictable.

race	[res]	*mirror*	[mɪwə]
berry	[bewi]	*correct*	[kɔwɛk]
parade	[pəwed]	*rain*	[ren]
ride	[raɪd]	*four*	[fɔ]
deer	[di]	*road*	[rod]
wrong	[rɔŋ]	*room*	[rum]

8. Examine the following data from W (3 years, 9 months), a child with phonological disorder, and determine the phonemic status of [k] and [t].

cage	[tedʒ]	*clean*	[tin]
call	[kɔl]	*neck*	[nɛt]

bike	[baɪt]		*car*	[kar]
book	[bʊk]		*back*	[bæt]
joke	[dʒok]		*cool*	[kul]
key	[ti]		*cake*	[tet]

9. Examine the data from the speech of another child with phonological disorder, T (3 years, 7 months), and determine whether the realizations of /k/ targets are predictable.

came	[kem]		*pick*	[pɪt]
duck	[dʌt]		*back*	[bæt]
clean	[kin]		*cap*	[kæp]
coat	[kot]		*come*	[kʌm]
cake	[ket]		*picky*	[pɪki]

10. Examine the following data from Japanese and determine whether [t], [tˢ], and [tʃ] are allophones of the same phoneme or represent two different phonemes, or three different phonemes. If allophones, state the complementary distribution; if phonemes, state the contrast.

1.	[te]	"hand"	9.	[tˢutʃi]	"earth"
2.	[takai]	"high"	10.	[ato]	"later"
3.	[tegami]	"letter"	11.	[kutˢu]	"shoe"
4.	[tˢukue]	"desk"	12.	[tʃitʃi]	"father"
5.	[utʃi]	"house"	13.	[matˢu]	"wait
6.	[tʃizu]	"map"	14.	[ita]	"board"
7.	[tatami]	"mat"	15.	[tomodatʃi]	"friend"
8.	[kata]	"person"	16.	[natˢu]	"summer"

On the basis of your findings, predict the most likely pronunciation of the following English target words by

a speaker of Japanese. You should concentrate on the realization of /t/ targets in these words, and ignore the
other potential problems.

city [   ],   *team* [   ],   *tear* [   ]
totem [   ],   *tune* [   ]

11. Examine the following data from Brazilian Portuguese
and determine the phonemic status of the suspicious
pairs [t - tʃ], and [d - dʒ]. If they are allophones, state the
complementary distribution; if separate phonemes,
state the contrast.

1.	[tʃinta]	"ink"	10.	[temer]	"to fear"
2.	[tokar]	"to touch"	11.	[dʒia]	"day"
3.	[dosi]	"sweet"	12.	[tarefa]	"task"
4.	[dexota]	"defeat'	13.	[dʒivida]	"debt"
5.	[donu]	"owner"	14.	[tomar]	"to take'
6.	[tarifa]	"fare"	15.	[tʃia]	"aunt"
7.	[ultʃimu]	"last"	16.	[durantʃi]	"during"
8.	[dozi]	"twelve"	17.	[dʒizer]	"to say"
9.	[dar]	"to give"	18.	[tempu]	"weather"

On the basis of your findings, predict the most likely
pronunciation of the following English words by a Portuguese speaker. You should concentrate on the /t/ and
/d/ targets in these words, and ignore the other potential problems.

city [   ],   *total* [   ],   *dinner* [   ]
desire [   ],   *teacher* [   ],   *dolphin* [   ]

Chapter 4

DISTINCTIVE FEATURES

Although segments have been discussed as individual units represented by a single symbol (e.g., /b/), the idea that sounds have internal structure has been introduced only implicitly. For example, while talking about the phonemic analysis of Korean in the preceding chapter, it was mentioned that /p/ was realized phonetically as [b] between two voiced sounds, and the same occurred with the realization of /t/ as [d], and /k/ as [g] in the same environment. From these examples, it was concluded that a group of sounds /p, t, k/ which are bilabial, alveolar, and velar voiceless stops, became voiced stops [b, d, g], respectively, in the environment between voiced sounds. In other words, the original phonemes, phonetic realizations, and the sounds representing the environment are all describable in terms of natural classes of sounds rather than as arbitrary combinations. Natural classes are groups of sounds in a language that share some articulatory, acoustic, or auditory features. The regularities that are found within a set of segments (natural classes) seem to relate to the features themselves rather than to the whole segments. In the case of the voicing of /p, t, k/, the natural class of voiceless stops became voiced, changing only in the feature [voiced].

Consider an example from English, the aspiration rule. As seen earlier /p/,/t/, and /k/ of English are realized as [pʰ], [tʰ], and [kʰ] respectively, in the initial position of stressed syllables. In this particular event, the sounds that are participating are bilabial, alveolar, and velar voiceless stops; however, it quickly becomes evident that the place of articulation is irrelevant, and what makes this group of sounds a natural class are the voiceless and stop characteristics.

As seen in these two examples, the /p, t, k/ of both English and Korean grouped themselves for a phonological event: voicing in the case of Korean and aspiration in the case of English. This grouping was cited as an example of a natural class, as these sounds were all voiceless stops. To compare these sounds with another set, consider the following three sounds [p, z, ŋ], and ask the question of whether a phonological event could be found where these three sounds are grouped together. The answer to this question is an unequivocal no. There is no phonological process or rule that requires the grouping of [p], [z], and [ŋ]. It can also safely be said that these three sounds will not be found to function together in any rule in any language. The reason for this is that [p] is a voiceless bilabial stop, [z] is a voiced alveolar fricative, and [ŋ] is a velar nasal. Consequently, unlike the natural class of voiceless stops /p, t, k/, this arbitrary set of sounds has nothing in common.

In order to make statements about classes of sounds, it is necessary to consider the features that comprise segments and to find the shared properties among the features. The descriptions of sounds given in Chapter 2, which also are exemplified in the above examples, have introduced the idea that a segment is a combination of certain phonetic properties. For example, in defining [z] as an alveolar voiced fricative, the articulatory components are denoted.

Although these labels seem adequate in providing the phonetic characteristics of sounds, they are problematic because they presuppose a fundamental division between consonants (defined in terms of place and manner of articulation and voicing) and vowels (defined in terms of tongue height, tongue advancement, lip rounding, and tense/lax distinction). These two classes of segments are described using different dimensions and treated in entirely different manners, implying that they have nothing to do with one another, which makes little phonetic sense. First, there are borderline sounds such as liquids and glides which have affinity with both vowels and consonants. Second, we cannot express phonological generalizations by using separate features. For example, a phenomenon such as palatalization reveals a certain commonality in both consonants and vowels. The data on Korean in Chapter 3 showed that /s/ becomes [ʃ] before [i]. With the background we have available up to this point, all that can be said is that an alveolar consonant becomes a palatal consonant before a high front vowel:

alveolar C → Palatal C / ___ high front V

where → indicates "become," / shows the environment, and the space bar indicates where this change will take place. But this notation, which describes a very common phonological event, is not very different from one in which an [s] becomes a [ʃ] before an [a], which describes a highly improbable, if not impossible, event:

alveolar C → Palatal C / ___ low back V

This is a defective form of notation in the sense that there is no way of distinguishing the common process of palatalization before a high front vowel from the highly improbable one before a low back vowel, because the labels we use to characterize the situation do not reveal anything about the commonality of sounds.

In order to express the phonological processes with the force of generality and to be able to distinguish the probable from the improbable, there is a need for a system of classification that views sounds as consisting of subsegmental componential features without making a separation between consonants and vowels. A system that would employ one set of features for both vowels and consonants would avoid the problem, and the similarity between [ʃ] and [i] in terms of tongue placement would be revealed by the feature [high], which is shared by these two sounds. The problems of the previous descriptions are not restricted only to this unjustifiable separation of consonants and vowels. Even within one major group, for example consonants, there are commonalities among sounds that are not indicated by the classifications available thus far.

For example, stops, affricates, and nasals make up a group sharing the feature [–continuant] in which the airstream through the mouth is stopped. This group is in contrast to other consonants, such as fricatives and liquids, in which the primary oral stricture allows continuous, although restricted, passage of the airstream [+continuant]. Another example is the group of [+anterior] consonants (labials, dentals, and alveolars), which have a stricture in front of the palato-alveolar region. Thus, all speech sounds fall into many different overlapping groups that are natural for some feature that may be relevant in some phonological events. This fact can best be expressed by analyzing each sound in terms of its constituent features. These features, and not the phonemes, are the smallest and most basic units of phonological analysis.

Features, like phonemes, are theoretical constructs, and there are many ways of analyzing a specific set of phonemes in terms of sets of features. There are different sets of features that search for the most suitable and efficient version. However, certain shared principles guide all feature systems despite their differences in details of features. All aim at providing a limited set of universal features that is adequate for describing the phonological contrasts of all languages of the world. In their descriptive function, features must accurately express the phonetic nature of a sound. In their contrastive function, they must permit one sound to be distinguished from another. In their classificatory function, features must define classes of phonemes that fall into groups with respect to their phonological behavior.

The first attempt at a distinctive feature theory was by the Russian linguist Roman Jakobson in 1928. Based on binary opposition, Jakobson tried to find a universal system of phonemic representation. Each phoneme was viewed as a bundle of distinctive features and was distinguished from all other phonemes in the language by its unique feature combination. The specification for any phoneme in terms of its distinctive feature content could be stated through one of a set of binary values [+/–] for each distinctive feature in the phonological system.

An elaborated version of the distinctive feature theory appeared with *Preliminaries to Speech Analysis* (PSA) by Jakobson, Fant, and Halle (1952). In this version, features were defined in acoustic terms. During the 1950s and 1960s, scholars found several shortcomings of the features of PSA and, to cure the ills of the Jakobsonian feature system, Chomsky and Halle proposed a new feature system in *The Sound Pattern of English* (SPE).

In this new system, like that of Jakobson, the principle of **universality** received considerable emphasis. Chomsky and Halle stated that, "the total set of features is identical with the set of phonetic properties that can in principle be controlled in speech; they represent the phonetic capabilities of man and, we would assume, are therefore the same for all languages" (pp. 294–295). They also upheld the Jakobsonian principle of **binarity**. This implies that features are assigned binary values and we can specify them by indicating whether a given attribute is present. This is done by assigning one of the two values, plus or minus, to the same feature [X], rather than having two separate labels such as nasal versus oral. For example, nasals would be specified as [+nasal] and oral sounds would be [–nasal].

The principle of binarity is a controversial one. Many phonetic specifications, such as aspiration, nasalization, and vowel height, can be described on a continuum and thus lend themselves better to a multivalued scale rather than to a two-way contrast of binarism. Although the debate about binarism regarding the phonetic details continues, it is generally assumed that the features that are used for phonological contrasts are essentially binary.

The fundamental difference between SPE and PSA, in addition to the changes in several features, is the shift from acoustically defined features to an almost exclusively articulatory defined set of features.

CHOMSKY AND HALLE FEATURES

In the following, the Chomsky and Halle feature classification will be surveyed. This system was chosen because of its wide distribution and use.

Major Class Features

The features [syllabic], [sonorant], and [consonantal] are called the major class features, as they distinguish basic groups of sounds such as vowels, glides, and obstruents.

[sonorant]: These are sounds that are produced with a vocal cavity configuration in which spontaneous voicing is possible. Nonsonorants (obstruents) have a vocal cavity configuration that inhibits spontaneous voicing.

[+]: vowels, nasals, liquids, glides

[–]: obstruents (i.e., stops, fricatives, affricates)

[syllabic]: Syllabics are sounds that function as syllable nuclei. Nonsyllabic sounds occur at syllable margins. This feature best specifies the contrast between consonants and vowels.

[+]: vowels, syllabic liquids, syllabic nasals

[–]: all others

[consonantal]: These are sounds that are produced with obstruction along the center line of the oral cavity. Nonconsonantal sounds are produced without such obstruction. This feature best specifies the contrast between glides and other consonants.

[+]: obstruents, nasals, liquids

[–]: vowels, glides, h, ?

With these three major class features, we can uniquely identify the major groups of sounds.

Table 4–1, in addition to distinguishing each class, also reflects the phonetic distance or similarity between the major groups of sounds. For ex-

Table 4–1. Classification of sounds in terms of the three major class features.

Class	Vowels	Syllabic Liquid & Nasals	Nonsyllabic Liquis & Nasals	Glides	Obstruent	*h,ʔ*
Syllabic	+	+	−	−	−	−
Sonorant	+	+	+	+	−	−
Consonantal	−	+	+	−	+	−

ample, vowels and obstruents, the two extremes, are maximally opposed to one another in that whatever value (+ or –) one group receives for a given major class feature, the opposite value is received by the other group. We can also see the similarities between the nonsyllabic liquids and nasals with syllabic liquids and nasals on the one hand, and with glides, on the other. The only feature that separates nonsyllabic liquids and nasals from syllabic liquids and nasals is [+/– syllabic]. The same group is distinguished from glides by [+/– consonantal]. The feature [syllabic] also makes the distinction between vowels and glides.

Manner Features

Continuant: Continuants are sounds that are produced with a primary constriction that allows the air to flow through the mid-sagittal region of the vocal tract. Noncontinuant sounds are made by completely blocking the flow of air through the center of the vocal tract. The best example of this feature is the contrast between stops and affricates versus fricatives.

[+]: fricatives, glides, liquids, h, vowels[1]

[–]: stops, affricates, nasals

Strident: Sounds that are produced with a constriction that forces the airstream to strike two surfaces, producing a high intensity noise are called stridents. This feature, which is acoustically defined, is retained from the original Jakobsonian system. It is used to distinguish strident fricatives and affricates from nonstrident fricatives and affricates.

[+]: labiodental, dental/alveolar, palato-alveolar and uvular fricatives. [f, v, s, z, ʃ, ʒ , X, ʁ]

[–]: bilabial, interdental, palatal and velar fricatives [ɸ, β, θ, ð, ç, j, x, ɣ]

In addition to fricatives, affricates can be [+/– strident]. The value of this feature for an affricate is determined by the fricative component of the affricate. For example [tʃ] is [+strident], whereas [tθ] is [–strident].

Delayed release: This feature is to specify the release of a consonant and separates stops from affricates. In stops, the release is abrupt (instantaneous), whereas in affricates it is gradual (delayed).

[+]: affricates

[–]: stops

Lateral: Laterals are sounds that are produced by a lowering of one or both sides of the tongue so that the air moves through the sides of the oral cavity. In nonlateral sounds, air flows out through the center of the mouth. This feature separates lateral liquids from nonlateral liquids.

[+]: l-sounds

[–]: all others

Nasal: These are sounds that are produced by lowering the velum and allowing the air to pass outward through the nose. Non-nasal (oral) sounds are produced with the velum raised so that access to the nasal cavity and is blocked and air is allowed to go out only through the mouth. This feature separates nasals from liquids.

[+]: nasal consonants, nasalized vowels and glides

[–]: all others

Cavity Features

Anterior: Sounds that are produced with a primary constriction located at or in front of the alveolar ridge are termed anterior. Non-anterior sounds are produced at or behind the alveopalatal region.

[+]: labials, dentals, alveolars

[–]: all others

Coronal: Coronals are sounds that are produced with the front part of the tongue raised from the neutral position. Noncoronal sounds are produced without this raising of the front part of the tongue.

[+]: dental/alveolar, palato-alveolar, retroflex, palatal[2]

[–]: all others

Distributed: Distributed sounds are those that are produced with a constriction that extends for a considerable distance along the direction of air flow. In nondistributed sounds, there is a smaller area of contact. This feature is basically used to separate apical from laminal fricatives.

[+]: bilabial, alveolar, palato-alveolar fricatives
      [β, ɸ, s, z, ʃ, ʒ]

[–]: labio-dental, dental, interdental, retroflex fricatives
      [f, v, s̪, z̪ θ, ð, ʂ, ʐ][3]

High: Sounds that are produced by raising the body of the tongue above the neutral position are called high. Nonhigh sounds are made without such raising of the body of the tongue.

[+]: high vowels, palato-alveolar, palatal, velar, palatalized and velarized anterior consonants, [w, j]

[–]: all others

Low: Low sounds are produced by lowering the body of the tongue below the neutral position. Nonlow sounds are produced without this lowering. This feature distinguishes uvulars from pharyngeals.

[+]: low vowels, pharyngeal, glottal, and pharyngealized consonants

[–]: all others

Back: Back sounds are produced by retracting the body of the tongue from the neutral position. Nonback sounds are produced without this retracting of the body of the tongue.

[+]: back vowels, velar, uvular, pharyngeal, velarized and pharyngealized consonants, [w]

[–]: all others

Round: Round sounds are produced with a protrusion of the lips. Nonround sounds are produced without a protrusion of the lips.

[+]: round vowels, labialized consonants, [w]

[–]: all others

In the literature, there is also the feature [labial]. There is a considerable overlap between [round] and [labial], but differences are clear: [labial] indicates a sound that has a stricture made with the lips. Rounded sounds are a subset of labial sounds, which also include consonants made with lip involvement such as bilabials and labiodentals.

Tongue Root Features

Advanced tongue root (ATR): These are sounds that are produced while pushing the tongue root forward, thus expanding the resonating chamber of the pharynx. Nonadvanced tongue root sounds are produced without this pushing forward of the tongue root. This feature is needed to distinguish vowels in some African languages.

Tense: Tense sounds are produced with a greater muscular activity at the root of the tongue, which creates a greater degree of constriction than is found in lax sounds. The English long vowels and diphthongs are [+tense], whereas the short vowels are [−tense]. It is worth noting that this feature is a very controversial one and is not known to co-occur with [advanced tongue root] distinctively in any language. It may be that these two features are variant implementations of a single category.

Laryngeal Features

Voiced: Voiced sounds are produced with a vibration of the vocal cords. Nonvoiced (voiceless) sounds are produced without vocal cord vibration.

Spread: These are sounds that are produced by a displacement of the arytenoid cartilages, creating a wide glottal opening. Nonspread sounds are produced without this configuration.

> [+]: aspirated, breathy voiced, murmured consonants, voiceless vowels and glides
>
> [−]: all others

Constricted: Constricted sounds are produced with a severe obstruction of the glottis inhibiting the free vibration of the vocal cords. Nonconstricted sounds are produced without such a configuration.

[+]: ejectives, implosives, glottalized or laryngealized consonants, vowels and glides

[−]: all others

In addition to these features, there are prosodic features such as
[+/−long], [+/−stress], and tone, which will not be detailed here.

Tables 4–2 and 4–3 summarize the above feature specifications for vowels and consonants.

Table 4–2. Distinctive feature matrix for English consonants.

Feature	j	w	m	n	ŋ	r	l	p	b	f	v	θ	ð	t	d	s	z	ʃ	ʒ	tʃ	dʒ	k	g	h
Syllabic	−	−	−	−	−	−	−	−	−	−	−	−	−	−	−	−	−	−	−	−	−	−	−	−
Sonorant	+	+	+	+	+	+	+	−	−	−	−	−	−	−	−	−	−	−	−	−	−	−	−	−
Consonantal	−	−	+	+	+	+	+	+	+	+	+	+	+	+	+	+	+	+	+	+	+	+	+	−
Anterior	−	−	+	+	−	−	+	+	+	+	+	+	+	+	+	+	+	−	−	−	−	−	−	−
Coronal	+	−	−	+	−	+	+	−	−	−	−	+	+	+	+	+	+	+	+	+	+	−	−	−
High	+	+	−	−	+	−	−	−	−	−	−	−	−	−	−	−	−	+	+	+	+	+	+	−
Low	−	−	−	−	−	−	−	−	−	−	−	−	−	−	−	−	−	−	−	−	−	−	−	+
Back	−	+	−	−	+	−	−	−	−	−	−	−	−	−	−	−	−	−	−	−	−	+	+	−
Continuant	+	+	−	−	−	+	+	−	−	+	+	+	+	−	−	+	+	+	+	−	−	−	−	+
Strident	−	−	−	−	−	−	−	−	−	+	+	−	−	−	−	+	+	+	+	+	+	−	−	−
Voiced	+	+	+	+	+	+	+	−	+	−	+	−	+	−	+	−	+	−	+	−	+	−	+	−
Nasal	−	−	+	+	+	−	−	−	−	−	−	−	−	−	−	−	−	−	−	−	−	−	−	−
Lateral	−	−	−	−	−	−	+	−	−	−	−	−	−	−	−	−	−	−	−	−	−	−	−	−
Round	−	+	−	−	−	−	−	−	−	−	−	−	−	−	−	−	−	−	−	−	−	−	−	−

Table 4–3. Distinctive feature matrix for English vowels.

Feature	i	ɪ	e	ɛ	æ	u	ʊ	o	ə	a	ɔ
High	+	+	−	−	−	+	+	−	−	−	−
Low	−	−	−	−	+	−	−	−	−	+	−
Back	−	−	−	−	−	+	+	+	+	+	+
Tense	+	−	+	−	−	+	−	+	−	+	−
Round	−	−	−	−	−	+	+	+	−	−	+

DISTINCTIVE FEATURES IN
DEVELOPMENTAL PHONOLOGY

In addition to their indisputable role in general phonology, distinctive features also have been used in the explanation of certain phenomena in applied phonology. An area that has been active with this inquiry is Child Phonology.

The obvious advantage of the use of distinctive features in child substitutions is the power of the generalization that occurs with different sounds. Consider the following uttered by a 4-year-old child with a phonological disorder:

[tʌn]	"sun"	[tɔk]	"sock"
[du]	"zoo"	[pit]	"feet"
[paɪb]	"five"	[nod]	"nose"
[bɛri]	"very"		

The following substitutions are observed:

/s/ → [t], /z/ → [d], /f/ → [p], /v/ → [b]

Although these substitutions affect four different sounds, they are really the mismatch of the two features [continuant] and [strident]:

Targets	*Substitutes*
+ continuant	– continuant
+ strident	– strident

Several studies have investigated phonological development from the perspective of features (Cairns & Williams, 1972; Crocker, 1969; Menyuk, 1968). Cairns and Williams (1972) examined a total of 200 substitution errors across grades 1 through 12. The researchers found that 148 of these substitutions involved just one feature value change, and 15 substitution errors involved a change of two feature values. In other words, in the majority of the commonly found substitutions, only one or two features changed. The authors also pointed out that the substitutions did not reveal any changes in the major classes of the sounds. [coronal] was the most likely to change in place of articulation features (in the form of [+coronal] → [–coronal]), and [continuant] was the most vulnerable in the manner of articulation features (in the form of [+continuant] →

[–continuant]). The investigators' explanations for the reasons behind the vulnerability of the features, [coronal] and [continuant], is related to ease of articulation. The suggestions that "lingual sounds [coronal] are among the most difficult to articulate" (p. 817), and "the production of a [+continuant] sound undoubtedly requires a greater amount of fine motor control than does the production of a complete stop" (p. 818) were offered as explanations for the crucial nature of two features.

There also have been several attempts in clinical phonology literature to use features to account for substitutions (Blache, Parsons, & Humpreys, 1981; McReynolds & Bennett, 1972; McReynolds & Engmann, 1975; Parker, 1976; Ruder & Bunce 1981; Singh, Hayden, & Toombs 1981; Stewart, Singh, & Hayden 1979; Toombs, Singh, & Hayden 1981).

Distinctive Feature Analysis of Developmental Data

McReynolds and Engmann (1975) provided the most detailed explanation of procedures of distinctive feature analysis. What follows is a very brief account of the basic principles of a feature analysis.

Consider the following data from M (4yrs, 8mos) who is phonologically disordered. The first task in a feature analysis is to write down the target phonemes and the number of occurrences in the data.

	Target	*M's Realizations*	*Changes*
1.	brush	[bwʌs]	r → w, ʃ → s
2.	that	[dæt]	ð → d
3.	pencil	[bɛndəl]	p → b, s → d
4.	sugar	[dugar]	ʃ → d
5.	dog	[dɔk]	g → k
6.	dish	[dɪs]	ʃ → s
7.	speak	[bik]	s → ∅, p → b
8.	scratch	[kwæt]	s → ∅, r → w, tʃ → t
9.	ring	[wɪŋ]	r → w
10.	chair	[dɛr]	tʃ → d
11.	window	[wɪndo]	-
12.	bridge	[bwɪt]	r → w, dʒ → t
13.	five	[baɪf]	f → b, v → f
14.	cow	[kaʊ]	-
15.	soup	[tup]	s → t
16.	sick	[dɪk]	s → d
17.	talk	[dɔk]	t → d
18.	shoe	[du]	ʃ → d

	Target	*M's Realizations*	*Changes*
19.	zoo	[du]	z → d
20.	black	[bæk]	l → ø
21.	finger	[bɪŋgər]	f → b
22.	trees	[dwis]	t → d, r → w, z → s
23.	sheep	[dip]	ʃ → d
24.	gun	[gʌn]	-
25.	chicken	[dɪkən]	tʃ → d
26.	car	[kar]	-
27.	brown	[baʊn]	r → ø
28.	flag	[bæk]	f → b, l → ø, g → k
29.	crash	[kwæs]	r → w, ʃ → s
30.	fish	[bɪs]	f → b, ʃ → s
31.	rabbit	[wæbɪt]	r → w
32.	teeth	[dit]	t → d, θ → t
33.	they	[de]	ð → d
34.	sky	[kaɪ]	s → ø
35.	neck	[nɛk]	-
36.	spoon	[bun]	s → ø, p → b
37.	ball	[bɔl]	-
38.	door	[dɔr]	-
39.	bread	[bwɛt]	r → w, d → t
40.	red	[wɛt]	r → w, d → t

Next, the number of correct renditions for these target phonemes should be determined. Sometimes this number will be zero for a particular target, as it will be rendered erroneously all the time. Following this, the substitutes for the targets in question with the number of times for each substitute (if there is more than one) will be recorded.

The next step is to list the features (+ and –) for the target and the substitute(s) and to compare the pluses and minuses of the features to come up with a number showing the instances in which each feature was used correctly. This is shown with reference to the target /s/:

	Target Correct /s/ 3	*Substituted* [t] 1	[d] 2	*Omitted* 1	*Correct Use*
sonorant	–	–	–		6
syllabic	–	–	–		6
consonantal	+	+	+		6
continuant	+	–	–		3
anterior	+	+	+		6
coronal	+	+	+		6

	Target Correct	*Substituted*	*Omitted*	*Correct Use*
nasal	–	–	–	6
high	–	–	–	6
voiced	–	–	+	4
strident	+	–	–	3

The same operation is performed for all of the targets and their substitutes. Looking at M's production, the following recurring feature mismatches are noted:

–anterior	→	+anterior	(ʃ → s, ʃ → d, tʃ → t, tʃ → d
			dʒ → t)
+high	→	–high	(ʃ → s, tʃ → t, tʃ → d, dʒ →t)
+continuant	→	–continuant	(f → b, s → t, s → d, z → d,
			θ → t, ʃ → d, ð → d)
+strident	→	–strident	(f → b, s → t, s → d, z → d,
			ʃ → d, tʃ → t, tʃ → d, dʒ →t)
–voiced	→	+voiced	(s → d, tʃ → d, p → b, t → d)
+voiced	→	–voiced	(dʒ → t, v → f, g → k, d → t)

Finally, the percentages of correct and incorrect use for each of the feature values are determined. In order to do this, the total number of possible occurrences for each feature value involved should be noted. This can be calculated through the segments in which the feature is present. For example, considering the feature [+continuant], the following picture emerges.

Phonemes That Are [+continuant]	*No. of Possible Occurrences*	*No. of Correct Occurrences*
f	4	0
v	1	1
θ	1	0
ð	2	0
s	7	3
z	2	0
ʃ	6	0
w	1	1
r	12	12
Total :	38	18
% incorrect :	54% (20/37)	

The object of this demonstration is to illustrate how evaluations can be made using distinctive features. There will not be any attempt to go through all of the other errors exemplified in M's erroneous productions, but it is not difficult to figure out, for example, that [+strident] would result in a high percentage of error too. The percentages found are important, because the targets for treatment would be the feature(s) that exhibits the highest error percentage.

Before concluding this section, it should be mentioned that the percentages that are calculated in feature analyses should be read with caution. The reason for this is that a certain value of a feature may be problematic only for a specific class of sounds and be irrelevant for another. For example, the [+continuant] examined from M above demonstrated an overall error pattern of 54% (20/37). However, if the segments involved are examined, it will be clear that the subject demonstrates this problem exclusively for the obstruents, [–sonorant]. Although M makes all 20 errors out of 25 possibilities in fricatives (80%), in sonorant targets there is no error regarding this feature value (0/13). A similar situation is found with regard to the feature [voiced]. As seen earlier, M exhibited difficulties in both directions with this feature. While some examples had [–voiced] → [+voiced], others had the reverse, [+voice] → [–voiced]. This fact is also explainable with reference to segment type and word position; all substitutions that show [+voiced] → [–voiced] are restricted to obstruents in the final position. M does not have a general problem with [+voiced]; rather, obstruents cannot be realized as [+voiced] in the final position. This important information is not reflected in the original analysis.

Another point that needs to be emphasized is the importance of the segment type or the specific word position in productions. For example, if the fricative targets in M's data are considered, it will be seen that the only correct productions are for /f/ (1/1) and /s/ (3/7) targets. In other words, on the surface there is a 50% correct (4/8) for these two targets and none for the other fricatives. However, this is rather misleading because the correct productions for these two targets are all in final position. The other target fricatives did not appear in final positions in M's data. This is an important variable that can be understood by looking at the erroneous productions for /s/ targets in the data; they all occur in nonfinal positions. Careful attention should be paid to where the incorrect production occurs before making any decisions about treatment planning.

Features and Intelligibility

In addition to having the capacity to provide generalizations for the seemingly different substitutions that have direct and important implications for therapy, the distinctive feature approach to child productions has also been used to measure the severity or intelligibility of errors. Pollack and Rees (1972) and Blumstein (1973) suggested that the number of feature errors co-occurring in the substitution of a target can provide an index of severity or intelligibility.

Although it is true, as suggested earlier by Cairns and Williams' (1972) work, that many commonly found child substitutions attested in the speech of both normally developing children and those with phonological disorders involve a change of only one or two features, certain other substitutions that are also very commonly found in normally developing children involve a large number of feature changes. Examples such as /r/ → [w], as in *rabbit* → [wæbɪt], Portuguese *branco* [branku] → [bwanku], or /l/ → [j] *line* → [jajn], or /r/ → [j] Turkish *para* [para] → [paja] clearly show that these common (thus nonsevere) errors involve multiple changes in features.

/r/	→	[w]	/l/	→	[j]
+sonorant		+sonorant	+sonorant		+sonorant
–syllabic		–syllabic	–syllabic		–syllabic
+consonantal		*–consonantal*	*+consonantal*		*–consonantal*
+continuant		+continuant	+continuant		+continuant
+anterior		*–anterior*	*+anterior*		*–anterior*
+coronal		*–coronal*	+coronal		+coronal
–high		*+high*	*–high*		*+high*
–low		–low	–low		–low
–back		*+back*	–back		–back
–nasal		–nasal	–nasal		–nasal
–strident		–strident	–strident		–strident
+voiced		+voiced	+voiced		+voiced
–lateral		–lateral	*+lateral*		*–lateral*
–round		*+round*	–round		–round

/r/	→	[j]
+sonorant		+sonorant
–syllabic		–syllabic
+consonantal		*–consonantal*
+continuant		+continuant
+anterior		*–anterior*
+coronal		+coronal
–high		*+high*
–low		–low
–back		–back
–nasal		–nasal

/r/	→	[j]
–strident		–strident
+voiced		+voiced
–lateral		–lateral
–round		–round

On the other hand, an unusual substitution such as /b/ → [v] as in *ban* → [væn] involves only two changes:

/b/	[v]
–sonorant	–sonorant
–syllabic	–syllabic
+conson.	+conson.
+anterior	+anterior
–coronal	–coronal
–continuant	*+continuant*
–strident	*+strident*
–high	–high
–low	–low
–back	–back
–nasal	–nasal
+voiced	+voiced
–lateral	–lateral
–round	–round

Clearly, simple feature counting is not the answer to the question of differentiating common errors from uncommon ones. As seen in the above examples there are common errors which involve six feature changes alongside unusual errors which have only two feature changes. This is an indication that, rather than counting the number of features, there is a need to look into the question of what feature(s) changed, and what values are involved. This point will be considered later in this chapter and will also be discussed in Chapter 10.

Implicational Feature Development

There is a great deal of similarity between the error patterns of children with phonological disorders and normally developing young children. For example, both groups use the features [+nasal] [+voice] and [–coronal] earlier and more frequently than the features [+continuant] and [+strident].

Some investigators have tried to delineate implicational feature developments by looking at the phonetic inventories of children. The underlying idea is whether the presence of a particular phonetic distinction implies the presence of another distinction. The establishment of an opposition depends on the use of different categories by the child. For example, the occurrences of [t] and [d] indicate a distinction for the feature [voice], the use of [b] and [m] indicates distinction for the feature [nasal]. Dinnsen, Chin, Elbert, and Powell (1990) studied 40 phonologically disordered children and found that, when the subjects made the distinction in [voice], there were also distinctions in the features [syllabic], [consonantal], [sonorant], and [coronal]. Distinctions in [continuant] occurred, then were followed by [nasal]. The distinctions in [strident] and [lateral] presupposed all of the above. These implicational distinctions seem to be the same for both normally developing young children and children with phonological disorders.

As for the application of distinctive features to therapy, there are two basic approaches. In the first approach, one or more target phonemes are used for training the feature. The second approach involves teaching all of the phonemes that have the given target feature at the same time.

In the first approach, phonemes that are involved in the +/– contrast can be used to demonstrate the feature. For example, the phonemes /t/ and /f/ can be used to teach the contrast of +/– of [continuant] to a child who does not use continuant consonants. It has been suggested by Parker (1976) that features cannot be separated from the context of phonemes in words. Parker stated that features are not a component of speech production but a component of language, and thus cannot be separated from words. Consequently, Blache et al. (1981) recommend the teaching of feature contrasts with minimal pairs such as *pea - bee*, and *sick - tick*. For example, a child with a phonological disorder who has difficulty with the feature [voiced] does not make a difference between the minimal pair *pea - bee* because these two words are produced homophonously. For this reason, the child's contact with the minimal pairs establishes the relationship between form and meaning and shows that the therapy cannot be restricted to articulation. This example demonstrates that there is a fundamental difference between articulation therapy and phonological therapy. A child who is exposed to phonological therapy receives sufficient information to make the necessary changes in his speech in order to reach communicative adequacy. This also demonstrates that phonological therapy addresses cognitive processing.

Another important aspect of therapy with distinctive features is the presupposition that features that are trained for one contrast with some sounds generalize to other sounds that share the same feature. For example, if there is a voicing problem with the fricatives, we do not need to work with all fricative pairs in voiced-voiceless distinction. If we introduce the contrast between one pair, for example /s/ and /z/, this will generalize to other pairs. There are some studies that support this view of generalization from words that were trained to other words that were not trained (Blache, Parsons, & Humpreys, 1981; Pollack & Rees, 1972; Weiner, 1981).

Other researchers have shown that there were generalizations of trained phonemes to other phonemes (Compton, 1970; Costello & Onstine, 1976; McReynolds & Bennett, 1972; Ruder & Bunce, 1981;). Generalizations seem to occur most effectively between phonemes that share features. Compton (1980) confirmed this in a 4-year-old child for whom the correction of /n/ resulted in the correction of other nasals without any effect for any other problematic consonants. Training of a segment will not have any effect on segments that do not share the same features. As was foreseen, McReynolds and Elbert (1981) showed that the training of /s/ did not change the production of /r/. It was found that, in the training of fricatives, generalization most frequently occurred between subgroups in terms of place of articulation. For example, generalization occurred in labiodentals (/f/ and /v/) and in coronals (/s/, /z/, /ʃ/, /ʒ/), but did not occur among all fricatives.

Several researchers have questioned the expectation that generalizations will occur across the board (Blache et al., 1981; Ingram, 1976; Weiner, 1981). They suggest that, in order to facilitate generalization, therapy should utilize several examples of a feature or a contrast instead of only one example.

Ruder and Bunce (1981) used a different therapeutic strategy for two children with severe disorders. One of these children consistently used only /m/, /b/, and /g/; the other child had only /g/, /n/, /ŋ/, and /d /. To increase their repertoire, Ruder and Bunce chose phonemes that the children produced in a limited fashion. In the first case, in addition to the regularly produced /m/, /b/, /g/, the child had a very limited production of /p/, /s/, and /k/. The investigators chose /s/ and /k/ for training to encourage the use of [+continuant], [+strident], [+coronal], [–voiced], and [+high]. The basic issue was whether the training of /s/ and /k/, the phonemes which together possess all features of /t/, would lead to a production of /t/. Following the traditional therapy through word level, the child was able to produce /t/, /f/, /ŋ/, /z/, and /ʃ/. On the basis of the concept of generalization, /f/, /tʃ/, and /ʃ/ were predicted. Ruder and Bunce's research shows that a careful selection of phonemes based on features that are lacking in the child's system can motivate the use of new features and thus result in a greater repertoire of sounds.

Despite the support cited above, the distinctive feature approach to therapy has had its share of criticism because of the questionable articulatory validity of the features (Parker, 1976; Walsh, 1974). However, Singh, Hayden, and Toombs (1981) showed that the feature system of Singh and Singh (1976) was useful for the establishment of a hierarchy of features for the errors of 1,077 public school children who underwent therapy. Moreover, Toombs, Singh, and Hayden (1981) suggested that the theory of markedness can give a better explanation than feature analysis for the substitutions of 801 students. The theory of markedness explains the relative complexity of phonemes on the basis of the number of features that are necessary for the production. According to the markedness theory, certain feature combinations are considered more natural than others. (See Chapters 7 and 10 for a detailed discussion of markedness.)

STEVENS AND KEYSER'S ENHANCEMENT THEORY

Distinctive features as they have been discussed so far present the sounds in terms of an unorganized bundle of features without any hierarchical arrangement among the features. Stevens and Keyser (1989), developing an earlier version of Stevens, Keyser, and Kawasaki (1986), presented a new look at distinctive features by proposing a hierarchical arrangement among features. Basing their evaluation on the acoustic characteristics of the Chomsky and Halle (1968) features, they proposed an enhancement theory with the following hypotheses: The acoustic manifestations of some distinctive features ([sonorant], [continuant], and [coronal]) are perceptually more salient than those of others; these are the primary features. In other words, the contrasting acoustic properties associated with the presence or absence of some features provide a stronger auditory response than those associated with other features. For example, in comparing the pairs /t, s/ (distinguished by the primary feature [continuant]) versus /t̪, t/ (distinguished by the secondary feature [distributed]), there is a striking difference in the acoustic or auditory domain between the properties that characterize these two features and the contrast characterized by [continuant], the more salient feature, is greater than the contrast of [distributed].

Stevens and Keyser (1989) suggested several reasons for the selection of the set [sonorant], [continuant], and [coronal] as primary features. One of the main reasons was that, among the features represented in sounds, each of these three features can be implemented independently of the presence or absence of other features. In other words, although the generation of the acoustic property associated with each of the primary features does not require that some other features have specific values, the feature values of the remaining features, called secondary features, may depend on the values of the primary features with which they are combined.

Other reasons for the choice of the three features as primary included the characteristics of these features being "especially closely tied to fundamental capabilities of the auditory system for processing temporal and spectral aspects of sound" (p. 87), and the use of these three features distinctively in a large majority of languages.

The strength of each of the primary features present in a sound is influenced by the combination of secondary features that co-occur with the primary features. As a result, certain feature combinations or segments are preferred over others because they provide the strongest representation of the contrast defined by the three primary features.

Another hypothesis of Stevens and Keyser (1989) was that a "given distinctive feature can be represented in a sound with varying degrees of strength, which in turn can be enhanced by its co-occurrence with other features" (p. 81).

The idea that segment X is preferred over segment Y has important implications for developmental phonology and phonological disorders. First, one can test the hierarchy and the enhancement relationships suggested by Stevens and Keyser in normally developing phonologies and determine findings from children's substitutions confirm their hypotheses. Second, one can examine data from phonological disorders and see in what sense substitutions that are labeled unusual or idiosyncratic violate Stevens and Keyser's suggested model. In short, it may be possible to determine if the hierarchy provides a principled way of distinguishing common substitutions from unusual ones. Yavas (1997a) examined developmental data through this model and found strong support for it. Below, some examples to illustrate the explanatory power of the model will be provided.

Child Substitutions: Normal Processes

First, we will look at common substitutions that are found in normally developing children as well as in individuals with phonological disorders. One such substitution is fricative stopping, as exemplified in *that* → [dæt]. The relationship between the target /ð/ and the substitute [d] is as follows:

ð	*d*
−sonorant	−sonorant
+*continuant*	−*continuant*
+coronal	+coronal
+consonantal	+consonantal
+anterior	+anterior
−strident	−strident
−back	−back
+voiced	+voiced
−distributed	−distributed
−high	−high

The two sounds in question share many characteristics, but differ in one primary feature value, [continuant]. This process is known as stopping and is cited very frequently for English-speaking children.

To explain why the stop is preferred over the fricative in this substitution, the feature [consonantal] for enhancement will be brought in. [+consonantal] works as an enhancing force for [−sonorant, −continuant]. The articulatory correlate of the positive value of [consonantal] is a narrow constriction at some point along the length of the vocal tract. Because this constriction is quite narrow, when the consonant is released into the following vowel, there is a quick movement of some formants. This formant movement results in a quick change in the spectrum over a portion of the frequency range. This is better achieved with a stop articulation rather than a fricative. Because of these factors, the substitute stop [d] has a clear advantage over the target fricative /ð/.

In addition to [consonantal], there are two other secondary features that enhance the primary feature [−continuant]. The first one is [distributed]. Stevens and Keyser argue that the feature "[continuant] in stops (i.e., [−continuant]) is enhanced if the length of the consonantal closure in the vocal tract is short and if the release is rapid. These attributes will give rise to an abrupt onset of acoustic energy at the release of the consonant" (p. 90). [−distributed] provides this short length of closure. Because both the substitute and the target sounds are [−distributed], the substitution of [−continuant] is favored and the resulting sound is more likely to be a stop rather than a fricative. In other words, [−continuant] is enhanced by [−distributed] and the stop is favored over the fricative.

The second feature that enhances [−continuant] is stridency. Being [−strident], the target and the substitute are affected differently. Because the generation of the frication noise is fundamental for [+strident] and can happen at a constriction, only [-sonorant] segments can be distinguished from each other with this feature. Stevens and Keyser argued that, in affricates, stridency weakens the strength of [−continuant] because the rate of release of the closure is limited due to the narrow constriction that must be maintained after the release. Consequently, segments that have the same values for [strident] and [continuant] would be preferred. In other words, [−strident] enhances [-continuant] (the stop substitute), but does not enhance [+continuant] (the target).

These examples, along with many other common substitutions (e.g., /r/ → [w] as in *rabbit* → [wæbɪt]; /ʃ/ → [s] as in *ship* → [sɪp]; /l/ → [j] as in *line* → [jajn]; /θ/ → [f] or [s] as in *thin* → [fɪn] or [sɪn]) permit us to make the following observations: First, the substitutions in this category require agreement in the feature value of two primary features. To be more specific, the feature value of [sonorant] plus [coronal] or [continuant] is required for any substitution in this category. Second, the substitutes reveal more preferred feature combinations than the targets based on the enhancement relationships. In other words, it is not how many features are changed from the target to the replacement that make a substitution normal or unusual. Rather, the question is which primary features, if any, are altered and which primary features are in an enhancement relationship with secondary features.

Child Substitutions: Unusual Processes

The validity of these observations receives support from another group of substitutions that are referred to as idiosyncratic or unusual substitutions. Cases such as f → [w] as in *fig* → [wɪg], /w/ → [b] as in *will* → [bɪl], /l/ or /r/ → [d] as in *lake/rake* → [dek], and /l/ → [ð] as in *lock* → [ðak] show some patterns that are not typically seen in normal development (Grunwell, 1987; Stoel-Gammon & Dunn, 1985).

In these unusual substitutions, the value of the feature [sonorant] is altered. In some, another primary feature is also altered.

f	→	*w*		*w*	→	*b*
−*sonorant*		+*sonorant*		+*sonorant*		−*sonorant*
+continuant		+continuant		+*continuant*		−*continuant*
−coronal		−coronal		−coronal		−coronal

r	→	*d*		*l*	→	ð
+*sonorant*		−*sonorant*		+*sonorant*		−*sonorant*
+*continuant*		−*continuant*		−continuant		−continuant
+coronal		+coronal		+coronal		+coronal

The change in [sonorant], which, in some cases, is accompanied by [continuant], seems to be the explanation for these unusual substitutions.[4–5]

SUMMARY

In this chapter, we have seen that segments can be broken down into sets of distinctive features. Each segment can be uniquely described and identified through the composition of features. The features assign a set of characteristics to each sound and uniquely describe the internal structure of the sound. By assigning a set of features to each segment, it is possible to make generalizations about a group of sounds that act together in phonological processes, such as assimilation. For language researchers, the use of distinctive features is a valuable component of phonological assessment. Normal and disordered phonological processes can be identified by conducting a distinctive feature analysis. By looking at the processes in terms of features, finer distinctions may be made in assessing the subject's productions of targets. Identifying the substitutions in terms of features allows the language researcher to recommend a more specific and targeted plan for remediation.

Some phonologists have proposed using a hierarchy of features based on articulatory or acoustic properties. Organizing the features in such a manner may provide a tool for explaining the naturalness or unusualness of substitutions made in developmental phonology and may give an explanation for preferences for certain sounds. We saw above how such a system can be utilized in developmental phonology by incorporating Stevens and Keyser's acoustically based hierarchy. The articulatorily based hierarchical model, Feature Geometry, will be discussed in Chapter 10.

NOTES

1. The classification of liquids as [+continuant] is controversial. First, the verdict on laterals is not unanimous. Although many agree with Chomsky and Halle in assigning [+continuant] to these sounds (Carr, 1993; Fromkin & Rodman, 1993; Giegerich, 1992; Hyman, 1975; Lass, 1984; O'Grady et al., 19913), others (Durand, 1991; Katamba, 1989,) are

expressly opposed to this and assign [−continuant]. The situation with *r*-sounds is not settled either. Here, the problem lies in the quality of the *r*-sound in question. Although general American (retroflex approximant) and British (alveolar approximant) English *r*-sounds are clearly [+continuant], the same cannot be said for trills, taps, and flaps.

2. The specification of palatals for the feature [coronal] is controversial. Although they are considered [−coronal] by some (Ladefoged, 1982; Sommerstein, 1977), there is overwhelming support for [+coronal] (Durand, 1990; Halle & Stevens, 1979; Katamba, 1989; Keating, 1990; Kenstowicz & Kisseberth, 1979; Stevens & Keyser, 1989).

3. Dentals and retroflex consonants are represented respectively by diacritics Ç and Ç placed under the alveolar symbols.

4. There are, however, some other substitutions that are also labeled idiosyncratic/unusual but do not show any changes in the value of [sonorant] between the substitutes and the targets, such as /b/ → [v] as in *ban* → [væn], and /t/ → [k] as in *pat* → [pæk]. These substitutions have one differing primary feature value between the target and the replacement, but keep the value of [sonorant] intact. They resemble the so-called common substitutions regarding the situation of the primary features. What makes them different, and thus unusual, comes from the counter-enhancement relationships between the primary and secondary features rather than from mismatches in the primary features.

5. It should be mentioned that in both normal and unusual substitutions, frequency in input should also be considered.

EXERCISES

1. Circle the segments that are

a. coronal	p	dʒ	d	k	l	h
b. anterior	p	dʒ	d	k	l	h
c. strident	X	tʃ	θ	k	β	v
d. sonorant	n	w	b	r	h	u
e. continuant	f	tʃ	ʃ	t	h	z

f. low		ʊ	æ	a	u	e	ə
g. back		ʌ	ʊ	o	ɔ	a	u
h. consonantal	a	j	l	ʔ	w	h

2. For each segment, if the value of the feature indicated is changed, what new segment will be derived?

Old Segment	Feature To Be Changed	New Segment
t	voiced	d
p	coronal	
o	high	
j	syllabic	
dʒ	voiced	
z	strident	
x	back	
s	high	
ʃ	continuant	

3. Natural classes: For each group of sounds listed below, circle the sound that does not belong to the group. Then identify feature(s) (in +/− value) shared by the remaining sounds in the group.

Example: p f ⓡ ð tʃ z   −sonorant

a.	p	t	w	k	b	d	g	_____
b.	f	θ	s	ʃ	h	z	d	_____
c.	p	t	g	k	f	θ	ʃ	_____
d.	d	t	s	z	k	l	n	_____
e.	f	b	v	p	t	k	g	_____
f.	f	s	ʃ	θ	h	tʃ	v	_____
g.	b	m	n	t	g	d	p	_____
h.	ʃ	f	z	tʃ	dʒ	s	d	_____

i.   a   e   u   o   ɔ   ʊ   _____

j.   i   o   u   j   ʃ   tʃ   dʒ_____

k.   dʒ   d   l   t   k   tʃ   ʃ _____

l.   p   d   l   g   m   n   t _____

m.   f   z   ʃ   b   v   θ   ð _____

n.   j   w   b   l   r   m   n _____

o.   f   z   h   p   tʃ   k   θ _____

p.   s   z   f   k   dʒ   ʃ   tʃ_____

4. Using M's data discussed in this chapter, calculate the percentages of errors regarding the features [anterior], [strident], and [voiced].

5. Identify the feature errors in the following common child substitutions:

   a.   v → b
   b.   θ → f
   c.   l → j
   d.   s → t
   e.   tʃ → t
   f.   ʒ → d
   g.   f → w
   h.   θ → s

6. Identify the error patterns in the following data utilizing generalizations based on features.

   a.   D (4;2)

gum	[dʌm]	big	[bɪd]
cat	[tæt]	walk	[wat]
sock	[tɔt]	go	[do]
come	[tʌm]	cow	[taʊ]

b. W (4;4)

sun	[tʌn]	*sick*	[tɪk]
soup	[tup]	*shoe*	[tu]
gas	[gæt]	*five*	[paɪb]
zoo	[du]	*miss*	[mɪt]
thick	[tɪk]	*save*	[teb]

Chapter 5

PHONOLOGICAL PROCESSES

Although it is possible to describe speech sounds in languages through features referring to place and manner of articulation, voicing, and nasality, features are elements of a dynamic system called phonology and thus are subject to change as they come into contact with other units in the system. To illustrate what is meant by this, a point made in the analysis of Korean in Chapter 3 will be revisited. The three sounds [s, z, ʃ] in Korean are in complementary distribution and are the positional variants of the same phoneme /s/. The phonetic manifestation of this phoneme before [i] is [ʃ]. The principle that sound units tend to be influenced by their environment is well illustrated here. The change we have illustrated is that of an alveolar sound (a fricative in this case) becoming a palato-alveolar (or palatal) before a high front vowel that is also articulated in the same area.[1] In other words, the consonant moved its place of articulation in accordance with the place of the following segment.

For another example, consider the relationship between [t] and [tʃ] in Portuguese:

[tal]	"such"	[tʃia]	"aunt"
[tempo]	"time"	[tʃirar]	"to take off"
[tentar]	"to try"	[tʃivi]	"I had"
[toaʎa]	"towel"	[tʃimi]	"team"
[tudu]	"all"	[vintʃi]	"twenty"

This limited 10-item list may seem inadequate for analysis, but it is representative of what occurs in the language. In this case of complementary distribution between [t] and [tʃ], we find [tʃ] before [i], and [t] in other environments. Here, similar to the Korean case studied earlier, there is an instance of an alveolar segment becoming a palato-alveolar before [i]. Although another change in the segment from a stop to an affricate has also taken place, this is irrelevant because Portuguese does not have a palatal stop, and the affricate [tʃ] is the closest segment to a stop in the palatal region.

The influence of the environment on a sound is not restricted to changing the place of articulation, and may occur in the changes of voicing and the manner of articulation as well. Regarding voicing, consider the relationship of [t] and [d] in the following data from Cree, an Algonquian language spoken in Ontario, Canada.

nisto	"three"	kodak	"another"
tahki	"all the time"	adim	"dog"
mibit	"tooth"	adihk	"caribou"
tagosin	"he arrives"	mihtʃet	"many"

The complementary distribution revealed by the data above points to intervocalic voicing whereby /t/ becomes [d] between two vowels. The underlying phonetic motivation can be shown with reference to the fact that vowels are voiced, and it is not surprising for a segment to become voiced when it is surrounded by voiced segments.

Finally, consider the Spanish example given in Chapter 3 to observe the effects of the environment on the change of the manner of articulation. As mentioned earlier, [d] and [ð], which belong to two different phonemes in English, are in complementary distribution in Spanish. The environment for the fricative [ð] is between vowels; otherwise, the manifestation of the phoneme is [d]. To explain why such a change takes place, it is necessary to look at the basic difference between stops and fricatives. This lies in the type of stricture involved. Stops are articulated with firm contact of the articulators, whereas fricatives involve only an approximation of the articulators without complete closure. The surrounding environment, vowels in this case, are open articulations and act as agents of relaxing the articulation. As such, they create a favorable environment for a more open articulation of the segment in between them. Thus, this may result in a change from a stop to a fricative between vowels. The processes seen in the above examples are not restricted to Korean, Portuguese, Cree, or Spanish; they are also found in other languages. Ultimately, such events seem to adhere to principles related to articulation or perception, and are shared by many languages.

It is important to note that all of the cases we have looked at up to this point were concerned with allophonic variations of certain phonemes modified in different environments. As such, they were necessarily confined to events that took place within a single morpheme.[2] However, phonological processes that are observed in languages are not restricted in their effects to allophonic variations and, in fact, most of these processes show up when different morphemes are put together. That is, the processes can occur within a single morpheme or across morpheme boundaries, as exemplified in the following:

impersonal	[ɪmpərsnəl]	*impertinent*	[ɪmpərtnənt]
indescribable	[ɪndɪskrajbəbl]	*indispensable*	[ɪndɪspɛnsəbl]
incapable	[ɪŋkepəbl]	*inconclusive*	[ɪŋkənklusɪv]

It can be observed in the above data, which is representative of the general pattern in English, that the nasal consonant of the negative prefix [ɪn], [ɪm], or [ɪŋ] agrees with the place of articulation of the first segment of the adjective it is attached to. The first pair has [ɪm] because of the initial bilabial stops of the adjectives *pertinent* and *personal*. The second pair has [ɪn], which is in line with the initial alveolar segment of the adjectives *describable* and *dispensable*. Finally, the third pair shows the agreement of the velar nasal in [ɪŋ] with the initial velars of the adjectives, *conclusive* and *capable*.

The phonetic motivation underlying this event, which is articulatory ease, is also evident, but the reason for variation is different from the earlier cases. In each of the previous cases, the changes that took place because of the environment were related to the allophones of one phoneme, and the modifications (variations) were allophonic in nature. The last case that was reviewed in relation to the negative prefix in English, however, does not deal with allophones of the same phoneme, but rather shows alternations among separate phonemes. That [m], [n], and [ŋ] are not allophones of the same phoneme but belong to separate phonemes in English can easily be shown by the following contrasting pairs of words: moon - noon, ham - hang, fan - fang. What is shown in this case is an alternation of different phonemes for the same morpheme with the same meaning. Such cases are traditionally called morphophonemic alternations, and the different phonetic manifestations of the same morpheme (morpheme alternants) are called the allomorphs.

To give a further example of an alternation between phonemes in a particular morpheme in a particular position, consider the following examples from Turkish.

[armut̠]	"pear"	[armud̠-u]	"his/her pear"
[tʃorap̠]	"sock"	[tʃorab̠-ɨ]	"his/her sock"

As can be seen, there is an alternation between root final consonants in these pairs: [p] alternates with [b] for the morpheme meaning "sock", and [t] alternates with [d] for the morpheme meaning "pear". Because the alternating sounds in each pair are in contrast in the language ([pak] "clean" vs. [bak] "look", [ter] "sweat" vs. [der] "he/she says"), these pairs constitute examples of morphophonemic alternations of the root final consonant.

Now that the difference between allophonic variations and allomorphic variation (morphophonemic alternations) has been made clear, we will see whether maintaining such a distinction is useful. We will do this by examining the case of Russian obstruents (Halle, 1965).

Among the phonemes of Russian are the following:

p	pʲ	t	tʲ	t	tʃ	k
b	bʲ	d	dʲ	-	-	g
f	fʲ	s	sʲ		ʃ	x
v	vʲ	z	zʲ		ʒ	

Most Russian obstruents come in palatalized/non-palatalized and voiced/voiceless pairs. /ts/, /tʃ/ and /x/ are exceptional in having no voiced phoneme counterparts. Although the language has [dz], [dʒ], and [ɣ], these are the respective allophones of the former set. There is a process at work in Russian which voices any obstruent if another voiced obstruent follows, as exemplified in the following:

[datʲli]	"should one give"
[dadʲbi]	"were one to give"
[zetʃli]	"should one burn"
[zedʒbi]	"were one to burn"

In the first and third examples, the morphemes /datʲ/ and /zetʃ/ are not modified when the suffix *li* is attached, because the first segment of the suffix is not a voiced obstruent. The situation, however, is different in the second and fourth examples when the suffix *bi* attaches. Because the initial sound of the suffix is a voiced obstruent, the root final voiceless obstruent is voiced. Now, because [tʲ] and [dʲ] belong to different phonemes, according to the distinction mentioned earlier, the forms in the first and second reveal a morphophonemic alternation, and the rule governing this is a morphophonemic rule.

Morphophonemic representation	/datʲ-li/	/datʲ-bi/
morphophonemic voicing rule applied		
Phonemic representation	/datʲli/	/dadʲbi/
allophonic voicing rule applied		
Phonetic representation	[datʲli]	[dadʲbi]

However, the forms in (3) and (4) will be subject to an allophonic rule, as [dʒ] is only an allophone of /tʃ/ and can be generated from the phonemic level to the phonetic level:

Morphophonemic representation	/zetʃ-li/	/zetʃ-bi/
morphophonemic voicing rule applied		
Phonemic representation	/zetʃli/	/zetʃbi/
allophonic voicing rule applied		
Phonetic representation	[zetʃli]	/zedʒbi/

To generate the *phonemic* representation above, it is necessary to break the obstruent voicing rule into two rules and to complicate one of them with an exception statement, that is,

(a) morphophonemic rule   [–son] → [+voiced] / _____ $\begin{bmatrix} -son \\ +voiced \end{bmatrix}$
   (except ts, tʃ, x)
(obstruents, with the exception of ts, t , and x, are voiced before voiced obstruents).

(b) allophonic rule   [–son] → [+voiced] / _____ $\begin{bmatrix} -son \\ +voiced \end{bmatrix}$

(obstruents are voiced before voiced obstruents)

The reader should read the prose versions of these rules and should not be concerned with the formalism at this point. The details of these formal representations will be dealt with later in this chapter.

Rule (a) generates the phonemic representation from the morphophonemic representations and then rule (b) generates the allophonic representations. That is, (a) is a morphophonemic rule, while (b) is an allophonic rule. But this analysis is definitely wrong. There is only one generalization that needs to be made here: voiceless obstruents are voiced when followed by a voiced obstruent. There is no reason to identify more than one process just to distinguish /ts, tʃ, and x/. The whole process can be simplified by writing one phonetically motivated rule that will account for all the variations.

$$[-\text{son}] \quad \rightarrow \quad [+\text{voiced}] \quad / \quad \underline{\qquad} \quad \begin{bmatrix} -\text{son} \\ +\text{voiced} \end{bmatrix}$$

(Obstruents are voiced before voiced obstruents)

This way of looking at things rejects the idea of having separate levels of morphophonemic representation and phonemic representation, and suggests a single level of representation above the phonetic level. This level is called the underlying representation and it is distinct from the surface (phonetic) level. The underlying form will have only the nonredundant (nonpredictable) properties. The predictable properties that appear in the surface form, in a similar fashion to what we saw in phonemic analysis earlier, will be supplied by rules. Going back to the Turkish example given earlier in this section, we can see that the underlying forms of the morphemes meaning "pear" and "sock" will be /armud/ and /tʃorab/, respectively. The surface forms of the nominative [armut] and [tʃorap] are predictable through the final devoicing rule. The alternative solution of voicing of p → b and t → d between vowels is made nonviable because of other forms such as [sepet] "basket" becoming [sepeti] "his/her basket," and [ip] "string" becoming [ipi] "his/her string" without any alternation in the root final consonant. The rules that map the underlying forms to the surface forms, regardless of whether they yield phonemically or allophonically distinct segments, are called phonological rules. These phonological rules are formal accounts of the phonological processes that have been considered. The model that is described here is known as generative phonology and will be dealt with later in this chapter. What follows is a description of these common phonological processes that are found in many languages.

PHONOLOGICAL PROCESSES

Assimilation

The term **assimilation** refers generally to the influence one sound may have on another when two are contiguous in time, as a result of coarticulation. Because assimilation is by far the most common type of process in language, our account of it will be more detailed than the description of other processes.

There are two necessary components that define assimilation: the sound that changes to become like the other sound, called the *conditioned sound*, and, the sound that creates the change, the *conditioning sound*. In several of the cases that have been mentioned so far in this chapter, assimilatory changes were exemplified. In the following, an examination of some of them in terms of the conditioning sound and the conditioned sound will be given.

In the case of Korean /s/ becoming [ʃ] before [i], and the Portuguese /t/ becoming [tʃ] before [i], the conditioning sounds are the vowels [i], and the conditioned consonants are /s/ and /t/. /s/ and /t/ became [ʃ] and [tʃ] (palatal) because of the high front vowel, which is articulated in the palatal area. Both of these cases are examples of consonants acquiring vowel features and changing their place of articulation.

The influence of one sound on the other in changing the place of articulation does not necessarily require the interaction of a consonant with a vowel. The change in the place of articulation of the nasal consonant of the negative prefix [ɪm, ɪn, ɪŋ] in English demonstrated this point well. The nasal consonant agreed in place of articulation with the following consonant. The first consonant of the adjective (the conditioning sound) determined the place of articulation of the nasal sound of the negative prefix (the conditioned sound). In this case, a consonant assimilates a feature, the place of articulation, from another consonant.

Coarticulatory effects of assimilation can go beyond the changes in place of articulation and can affect voicing and manner of articulation. In the Russian example given earlier, an obstruent (conditioned sound) became voiced before a voiced obstruent (conditioning sound). This is an example of an assimilation in voicing; it is also another example of a consonant acquiring consonant features.

An example of a vowel acquiring consonant features can be seen in vowel nasalization in English. As the following examples show, the differences between the following pairs of English words go beyond the change in the final consonant; the vowels before the final consonants also are different.

bean	[bĩn]	*bead*	[bid]
green	[grĩn]	*greed*	[grid]
can	[kæ̃n]	*cat*	[kæt]

In the left column of words, the vowels are nasalized because of the following nasal consonants. The nasal consonant is produced with the velum lowered, which allows air to escape through the nasal cavity. In the production of these words, speakers lower their velum before they terminate producing the vowel as they get ready for the nasal consonant. This creates the nasalization of the vowels. The nasalization of vowels before nasal consonants serves as an example of a vowel acquiring consonant features.

In the cases reviewed so far, the later sound conditioned the earlier sound. The force of the change operates backwards in the word. This can be shown by AX → XX where the first sound becomes more like the second sound, and where "becoming more like" means acquiring some phonetic feature(s)—place of articulation, manner of articulation, or voicing—from the conditioning sound. The process is called a *regressive assimilation* or *anticipatory coarticulation* when the direction of influence is from the later sound to the earlier sound.

If a given sound produces changes in the sound that follows it, the assimilation is *progressive (perseverative coarticulation)*. Consider the following data from Turkish, which illustrate two cases of progressive assimilation:

1.	[konuʃ]	"talk"	[konuʃtu]	"s/he	talked"
2.	[gør]	"see"	[gørdy]	" "	saw"
3.	[kɨz]	"be angry"	[kɨzdɨ]	" "	got angry"
4.	[as]	"hang"	[asti]	" "	hung"
5.	[oku]	"read"	[okudu]	" "	read"
6.	[øp]	"kiss"	[øpty]	" "	kissed"
7.	[gel]	"come"	[geldi]	" "	came"
8.	[itʃ]	"drink"	[itʃti]	" "	drank"

The past tense morpheme can assume one of the following phonetic manifestations: [ti, tɨ, tu, ty, di, dɨ, du, dy]. These eight allomorphs can be summarized as an alveolar stop followed by a high vowel. What is really interesting in these examples, however, is that the voicing of the alveolar stop is entirely dependent on the last sound in the verb root. If the last sound of the verb root in the left column is voiceless, then the consonant of the past tense suffix is the voiceless [t] (as in examples 1, 4, 6, and 8). If, however, the last sound of the verb root is voiced, then the consonant is the voiced [d] (examples 2, 3, 5, and 7). In addition to the changes in voicing in the consonants, these examples demonstrate another assimilatory change that affects the vowels. As noted earlier, the vowel of the past tense suffix must be a high vowel. The choice among the four candidates [u, y, i, ɨ], however, is not arbitrary and is governed by the vowel harmony rule, which is also a progressive assimilation process. The two rounded vowels [u, y] are used whenever the last vowel of the root was round and the two unrounded vowels [i,ɨ] are used whenever the last root vowel was unrounded. The choice between the two candidates in each group after the rounding is decided is determined by the front/back dimension of the vowels. When the last root vowel is a back vowel, the suffix vowel must be back. Likewise, when the root vowel is front, then the suffix vowel is front.

These principles will be illustrated with an example. In example 1 we have the form [konuʃ-tu]. Because the root ends in a voiceless sound [ʃ], the consonant of the past tense suffix must be the voiceless one, [t]. The determination of the suffix vowel will be made on the basis of the last vowel of the root in the two dimensions of roundness and backness of the vowel. Because the vowel in question is [u], a round back vowel, the suffix will need to contain a round back vowel. Among the four available high vowels for this suffix, only [u] fits this description, and the form comes out as [konuʃtu]. Although the conditioning and the conditioned sounds are adjacent for the initial consonant of the past tense suffix, they are not adjacent for the agreement between the vowels, and this assimilation is made at a distance. This example demonstrates that vowels can influence each other at a distance which is not typically seen in consonants. However, because the force of the change operates forward in the word in both cases in the above examples, they both qualify for progressive assimilation. The harmony of the vowels is an example of a vowel acquiring vowel features.

What has been shown so far makes the point that assimilation can be responsible for changes in many dimensions of sounds, such as place of articulation, manner of articulation, and voicing. Also, it has been shown that consonants can acquire feature(s) from consonants or from vowels, vowels can do the same, and the direction of the assimilation can be progressive or regressive.

Other cases of assimilation, however, cannot be classified as progressive or regressive as the conditioning environment is not restricted to the preceding or the following environment but provided by both simultaneously. In Chapter 3, it was mentioned that the sounds [d] and [ð] in Spanish are allophones of the same phoneme /d/, and [ð] occurs between two vowels. The change from /d/ to [ð] (from stop to fricative) is conditioned by both the preceding and the following environments. This can be viewed as assimilation to the surrounding vowels. Vowels, as well as fricatives, liquids, and glides, carry the feature [continuant], which means that these sounds can be continued as we pronounce them. Stops, on the other hand are noncontinuant sounds. The change from a stop to a continuant between two other continuant sounds is a clear case of assimilation in the manner of articulation.

Another case that involves both the preceding and the following environment is the Cree example given at the beginning of this chapter. In this case, a voiceless stop turns into a voiced stop between two vowels. In other words, the stop becomes voiced to match the feature of voicing for the vowels.

Some types of assimilation are better known by their specific names rather than the general label "assimilation." For example, the changes that are known as **palatalization**, (Korean /s/ → [ʃ] before [i], Portuguese /t/ → [tʃ] before [i]), **labialization**, and **weakening** (Spanish /d/ → [ð] between two vowels) are all assimilatory changes.

Another very common type of change that can also be viewed as a special kind of assimilation is that of **final devoicing**. Sounds at the end of a word, especially obstruents, often change from voiced to voiceless. In several languages (e.g., German, Polish, Russian, and Turkish), stops come in voiced and voiceless pairs /p, b/, /t, d/, /k, g/, and they occur freely in initial and medial positions of the word. However, in final position, the voiced-voiceless contrast is not found, and we find only the voiceless ones. The reason for this is that the sound matches the voicelessness of the silence following the end of the word.

All of these assimilations are examples of partial assimilation, because the changed sound retains at least one of the original features that distinguishes it from the unchanged sound. If all of the features are changed to match those of another sound, then two sounds end up being identical. When the assimilation process results in contiguous identical consonants, these are called geminates, and the assimilation is total. Some common examples of gemination are *give me* [gɪmmi], and *let me* [lɛmmi].

Dissimilation

The assimilatory changes that were looked at in the preceding section were rather phonetically transparent cases relating to the principle of ease of articulation. Although these processes make the job of the speaker easier by facilitating speech production, they are not as friendly to the hearer as they are to the speaker. The more similar the sounds are, the greater the difficulty the hearer has in discriminating among them. Dissimilation, a process in which segments change to become less like a neighboring segment, ensures easier discrimination and perception. Although it is much rarer than assimilation, examples of dissimilation are observed in both historical changes as well as in present day data. The cases of Latin *anma* becoming Spanish *alma* and Latin *arbor* becoming Spanish *arbol* illustrate the point well. In the first pair, the Latin word has two nasals which turn into one lateral and one nasal sequence in the Spanish word. In the second pair, the Latin word *arbor* has two identical liquids /r/, whereas the Spanish word turns one of these into a lateral liquid, making it less similar.

Another case of dissimilation concerns the adjectival suffixes in English that are manifested phonetically as [əl] or [ər]:

[əl]	[ər]
anecdote - anecdotal	angle - angular
spirit - spiritual	circle - circular
culture - cultural	single - singular
region - regional	circle - circular

As these examples demonstrate, [ər] is found only when the last sound of the noun is [l], otherwise we have the ending as [əl].[3] Examples such as *library* [laɪbɛri] (the elimination of the first [r]) and *February* [fɛbjuɛri] (the changing of the first [r] to [j]) can also be cited for dissimilation (although deletion is occurring).

Deletion

When morphemes are strung together to form words, there are phonological phenomena other than assimilation and dissimilation that can take place. A common phonological change is deletion whereby a vowel or a consonant is lost. In many cases, deletion changes the syllable structure of a word.

Consonant Loss

French words may end in a consonant. For many words, this final consonant is dropped when the following word starts with a consonant:

je parle a mes amis [zə pærl a mez æmɪ] "I speak to my friends"
je parle a mes parents [zə pærl a me pərã] "I speak to my parents"

un petit animal [œ̃ pətit əniməl] "a small animal"
un petit garçon [œ̃ pəti gərsɔ̃] "a little boy"

In English, consonant clusters at the end of a word lose a consonant if the next word starts with a consonant. For example, *best friend* and *most people* are pronounced [bɛs frɛnd] and [mos pipl], respectively. However, the same deletions are not observed in *best apples* or in *most areas*, as the final consonant clusters are followed by a vowel in these sequences.

Vowel Loss

There are several processes referring to vowel loss in different word positions. **Aphesis**, or aphaeresis, is the deletion of the initial unstressed vowel, exemplified by [baʊt] for *about*, or [rɪəmɛtɪk] for *arithmetic*. **Apocope** refers to the loss of word final vowels. Historically, this was observed in English. Old English *mona* became *moon* [mun] and *nama* became *name* [nem] in Modern English. If the loss refers to the medial vowel, then the process is called **syncope**. Some midwestern American speakers drop the pretonic vowels (the unstressed vowel before the stressed vowel) before a liquid, as in *policeman* [plismən], *believe* [bliv], *Columbus* [klɔmbʊs], and *terrific* [trɪfɪk]. Examples of syncope in post-tonic syllables (the unstressed syllable after the stressed syllable) are *family* [fæmli], *interest* [ɪntrɛst], and *vegetable* [vɛdʒtəbl].

A special case of deletion, **haplology**, refers to a situation in which the entire syllable is deleted when it is identical (or similar) to another syllable. Latin *stipipendium* "tax contribution" became *stipendium*, and *nutritrix* "nurse" became *nutrix*. The word *England* was originally *Angleland*, meaning the Land of Angles in Modern English. The two syllables are reduced to one through haplology. The word haplology sometimes suffers the same process and becomes haplogy.

Coalescence

Sometimes, a process may have a mixture of both assimilation and deletion, and the two segments are replaced by one segment that shares the characteristics of each of the original segments. This process, known as **coalescence**, is responsible for the forms like

| Latin | *aidifikum* | to | Spanish | *edificio* | "building" |
| Latin | *aikwalem* | to | Spanish | *egual* | "equal" |

In these examples we see that Latin [aɪ] (a low vowel-high vowel combination) resulted in [e] (mid vowel).

A special case of coalescence is the deletion of one of the two identical consonants, which is called **degemination**:

| Latin | *terra* | to | French | *tɛrə* | "earth" |
| Latin | *gutta* | to | French | *guta* | "drop" |

Epenthesis

Although it is less common than deletion, we also observe insertion of segments in languages, which is called **epenthesis**. As in deletion, the segments in question may be consonants or vowels.

In English, a short voiceless stop is inserted after a nasal and before a voiceless fricative followed by an unstressed vowel. This accounts for the fact that many people do not distinguish between the pairs *prince* and *prints*, *sense* and *scents*, or *cents*, *mince* and *mints*, or *dense* and *dents*. Also, the pronunciations of words such as *presence*, *France*, and *answer* all have a short [t] after the nasal and before the voiceless fricative. The motivation for this can be shown with reference to the composition of the neighboring segments and the intruding segment. As we saw earlier, nasals are [+sonorant, –continuant], and the following fricative is [–sonorant, +continuant]. In other words, these neighboring segments are diametrically opposed with regard to these two features. The intrusive [t], on the other hand, having the [-sonorant, –continuant] combination, shares one property with each of the two opposing segments and, as such, it serves as a compromise, or bridge, during the transition.

Vowel epenthesis is a commonly seen process in which a language that does not permit a specific consonant cluster borrows words from another language and modifies according to its own phonological patterns. For example, Turkish does not permit any initial consonant clusters. When words are borrowed from languages in which these sequences are permitted, epenthetic vowels are used to modify the clusters:

train	tiren
sport	sipor
traffic	tirafik

Note that the syllable structure is modified and the resulting Turkish words have one more syllable.

Portuguese, like Spanish, does permit initial clusters, but the range of combinations of segments is not as wide as in English. For example, words cannot start with [s] plus another consonant in Portuguese. Thus, when English words such as *sport*, *score*, and *stress* entered the language, they were assimilated in the form of [ɛspor tʃi], [ɛskor], and [ɛstrɛs], respectively.[4] These examples show that, in Portuguese, the epenthetic vowel occurs before the first element of the cluster rather than in between the cluster as we saw in Turkish. The end results, however, are the same: Undesired clusters are modified and the modified words have an extra syllable.

Metathesis

We have seen that processes such as deletion and epenthesis can change the syllable structure of the word. Another process which can modify the shape of a word, though this time not in the form of deleting or adding, is **metathesis**. In metathesis, the linear order of segments changes by the transposition of two elements. Historical changes illustrate this process well:

Old English	*hros*	to	Modern English	*horse*
Old English	*brid*	to	Modern English	*bird*
Latin	*periculum*	to	Spanish	*peligro* "danger"
Latin	*parabola*	to	Spanish	*palabra* "word"

Synchronically, this process is observed in the following examples, in which in some varieties of English *ask* are pronounced as [æks], and *prescribe* is pronounced as [pərskraɪb].

Neutralization

Finally, mention should be made of neutralization, which refers to the collapse of a phonemic contrast between sounds in certain environments. For example, final devoicing of obstruents in German, Russian, Polish, and several other languages, which was mentioned during the discussion of assimilation, is a good example. Here, the voicing distinction between /p, b/, /t, d/, and /k, g/, which is observed in word-initial and word-medial positions, is lost in final position. Thus, the voicing contrast is neutralized in final position. Neutralization of a contrast creates a many-to-one mapping between phoneme and phone:

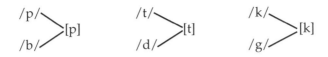

GENERATIVE PHONOLOGY AND
CLINICAL IMPLICATIONS

Previously in this chapter, it was stated that having separate levels of morphophonemic representation and phonemic representation is not justified and facts dictated that a single level of representation, apart from the phonetic level, should be utilized. This way of representing things describes a model which is called **generative phonology**. Generative phonology espouses the idea that we operate on a highly organized system of phonological rules in putting together the morphemes of language.

Taking the morpheme as the basic unit, this model assigns a single underlying representation for one meaning (morpheme) even if there are multiple forms (allomorphs) representing this meaning at the phonetic level. To understand this point, the possible relationships between forms and meanings in language will be considered. The following three relationships are possible:

a. one form with multiple meanings.
    example: *bank* 1. financial institution
                  2. a slope especially at the side of a river
           bat   1. a wooden implement for striking the ball in baseball
                  2. flying mammal with a mouselike body
b. one form with one meaning.
    example: *sun, moon*
c. multiple forms with one meaning
    negative prefix [ɪm,ɪn, ɪŋ] as in *impossible, intolerant,* and *incompetent,* respectively.

The cases in b are very straightforward and do not require any further comment. The cases in a represent **homonymy**, which is very common in languages. Because the homonymous forms are normally used in different contexts, they do not create any problems and no further elaboration for these is needed.

The real focus is on the cases exemplified in c, whereby the same meaning (morpheme) has different phonetic manifestations. It is the assumption of generative phonology that the most economical way of storing and operating on language is by way of one-to-one relationship between the form and the meaning. Thus, despite its phonetically multiple surface forms, a morpheme will be assigned one unique underlying form and the surface alternations (allomorphs), which are functions of different contexts, will be accounted for by phonological rules. The claim is that a speaker of English, for example, must learn only one underlying representation for the negative prefix, and phonological rules will convert that representation into the different surface forms [ɪm, ɪn, ɪŋ]. In doing this, there must be phonetic similarity among the allomorphs, so that phonological rules can convert one into another.

Identifying the specific underlying form is probably the most important task and deserves much attention. In Chapter 3, in which we examined phonemic representation and its differences from phonetic representation, it was concluded that the phonemic representation should include information that is not predictable by rules. For example, the English word *pit* was represented as /pɪt/, but its phonetic representation is [pʰɪt]. The aspiration of the initial [p] is a predictable property of English voiceless stops in that particular context and was excluded from the phonemic representation. Similarly, in the underlying forms for morphemes, predictable properties will be excluded. These include allophonic variation as well as allomorphic variation in which we have different surface manifestations of the same morpheme.

For example, three different surface manifestations, [s, z, əz], of the English plural as exemplified in *cats* [kæts], *dogs* [dɔgz], and *buses* [bʌsəz], respectively, is reduced to one underlying form /z/, as the others are derived through the phonological rules. Phonological rules utilize the information given in the underlying representation to further specify the predictable properties in the surface phonetic forms. In accounting for these, phonological rules perform operations that are exemplified in the previous section on phonological processes, which include changes, addition, deletion, and transposition of segments. Before explaining the strategy for the decision of the underlying forms, we will digress here a little and show how phonological rules are formulated to describe these processes. Because these operations are not restricted to normal language data and are also found in young children and in disordered phonology, examples from those areas will be used to show the clinical relevance.

Distinctive features are used for the phonological rule format of generative phonology. These allow segments to be grouped in natural classes. As seen in the last chapter, distinctive features are used to show context-free changes in children's substitutions in comparison to adult targets. Context-sensitive changes, insertions, and omissions are automatically excluded. In generative phonology, distinctive feature analysis is taken one step further by including context-sensitive information as well as noting deletions and insertions that contain segments with no feature specifications. This way, a more adequate framework for analysis of child speech can be offered. The formalized rule statements identify the contextual motivation for the child's productions in terms of its differences from adult targets.[5] Although the formal representation of phonological rules will not be detailed here, the basics will be examined.

A common substitution found in young children and in the clinical population is voicing of word-initial consonants before vowels, such as *toe* → [do], *pea* → [bi], which is shown by the following rule notation:

[–syl] → [+voiced] / # _____ [+syl]

which reads "consonants become voiced in word-initial position before vowels." First, there is the input which is affected by the process. This is given on the left of the arrow. The feature specification describes the segment(s) in this input. In the above case, this refers to consonants. The specification to the immediate right of the error is the output of the rule, and indicates the change. The arrow is to be read as "becomes" or "is changed to." In the output, only the changed feature specifications are shown; the feature values that remain the same are not repeated. The diagonal bar (/) should be read as "in the context of," which indicates the environment in which the change occurs. The environment bar (___) shows where the input is placed. The relevant environment for the change is put before or after the input depending on the rule. In the above rule, in which voicing took place in initial position before a vowel, the input is placed between the word boundary symbol (initial position) and the vowel. In this case, then, both the preceding and the following environments are relevant.

M's data, presented in the previous chapter, provided several substitutions in which segments were changed. One of these was the fronting of the palatal fricative to alveolar position in final position, as in *brush* → [bʌs], or *dish* → [dɪs], which is shown in the following:

$$
\begin{bmatrix} +\text{cons} \\ +\text{cont} \\ +\text{high} \\ -\text{ant} \end{bmatrix} \rightarrow \Big/ \begin{bmatrix} -\text{high} \\ +\text{ant} \end{bmatrix} \quad \underline{\hspace{2cm}} \quad \#
$$

(palatal fricatives become alveolar in word-final position)

As mentioned earlier, phonological rules perform other operations in addition to changing feature values. Deletion is another process that is commonly found in young children and in the clinical population. For example, deletion of final consonants in word final position (*dog* → [da], *kid* → [kɪ]) is shown in the following representation:

$$[\text{–syl}] \quad \rightarrow \quad \emptyset \quad / \quad \underline{\hspace{2cm}} \#$$

"consonants are deleted in word-final position."

Here, the null symbol, $\emptyset$, indicates that the entire segment is deleted. In this case, only the following environment is relevant for the rule.

Another deletion rule can be cited from M's data. Recall that the lateral liquid was deleted in initial consonant clusters, as exemplified in *black* →[bæk], and *blue* → [bu]. This is shown in the following:

$$\begin{bmatrix} \text{–syl} \\ \text{+ cons} \\ \text{+ lat} \end{bmatrix} \quad \rightarrow \quad \emptyset \quad \Big/ \quad \# \, [\text{–syl}] \, \underline{\hspace{1.5cm}}$$

"lateral liquid is deleted in word-initial consonant clusters."

In this particular deletion process, the preceding environment is crucial for the application.

Insertion rules are the opposite of deletion in that we find the null symbol as the input. Examples of the epenthetic vowels in the productions of young children and the clinical population, such as *blue* → [bəlu], and *play* → [pəle], are shown in the following:

$$\emptyset \quad \rightarrow \quad \begin{bmatrix} \text{+syl} \\ \text{–high} \\ \text{–low} \\ \text{–round} \\ \text{–tense} \end{bmatrix} \quad \Big/ \quad \# \quad \begin{bmatrix} \text{–syl} \\ \text{+cons} \end{bmatrix} \, \underline{\hspace{1cm}} \, \begin{bmatrix} \text{–syl} \\ \text{+cons} \end{bmatrix}$$

Metathesis can also be represented by phonological rules. Although it is not very frequent in child phonology, examples are cited in the literature (Smith 1973). Permutations such as *milk* → [mlɪk], and *self* → [slɛf] are accounted for by the following formalization:

V	[+lat]	C	→	[+lat]	V	C
		–cor				–cor
1	2	3		2	1	3

"the sequence 1 2 3 becomes 2 1 3."

In previous examples, segments were added, deleted, or changed, but were not allowed to change the overall linear sequence of the segments in a word. In order to show this transposition process, the different type of rule format shown above is used. The segments are numbered and the order is changed to represent the output. The use of V and C indicates vowel and consonant, respectively.

Finally, another process occurs, coalescence. Here, the realization as the combination of the two elements in the target is considered. It is common to find examples of coalescence in young children, especially when they attempt certain consonant clusters. For example, *swim* → [fɪm] will be accounted for as in the following:

$$
\begin{array}{ccc}
\text{s} & \text{w} & \text{f} \\
\begin{bmatrix} +\text{cor} \\ +\text{ant} \\ +\text{cont} \\ +\text{strid} \\ -\text{voice} \\ -\text{labial} \end{bmatrix} &
\begin{bmatrix} -\text{syl} \\ -\text{cons} \\ -\text{cor} \\ +\text{cont} \\ +\text{lab} \\ -\text{cor} \end{bmatrix} \rightarrow &
\begin{bmatrix} +\text{cont} \\ +\text{strid} \\ -\text{cor} \\ +\text{ant} \\ -\text{voice} \\ +\text{labial} \end{bmatrix}
\end{array}
$$

As seen in this example, the child's production is a combination of the components of the adult target.

Having shown the basics of the rule formulations, we are ready to go back, examine again the case of the negative prefix [ɪm, ɪn, ɪŋ] in English, and resume the discussion of the underlying forms. As described earlier, the alternant with the bilabial nasal occurred with adjectives that start with a bilabial consonant (*impossible, impertinent*), the alveolar nasal with adjectives that start with alveolar consonants (*indecent, intolerant*), and the velar nasal with adjectives that start with a velar consonant (*incongruent, incapable*). When a morpheme such as this has several different phonetic manifestations, it is reasonable to expect that one of the phonetically occurring allomorphs can be taken as the underlying form. The way this situation has been described so far does not allow us to make a choice among the three allomorphs (alternants) as the underlying form, because the distribution of the three appears equal. However, if adjectives starting with vowels (*inoperable, inactive*) are considered, then it will be clear that the form with the alveolar nasal [ɪn] is the one that enjoys greatest freedom of occurrence and is the least restricted. Thus, the choice for the underlying form will be this particular allomorph,/ɪn/, and the two other allomorphs, [ɪm, ɪŋ] at the surface, will be derived by the phonological rules converting the alveolar nasal to bilabial and velar nasals in the phonetic representation. Thus the following rule describes the process:

$$\begin{bmatrix} C \\ [+\text{nasal}] \end{bmatrix} \rightarrow \begin{bmatrix} \alpha\ \text{ant} \\ \beta\ \text{cor} \end{bmatrix} \Big/ \underline{\hspace{2cm}} \begin{bmatrix} -\text{son} \\ \alpha\ \text{ant} \\ \beta\ \text{cor} \end{bmatrix}$$

This rule changes the specifications for [anterior] and [coronal] in an un-derlying /n/ to those of the following obstruent. Greek letters show the agreement between the obstruent and the nasal by demanding the iden-tical values for the features [anterior] and [coronal]. According to the alpha rule, if the specification for [anterior] is +, then that of the output will be +. If [anterior] in the context is –, the output will be –. The same is true for coronal, too. Application of this rule to the underlying forms re-sult in the following derivations:

Underlying form	/ɪn-peʃənt/	/ɪn-kepəbl/
Phonological rule	ɪmpeʃənt	ɪŋkepəbl
Phonetic rep.	[ɪmpeʃənt]	[ɪŋkepəbl]

To give one more example, we can review the plural morpheme alter-nants [s, z, əz]. As mentioned earlier, one of these allomorphs, /z/, is cho-sen to represent the underlying morpheme, and the multiple surface forms are derived from it via phonological rules. The facts for plural for-mation are as follows: If the last sound of the noun is a sibilant (i.e., s, z, ʃ, ʒ, tʃ, dʒ), the plural allomorph is [əz] (e.g., *churches* [tʃərtʃəz], *bushes* [bʊʃəz], *buses* [bʌsəz]). If the noun ends in one of the remaining sounds, which are all nonsibilant, the voicing is the determining factor. If it is voiced, then the plural is [z] (e.g., *bags* [bægz], *beds* [bɛdz]). If voiceless, the plural is [s] (e.g., *cats* [kæts], *caps* [kæps]). The reason that /z/ is cho-sen from among the three alternants is that the derivation of the other two is made easier than choosing either one of the two and deriving the phonetic representation. Specifically, the derivation of [s] is achieved by a single rule of assimilation whereby the plural assimilates the voicing of the non-sibilant voiceless:

Underlying form	/kæt-z/	*cats*
Phonological rule	kæts	
Phonetic form	[kæts]	

The derivation of [əz] is also arrived at via single phonological rule of schwa insertion between the two sibilants:

Underlying form	/bʌs-z/	*buses*
Phonological rule	bʌsəz	
Phonetic form	[bʌsəz]	

If we choose any one of the other allomorphs for the underlying form, there will be a need for a more complicated two-rule derivation for the correct surface forms:

	cats /kæt-əz/		*buses* /bʌs-s/
Schwa-deletion	kætz	schwa-insertion	bʌsəs
Voicing assimilation	kæts	s → z	bʌsəz
Phonetic form	[kæts]		[bʌsəz]

It is important to keep in mind that the underlying representation is a theoretical construct. As such, it is a claim about how a native speaker of a language stores this particular morpheme in his or her lexicon.

The above situation in which the underlying representation is identical to one of the alternants (allomorphs) illustrates a concrete analysis. Sometimes, the postulated underlying representation differs from any of the surface manifestations of the morpheme that speakers utter, and is judged to be abstract. Linguistics literature is very rich on the abstractness controversy. This introductory text will not go into that problem in detail, but will consider its implications for the clinical population.

Consider the data from Mikey:

bed	[bɛt]	wet	[wɛt]
egg	[ɛk]	bake	[bek]
bag	[bæk]	back	[bæk]
cab	[kæp]	cap	[kæp]
go	[go]	door	[dɔr]

These and many other similar words show that Mikey produces all stops, but the production of the final stops is restricted only to the voiceless set [p, t, k], and the voiced set [b, d, g] is never found in this environment. The traditional interpretation of the data would assign the underlying forms of the morphemes *bed*, *egg*, *bag*, and *cab* with final voiced stops. Then the phonological rule of final devoicing would convert the voiced stops into voiceless ones in final position:

$$\begin{bmatrix} -\text{sonorant} \\ -\text{continuant} \\ -\text{del. release} \end{bmatrix} \rightarrow [-\text{voice}] \Big/ \underline{\hspace{1cm}} \#$$

What this rule says is that a stop (–sonorant, –continuant, –delayed release) is voiceless in final position. This way of looking at things, which is called the relational account, claims that there is a systematic relationship between the target system the child is trying to acquire and his or her erroneous production. It assumes that the child's underlying representation of these words is correct (i.e., adultlike).

Although this interpretation is not implausible, it does imply that the child has internalized the underlying forms that are not found in the forms she or he produces. This necessarily results in an abstract representation that is disputed by some scholars. The independent account advanced by Dinnsen and Chin (1994), Chin (1993), Gierut (1985), and Maxwell (1979, 1981) maintains that the underlying forms should be based on facts evident only in the child's productions without any a priori assumption that they are in agreement with the ambient language. This means that, if there is no indication that the child uses morpheme final voiced stops, the underlying forms cannot be presumed to be adultlike. If, on the other hand, there is evidence that the child has voiced/voiceless alternations in morphologically related forms of the morphemes in question, then the correct (adultlike) underlying form can be supported.

To illustrate this, consider the following morphologically related forms of the words we saw above:

cabby	[kæbi]	eggy	[ɛgi]
baggy	[bægi]	bedding	[bɛdɪŋ]

Because there is evidence that the child uses the voiced stops in relation to the morphemes in question, correct underlying forms are supported.

The issue of correct underlying forms is not merely a discussion at the theoretical level, but has consequences regarding the clinical population. There are arguments suggesting the postulation of incorrect underlying forms for some phonologically disordered children. The first argument comes from cases in which there is a need to differentiate among the seemingly identical error patterns observed in different children. To exemplify this, let us consider some well-known cases in which there is final consonant omission in children's speech. This will be demonstrated by using the same words we cited for Mikey earlier:

	Child I	*Child II*
bed	[bɛ]	[bɛ:]
wet	[wɛ]	[wɛ]
bag	[bæ]	[bæ:]
back	[bæ]	[bæ]
cab	[kæ]	[kæ:]
cap	[kæ]	[kæ]

As can be seen in these examples, both children have final consonant omission, but their renditions are different when the target word has a final voiced stop. While Child I simply omits the final consonant for all words, Child II lengthens the vowel if the target ends in a voiced stop. By doing so, Child II manifests his or her awareness about the final voiced stops in *bed, bag,* and *cab.* Thus, Child I does not show any indication of contrast between final voiced and voiceless stops, and he or she will be assigned incorrect underlying representations for the three words in question. However, Child II reveals the knowledge about the final voiced stops and will be assigned the correct underlying form.

Another argument advanced for differentiating between the children with incorrect and correct underlying representations comes from the differences in children's learning patterns. During therapy sessions, the greatest improvements are sometimes observed in errors associated with correct underlying representations. Also, treatment directed at errors associated with incorrect underlying representations results in improvements in the child's entire system, whereas treatment directed at errors associated with correct underlying representations results in improvements limited to that class of errors (Dinnsen & Elbert, 1984; Gierut, Elbert, & Dinnsen, 1987).

It has also been suggested that variability (mean number of substitutions) can be an indicator of correctness of underlying representations. Barlow (1996) analyzed data from 40 children with nonorganic speech disorders to find out if variability in substitution errors corresponded with the nature of underlying representation. Her results suggested that variability correlates with correctness of the underlying form in that more variability occurred for sounds that were considered to be underlyingly incorrect in a given child's system than for sounds that were considered to be underlyingly correct. It was concluded that greater overall variability would occur in systems with more incorrect underlying forms.

The existence of nonsystematic correspondences between the target system and the child's system is another type of situation in which underlying representations cannot be assumed to be correct. The reason for this is that, if the underlying representations are assumed to be correct in nonsystematic correspondences, then contradictory processes will have to be posited to account for the variability in production.

Finally, certain allophonic phenomena seem to require the assumption that the subject has at least some incorrect underlying forms. For example, the case from Camarata and Gandour (1984) presented the end of Chapter 3, in which [b] and [d] contrasted but [d] and [g] were in complementary distribution, exemplifies this well. If the child's underlying forms were assumed to be correct in this case, then the nontarget complementary distribution of sounds would have had to be considered accidental.

It should be pointed out that these interpretations assume the one-lexicon model in which the underlying form is viewed as the representation handling both recognition and production. This, however, is not the only possible model for child representations, and some investigators have proposed that a word can have two different types of representations. The two-lexicon model advanced by Kiparsky and Menn (1977) and Menn (1976, 1978, 1983) makes a distinction between the input lexicon, which contains the information necessary for the child to recognize the word, and the output lexicon, which contains the child's stored information about how the word should be pronounced. The output lexicon, which corresponds to the underlying form in the one-lexicon model, may be quite a bit less accurate than the child's knowledge of input words (Chiat, 1994). Thus, in a two-lexicon model, the situation in which the two children had no final stops that was mentioned above would be interpreted differently. The correctness of the underlying form would be irrelevant and Child II, who had vowel lengthening before the deleted final voiced stop targets, would be considered advanced relative to production of codas. Child I would need more systematic remediation because of greater limitations on output. Developmental data supporting the two-lexicon model have been reported by McGregor and Schwartz (1992), Schwartz and Leonard (1982), and Schwartz, Leonard, Loeb, and Swanson (1987).

SUMMARY

In this chapter, we have looked at several phonetically motivated phonological processes that may help to explain allomorphic variation (different phonetic representations for the same meaning). It was shown that the separation of allomorphic variation from allophonic variation (predictable variation between the allophones of the same phoneme) is not justifiable, because it duplicates the same rules in many cases. This has the natural result of rejecting the idea of separate phonemic and morphophonemic levels and suggests a single underlying level of representation that is distinct from the surface phonetic representation. The rules that map the underlying forms to the surface forms, regardless of whether they yield phonemically or allophonically distinct segments, are called phonological rules. These rules are accounts or representations of phonological processes we examined. This model of phonology, known as generative phonology, has influenced the analysis of clinical data and has implications for therapy. The nature of the child's representations and the interpretation of the data might be different depending on whether one espouses a one- or two-lexicon model.

NOTES

1. Although the labels such as palato-alveolar or palatal are not used for vowels, the point that [i] is made corresponds to the palato-alveolar region.

2. Morpheme can be defined as the minimal grammatical unit that has meaning. For example, *cats* has two morphemes: *cat* and *s* of plural.

3. Like many other rules, this has exceptions too. *column-ar* and *line-ar* illustrate that the last sound does not need to be [l] for the ending to become [ər].

4. The first example also has an inserted vowel [i] at the end. This is due to the fact that no Portuguese words can end with a stop sound. When a conflicting case such as this one arises, then an epenthetic [i] is inserted. The insertion of [i] provokes the palatalization of [t], and we get the resulting [tʃ].

5. This way, the assumption is made automatically that the child's underlying representation is a replica of the adult phonemic form, which is questionable. This point is taken up in greater detail later in this chapter.

EXERCISES

1. Identify the processes that are exemplified in the changes below:

governor	[gavərnər]	→	[gavənər]	_____
evening	[ivənɪŋ]	→	[ivnɪŋ]	_____
hundred	[hʌndrəd]	→	[hʌndərd]	_____
comfort	[kʌmfərt]	→	[kʌmpfərt]	_____
electrician	[ɛlɛktrəʃən]	→	[lɛktrəʃən]	_____

2. Identify the phonological processes given in the following.

   a. f becomes v before a voiced sound.   _____

   b. s becomes ʃ before i   _____

   c. t becomes tʃ before j   _____

   d. b becomes p word finally.   _____

   e. d becomes ð between two vowels   _____

   f. Word final ə is deleted in an
       unstressed syllable   _____

   g. sk becomes ks   _____

   h. d becomes g when following z   _____

   i. t becomes s when followed by s   _____

3. Identify the phonological process that accounts for the change from A to B:

A	B	
[most pipl]	[mos pipl]	_____
[ərɪθmətɪk]	[rɪθmətɪk]	_____
[laɪbrɛri]	[laɪbri]	_____
[sʌmθɪŋ]	[sʌmpθɪŋ]	_____
[blaɪnd mæn]	[blaɪn mæn]	_____
[vɛdʒətəbl]	[vɛdʒtəbl]	_____
[sɛns]	[sɛnts]	_____
[hʌndrɪd]	[hʌndɪrd]	_____
[mɪs ju]	[mɪʃ ju]	_____
[sɛkrətɛri]	[sɛkrətri]	_____

4. Match the following descriptions with the changes shown with the phonological rules:

   ___ /θ/ and /ð/ are replaced by /t/ and /d/, respectively, in word-final position.

___ /tʃ/ and /dʒ/ are replaced by /ʃ/ and /ʒ/, respectively, in word-initial position.

___ /d/ is dropped following /n/ in word final position.

___ /b/ is dropped following /m/ in word final position.

___ /g/ is dropped following /ŋ/ in word final position.

a.
$$\begin{bmatrix} +\text{strident} \\ \\ +\text{coronal} \end{bmatrix} \rightarrow [+\text{continuant}] \Big/ \# \underline{\hspace{2cm}}$$

b.
$$\begin{bmatrix} -\text{continuant} \\ -\text{nasal} \\ +\text{anterior} \\ +\text{coronal} \\ +\text{voice} \end{bmatrix} \rightarrow \emptyset \Big/ \begin{bmatrix} +\text{nasal} \\ +\text{anterior} \\ +\text{coronal} \end{bmatrix} \underline{\hspace{2cm}} \#$$

c.
$$\begin{bmatrix} -\text{continuant} \\ -\text{nasal} \\ -\text{anterior} \\ -\text{coronal} \\ +\text{voice} \end{bmatrix} \rightarrow \emptyset \Big/ \begin{bmatrix} +\text{nasal} \\ -\text{anterior} \end{bmatrix} \underline{\hspace{2cm}} \#$$

d.
$$\begin{bmatrix} +\text{continuant} \\ +\text{anterior} \\ -\text{strident} \end{bmatrix} \rightarrow [-\text{continuant}] \Big/ \underline{\hspace{2cm}} \#$$

e.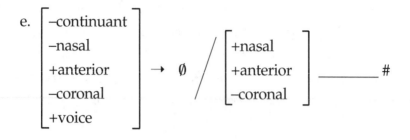

5. Identify the child substitutions of affricates and write the phonological rule:

chicken	[tɪkən]	*church*	[tərtʃ]
jam	[dæm]	*june*	[dun]
teacher	[titʃər]	*torch*	[tɔrtʃ]
child	[tald]	*fudge*	[fʌdʒ]
large	[lardʒ]	*lunch*	[lʌntʃ]

6. Identify the child substitutions of the voiceless alveolar fricatives and write the phonological rule:

sun	[tʌn]	*soup*	[tup]
save	[tev]	*sick*	[tɪk]
sock	[tɔk]	*kiss*	[kɪs]
glass	[gæs]	*basket*	[bæskət]
goose	[gus]	*see*	[ti]

7. Identify the child substitutions of fricatives and write the phonological rule:

suffer	[sʌpər]	*coffee*	[kapi]
voice	[vɔis]	*filling*	[fɪlɪŋ]
sitting	[sɪtɪŋ]	*support*	[səpɔrt]
seven	[sɛbən]	*four*	[fɔr]
lazy	[ledi]	*zipper*	[zɪpər]

8. Identify the child substitutions of voiceless stops and write the phonological rule:

supper	[sʌbər]	*pig*	[pɪg]
pickle	[pɪkl]	*pupy*	[pʌbi]
tail	[tel]	*tickle*	[tɪkl]
letter	[lɛdər]	*pecking*	[pɛgɪŋ]
coat	[kot]	*pick*	[pɪk]

Chapter 6

PHONOLOGICAL DEVELOPMENT AND DISORDERED PHONOLOGY

The previous chapters of this book have been concerned with the elements of phonological description and analysis and their relevance to the clinical population. At the same time, some aspects of normal phonological development in children were discussed. In this chapter, first the acquisition of phonology will be dealt with in greater detail and a more systematic account of it will be given. Following this, children's incorrect productions will be examined. Finally, the similarities and differences between normal and disordered phonological development will be looked at.

The topic of phonological acquisition is crucial to practitioners of language pathology and special education, as a disorder can only be defined if knowledge about normal development is provided. What follows is a description of the stages of phonological development and its relevance to clinical phonology.

PRELINGUISTIC STAGE (1 MONTH–1 YEAR)

The prelinguistic stage normally lasts through the first year of life. The label prelinguistic (sometimes preverbal or prelexical) denotes the fact that the child's vocalizations lack stable sound-meaning relationships. Sound production during this 1-year period is best described by Oller (1980) in terms of the following five stages.

Phonation Stage (Birth–1 Month)

This stage is characterized by reflexive vocalizations (crying, burping, etc.). There are, however, some nonreflexive vocalizations termed quasi-resonant nuclei (hereafter QRN) sound like syllabic nasals or nasalized vowels.

Goo Stage (2 Months–3 Months)

This stage is characterized by the addition of back (velarlike) sounds to QRN to form some kind of CV sequences. However, Oller (1980) is quick to point out that the timing of these syllables is irregular and not adultlike.

Expansion Stage (4 Months–6 Months)

This is often described as a period of vocal play. We see the addition of productions that are called fully resonant nuclei (vowel-like elements), raspberries (labial trills), squeals (high-pitched sounds), growls (low-pitched creaky sounds), and yells. Toward the end of this period, the child produces marginal babbling which consists of consonant closures alternating with fully resonant nuclei. Similar to the Goo stage, however, the timing of these sequences is slower and not adultlike (Oller, 1980). Kent (1984) relates the changes at this stage to the changes in the vocal tract anatomy of the child, which include the disengagement of the larynx and nasopharynx and the descent of the larynx.

Canonical Babbling Stage (7 Months–9 Months)

This stage is characterized by a change in the timing of CV sequences that approximates adult speech. The babbling and reduplicated babbling (e.g., dada) with mature timing leads many parents to believe that their children are uttering real words. In terms of sound classes, stops, nasals, glides, and lax vowels are most common. There is also a shift in the place of articulation of the consonants; a sharp decline in velars is accompanied by an increase in labials and especially in alveolars (Smith & Oller 1981).

Variegated Babbling Stage (10 Months–1 Year)

The last period of the prelinguistic stage is characterized by variegated babbling (combination of nonreduplicated syllables) and a wider variety of consonants and vowels. Children also produce long strings of syllables with different stress and intonation. However these productions, called gibberish, do not contain any real words in them.

Several studies have looked at cross-linguistic patterns of early babbling and found tendencies independent of the particular language to which children are exposed. Locke (1983) examined several studies conducted on different languages and found that 90 percent of the sounds produced by children aged 11–12 months can be summed up in stops [p], [b], [t], [d], [k], [g], nasals [m], [n], glides [w], [j] and [h], and the fricative [s]. Vihman (1992) revealed similarities in babbling among infants acquiring French, English, Japanese, and Swedish. However, there are also some studies that have suggested that there are language-specific differences in babbling beginning as early as 10 months (Boysson-Bardies & Vihman, 1991; Boysson-Bardies et al., 1992).

FROM PRELINGUISTIC PRODUCTION TO THE FIRST WORDS

The transition from babbling to meaningful speech has been described in a maximally opposing fashion by two well-known views in literature. Brown (1958) advanced the babbling drift view, which claims that the prelinguistic vocalizations that are similar to adult utterances are reinforced by the caretaker of the child, and these productions gradually conform to the language being learned. The opposing view, called the discontinuity view (Jakobson, 1968), claims that there is no relationship between babbling and meaningful speech. Babbling is characterized by an incredible variety of sounds that are found in all languages, whereas meaningful speech shows a remarkable loss of ability to produce many of these sounds. Jakobson argued that there is an actual silent period between the prelinguistic and linguistic periods.

Recent research supports neither of these two views. Contrary to the patterns that are expected by the babbling drift view, children from different language backgrounds do not differ in their productions at the end of their first year. Also, contrary to Jakobson's discontinuity view, there does not seem to be a clear break, or a silent period, between babbling and meaningful speech. Rather, there are similarities found between patterns of babbling and of meaningful speech (Stoel-Gammon & Cooper, 1981; Vihman et al., 1981).

The end of the first year generally is marked by the increase in frequency of babbling and the beginning of the first real words. Apart from these, however, another type of production, called vocables or proto words, may complicate the picture. Vocables are productions with some phonetic and semantic consistency and, thus, are different from babbling. What sets them apart from real words, however, is that, although vocables have phonetic and semantic consistency, they do not have any relationship with the adult target words. Thus, these three types of productions—babbling, vocables, and real words—may overlap at the end of the first year.

1 YEAR TO 1 YEAR 6 MONTHS

The first 50 word period, which corresponds approximately to age 1 year–1 year, 6 months is recognized by many as a distinct stage in phonological development because it has characteristics that are different from the earlier prelinguistic stage (birth–1 year) and the following stage of phonemic development (1 year 6 months–4 years). Although there may be some differences among scholars as to how to define this period, it is generally considered presystematic, that is, it lacks sound contrasts and/or consistent rules or processes, and it has great phonetic variability. Children appear to produce whole words rather than dividing words into their phonemes. As documented by Ferguson and Farwell (1975), during the early word productions, children produce different sounds phonetically but their contrastive use is lacking. For example, we might hear [ba] and [da] and conclude that the child has mastered the phonemic contrast between /b/ and /d/. However, further observation may reveal that this child is using the two phones interchangeably when referring to the same object, for example [ba] and [da] for *daddy*.

Phonologically, the first words are characterized by simple syllable structures, typically CV and VC, but also CVC. Some children show a great deal of syllable reduplication in CVCV. The repertoire of sound segments is relatively limited, consisting primarily of the stops, nasals, and glides that dominated the late babbling period. In terms of place of articulation, labials and alveolars seem to be much more common than palatals and velars. The preferred vowels seem to be concentrated on the basic vowel triangle of [i], [a], and [u].

A second characteristic of this period that also emphasizes the importance of particular words is the existence of **progressive idioms** (Ferguson & Farwell, 1975; Moskowitz, 1971). In these, we find a word that is produced with phonetic accuracy and is different from the other words produced by the child. Therefore, the production in question shows a more advanced form than the child's other words. The best known example of a progressive idiom is Hildegard's (Leopold, 1939) correct production of *pretty* at 10 months. At this point in development, Hildegard did not have any other production with [pr] cluster, and targets with such clusters were not realized correctly. That this correct production was more advanced than the child's stage was proven by her later productions of [pɪti] and then [bɪdi] for *pretty*.

Another commonly cited aspect of this early development is the existence of phonological **selectivity** or **avoidance** patterns. As several researchers (Drachman, 1973; Ferguson & Farwell, 1975; Kiparsky & Menn, 1977; Schwartz & Leonard, 1982; Macken & Ferguson, 1983; Shibomoto & Olmsted, 1978; Vihman, 1981) have stressed, children appear to be selective in the adult words they attempt during this period. Selection is based on the words' phonological characteristics. As early as 1927, Holmes described his daughter Mollie's avoidance of difficult sounds. Velten (1943) described her daughter Joan's avoidance of final voiced stops. Waterson (1971, 1978) reported selectivity in terms of the length of target words. Ingram (1978) described the avoidance of initial fricatives, whereas Ingram (1979) focused on avoidance of consonant clusters. Avoidance of words with particular phonemes was noted by many other researchers in the literature of phonological development. Evidence for this behavior also comes from languages other than English (Itkonen, 1977, Finnish; Macken, 1979, Spanish; Vihman, 1981, Estonian). Thus, the patterns of selection and avoidance appear to be regulated by particular phonemes, consonant clusters, or the length of target words.

Schwartz and Leonard (1982) studied selection/avoidance patterns and found that children tended to select words with sounds and syllable shapes they could produce, forming a group of **in-phonology** words, and avoid words with sounds and structures that are outside their repertoire, **out-phonology** words.

It should be kept in mind that what we have discussed thus far should be treated as tendencies rather than absolute patterns for all children. As is obvious from the selection/avoidance patterns, different children base their preferences on different targets. Also, the presystematicity and variability in production may be different from child to child. In this respect, it is worth pointing out that in at least some late talkers—children who go through the first 50 words period after age 1 year 4 months—phonetic variability is much less common. This suggests that variability might be related to age rather than to the linguistic period of first 50 words (French 1989; Yavas 1995).

SYSTEMATIC DEVELOPMENT

Following the 50 word stage, which is characterized by presystematicity and variability, the child enters the next stage in development with a rapid growth in vocabulary. During this growth in vocabulary, the child's productions become less variable and a more consistent relationship of these phonetic forms can be established with the adult targets. When the child has more vocabulary to deal with, she or he is forced to develop a rule-governed system based on phonemes, as the word-by-word approach becomes nonviable. By age 4 years, the child forms a phonological system in which most phonemes are established.

Phonemic Development (1 year 6 Months–4 Years)

The order of acquisition of phonemes and age norms in development have been the subject of many studies as they pertain to the area of clinical phonology. Speech-language pathologists would like to know the order of normal acquisition so that they can detect phonological disorders and plan therapy. Generally, large group studies have focused on the articulatory correctness of sounds. Investigators usually test the consonantal phonemes and report the percentage of children that produce the adult target sounds accurately at a specific age. As seen in the Tables 6–1 and 6–2, the order of acquisition of sounds demonstrates the same pattern over and over again: stops, nasals, and glides are mastered earlier and are followed by liquids, fricatives, and affricates.

Although there are remarkable similarities in the order of acquisition of sounds among these studies, differences in terms of the age norms are also observed. This lack of agreement among the studies is partly due to the criteria used to define acquired. Some studies (Templin, 1957; Prather

Table 6–1. Age of customary mastery of consonantal phonemes.[a]

Age	Phoneme
3;0	p, m, n, ŋ, f, w, h
3;6[b]	j
4;0	b, k, g, r̩, d
4;6	s, ʃ, tʃ
5;0	
6;0	t, l, θ, v
7;0	ð, z, ʒ, dʒ

Source: From *Normal and Disordered Phonology in Children* (p. 30), by C. Stoel-Gammon and C. Dunn, 1985, Austin, TX: Pro-Ed. Reprinted by permission.

[a]A phoneme is "mastered" when produced correctly by 75% of the subjects.

[b]The phonemes are listed cumulatively by age; only newly mastered phoneme are shown for each age.

Table 6–2. Age of customary production and mastery of consonantal phonemes.

Age	Consonants Customarily Produced	Consonants Mastered
Before 2;0	p,b, m, n, w, h[a]	
2;0[b]	t, d, k, g, ŋ	
3;0	f, s,r, l, j	p, m, n, w, h
4;0	v, z, ʃ, tʃ, dʒ	b, d, k, g, f, j
5;0	θ, ð	
6;0	ʒ[c]	t, ŋ, r, l
7;0		θ, ʃ, tʃ, dʒ
8;0		v, ð, s, z

Source: From *Normal and Disordered Phonology in Children* (p. 31), by C. Stoel-Gammon and C. Dunn, 1985, Austin, TX: Pro-Ed. Reprinted by permission.

[a]These consonants exceeded 70% correct production at 2;0, the youngest level tested.

[b]The phonemes are listed cumulatively; only new phonemes are shown for each age.

[c]This consonant was not "mastered" by 8;0 and thus does not appear in the right-hand column.

et al., 1975) considered a sound as acquired when it is produced correctly by 75% of the subjects at any age level. On the other hand, Poole (1934) required 100% as the criterion.

Another reason for the differences observed is the word positions considered. For example, Templin (1957) required accuracy in all three word positions (initial, medial, and final), whereas Prather et al. (1975) looked at only initial and final positions.

Yet another reason for the divergences comes from the fact that different researchers require different degrees of phonetic accuracy of the production. As mentioned by Ingram (1978), /s/ provides a good example: If strict criterion for phonetic accuracy were applied, /s/ would be considered a late acquisition, as children take some time for a fully accurate production of this phoneme. On the other hand, children reveal their awareness of this phoneme rather early despite their difficulties in its phonetic implementation. Thus, it might be considered an early acquisition if we disregard the imperfections in the productions. This is in accordance with Moskowitz' (1975) suggestion that phonemic acquisition is ahead of phonetic acquisition for fricatives. That is, children are aware of the meaning contrasts before they produce them accurately.

The variables that may contribute to the lack of agreement among studies are not exhausted in the above discussion. The types of utterances used in testing—isolated words, connected speech, length of words, stress patterns, word familiarity, number of words tested for each word position, the effects of sounds in words such as consonant harmony, and conditions of data collection—are all potentially influential factors in the resulting generalizations.

Although general tendencies in the order of acquisition of sound classes are mentioned, it is worth noting that there seem to be differences due to the position of the sound in the word. For example, it has been suggested (Edwards, 1979; Ferguson, 1975) that the acquisition of stops is favored in the initial position, whereas, for the fricatives, final position seems to be the most favorable environment. Yavas (1988) brought supporting evidence for both of these observations from Brazilian Portuguese. However, Stoel-Gammon (1984) did not find any evidence supporting the final position for earlier fricative acquisition. What does seem to hold is that prevocalic position is favored by voiced sounds and final position is favored by voiceless sounds.

In connection with this, it should be pointed out that a four-way word position distinction, in place of the traditional three-way (initial, medial, and final position) distinction, may be more appropriate. Grunwell (1981, 1985) suggested that the traditional medial position should be divided into two: syllable final within word and syllable initial within word. She argued that this separation is justified, as data from normally developing and phonologically disordered children reveal different tendencies for the same phoneme in these two positions. Yavas (1988) found supporting evidence for this from data on the acquisition of Portuguese: A significant number of children showed acquisition of /r/ in Brazilian Portuguese in syllable initial within word position long before they acquired the same sound in syllable final within word position. Had the data been analyzed only in terms of medial position, this significant difference would not have been revealed. This example is instructive, as it comes from a basically open-syllable language.[1] In a language with more syllable final consonants, the distinction between syllable final within word and syllable initial within word could be much more significant.

Consonant Clusters

The combination of two or more consonants in initial or final position is generally a late development in the phonological system. It has been noted (Templin, 1957) that certain clusters develop earlier than others.

As seen in Table 6–3, /s + nasal/, /s + stop/, and /stop + liquid or glide/ clusters are acquired earlier in the initial position. The final position generally favors the combinations of /nasal or liquid + voiceless stop/ and /stop + stop/ or /stop + fricative/. In general, two-member clusters are acquired earlier than three-member clusters. Beyond these, however, the extremely rich variety of clusters in English makes any attempt to generalize the order of acquisition in terms of sound classes rather difficult.

Finally, mention should be made of vowels. Historically, vowel development has been the step-child of the field of phonological development. Very few studies have concentrated on vowel development and they suggested that children acquire the system accurately by 3 to 4 years of age (Templin, 1957). As for the relative order of vowel acquisition, diary studies have given some partial answers. Wellman et al. (1931) found that /i, a, u, o, ʌ, and ə/ were acquired by 2 years. To these, /ɛ/ and /ɔ/ were added by 3 years of age. /ɪ, e, æ, ʊ/ were acquired by 4 years. The r-colored vowels were acquired later. With some discrepancies, especially for /æ, ɛ, and ɪ/, the above order was supported by Hare (1983) and Paschal (1983). Also, Stoel-Gammon (1985) and Dyson (1988) found that r-colored schwa /ɚ/ was present in many of their subjects by 2 years of age. Here, again, different criteria used in different studies could explain the divergences.

Table 6–3. Age of mastery of consonantal clusters.

Age	Initial Clusters	Final Clusters
4;0	pl, bl, kl, gl	mp, mpt, mps, ŋk
	pr, br, tr, dr, kr	lp, lt, rm, rt, rk
	tw, kw	pt, ks
	sm, sn, sp, st, sk	ft
5;0[b]	gr, fl, fr, str	lb, lf
		rd, rf, rn
6;0	skw	lk
		rb, rg, rθ, rdʒ, rst, rtʃ
		nt, nd, nθ
7;0	spl, spr, skr	sk, st, kst
	sl, sw	lθ, lz
	ʃr, θr	dʒd
8;0		kt, sp

Source: From *Normal and Disordered Phonology in Children* (p. 33), by C. Stoel-Gammon and C. Dunn, 1985, Austin, TX: Pro-Ed. Reprinted by permission.

[a]A cluster is "mastered" when produced correctly by 75% of the subjects.

[b]The clusters are listed cumulatively; only newly mastered clusters are listed for each age.

PATTERNS OF ERRONEOUS PRODUCTIONS

When the productions of children's speech are analyzed, clear systematic patterns are found in their erroneous approximations to adult target words. The errors are quite similar across children and across languages, suggesting that all children develop similar organization patterns of their phonologies. One of the most common ways of describing these error patterns in children has been with reference to phonological processes.

Process analysis is probably the simplest and most economical way of describing the differences between the adult targets and the realization of these targets by children. The phonological processes that are used here are not the same processes that were dealt with in Chapter 5 in relation to generative phonology. Rather, as described by Stampe (1969, 1973) and Donegan and Stampe (1979), they are innate simplification tendencies. According to this model, known as Natural Phonology, humans are born with an innate system of natural phonological processes such as consonant cluster simplification and stopping of fricatives. These processes reflect natural restrictions in the human speech capacity and result in systematic simplifications of adult forms by children. Stampe described processes as mental operations that are gradually suppressed or limited as children acquire the phonological system. Several researchers disagree with Stampe and do not attribute psychological reality or explanatory power to processes (Grunwell, 1985; Ingram, 1981; Stoel-Gammon & Dunn, 1985). The general consensus is that processes provide a good descriptive device for the relationship between the adult targets and the children's erroneous production of them. This book follows suit and treats processes as a mere descriptive apparatus.

It is generally agreed that children's simplification patterns fall into the following three groups: (1) syllable structure processes, which modify the syllabic structure of the adult target word, (2) substitution processes that replace one class of sounds for another, and (3) assimilation processes in which one sound becomes more similar to another.

Syllable Structure Processes

Unstressed/Weak Syllable Deletion

This refers to the child's deletion of unstressed syllable(s) of a multisyllabic word. The rationale for this process is that stressed syllables are more perceptible and unstressed syllables are prone to deletion in trisyllabic and longer words:

banana	[nænə]	*potato*	[tedo]
telephone	[tɛfon]	*tomato*	[mado]

In these examples, pretonic syllables (unstressed syllables occurring before the stressed syllable) are omitted. Post-tonic syllables (unstressed syllables occurring after the stressed syllable) can be deleted too:

elephant   [ɛfənt]

Examples of unstressed syllable deletion are widely available from other languages:

Turkish :	[ɨspanak]	"spinach"	→	[panak]
Portuguese:	[edʒifisju]	"building"	→	[fisju]
Spanish :	[eskoβa]	"broom"	→	[kowa]

Final Consonant Deletion

This process refers to the deletion of word-final consonants or consonant clusters in the adult target. Because the most basic syllable type is, universally, CV (see Chapter 7 for more on this), children tend to delete final consonants that require more articulatory control than open articulations such as vowels:

kid	[kɪ]	*dog*	[da]
desk	[dɛ]	*milk*	[mɪ]

Examples from other languages abound:

Spanish:	*arbol*	[aɾbol]	"tree"	→	[abo]
Turkish:	*otur*	[otur]	"sit"	→	[otu]
Portuguese:		[lapis]	"pencil"	→	[lapi]

Reduplication

Reduplication refers to the complete repetition of one of the adult target syllables in a word. It is a way of maintaining the number of syllables in the target word while avoiding more difficult combinations:

bottle	[baba]	*dog*	[dada]
cat	[kaka]	*water*	[wawa]

Reduction of Consonant Clusters

This is the simplification of the consonant cluster by deleting one of its members. This is done to avoid the difficulty of putting two consonants in a row in the same syllable, and it results in a preferred CV syllable type. Typically, the member that is deleted is the one that is thought to be more difficult to produce in that it generally belongs to one of the later acquired sounds:

1. stop + approximant, or fricative (other than /s/) + approximant: Typically, the approximant is deleted and the stop or fricative is retained:

blue	[bu]	*bread*	[bɛd]
free	[fi]	*play*	[pe]

2. /s/ + stop or nasal: Typically, /s/ is deleted and the stop or the nasal is retained:

stop   [tap]   *snail*   [nel]

3. /s/ + approximant: Here, either reduction is possible. Sometimes, /s/ is deleted and the approximant is retained and other examples show retention of /s/ and deletion of the approximant:

slip   [lɪp]   or   [sɪp]

Sometimes, we observe a production which is the result of a feature combination coming from two sounds. For example, the word *swim* is realized as [fɪm] in which /f/ is a representative of the fricative of /s/ and the labial of /w/.

In the case of three-member clusters that have the combination of /s/ + stop + approximant, the typical reduction pattern is the elimination of /s/ and the approximant and the retention of the stop:

street   [tit]   *splash*   [pæʃ]

Occasionally, instead of the elimination of one member, an epenthetic vowel is inserted to break up the unmanageable cluster. The vowel is almost always a [ə]:

blue   [bəlu]   *play*   [pəle]

The reduction of consonant clusters is a very common process in all languages that permit such sequences:

Spanish: [krus]   "cross"   →   [kus]
Portuguese: [bruʃa]   "witch"   →   [buʃa]
German: [ʃpigəl] "mirror" →   [pigəl]

Literature is also available on Norwegian (Vanvik 1971), French and German (Lewis, 1936), Slovenian (Kolarič, 1959), and Czech (Pačesova, 1968).

Substitution Processes

Substitution processes relate the child's utterances to adult targets in which a class of phonemes is replaced by another class of phonemes. In this group of changes, we find the following processes.

Stopping

Stopping is the use of a stop sound in place of a fricative or an affricate target. The rationale for this process refers to the complexity of the fricative target in which a relatively long period of narrowed approximation of the articulators demanding great muscular control is required. As opposed to this, stops involve very straightforward contact of the articulators:

van	[bæn]	*that*	[dæt]
sun	[tʌn]	*jam*	[dam]

Stopping is another very common process cross-linguistically:

Spanish:	[sopa]	"soup"	→	[topa]
Portuguese:	[sapu]	"frog"	→	[tapu]
Turkish:	[sen]	"you"	→	[ten]

Also cited are Hindi (Srivastava, 1974), Slovenian (Kolarič, 1959), Czech (Pačesova, 1968), Mandarin (Chao, 1951), Norwegian (Vanvik, 1971), and Estonian (Vihman, 1971).

Fronting

Fronting refers to a process whereby palatal or velar sounds are replaced by alveolar or dental sounds. The apex (tip) of the tongue has greater mobility and is considered the easiest to control of all active articulators. Thus, dental/alveolar articulations are more frequent (see Chapter 7 for more on this). Articulations that demand the involvement of more posterior parts of the tongue are avoided by this process.

fish	[fɪs]	*key*	[ti]
shoe	[su]	*go*	[do]

Following are some examples of palatal[2] and velar fronting cross-linguistically:

Spanish:	[tʃikle]	"chewing gum"	→	[sikle]
Portuguese:	[ʃapew]	"hat"	→	[sapew]
Turkish:	[ʃu]	"that"	→	[su]

This process is also noted in German (Mohring, 1938), Hindi (Srivastava, 1974), Czech (Pačesova, 1968), Arabic (Omar, 1973), Estonian (Vihman 1976), and French (Lewis, 1936).

Liquid Gliding

This term refers to the replacement of target liquids by glides. This process involves a change from a consonant production to a more vowel-like production. Because glides have a greater degree of opening of the articulators, they require less articulatory control.

carrot	[kæwət]	*rabbit*	[wæbɪt]
look	[wʊk]	*line*	[jajn]

In English, /r/ is generally replaced by [w], whereas /l/ is replaced by either [w] or [j], depending on the following vowel. The replacements of these targets, especially the /r/, may be different in different languages. As the following examples show, /r/ is replaced either by [j] or [l]:

Spanish:	[paɾeð]	"wall"	→	[pale]
Portuguese:	[amaɾɛla]	"yellow"	→	[amajɛja]
Turkish:	[para]	"money"	→	[pala] or [paja]

This common process is also cited for Mandarin (Chao, 1951), Estonian (Vihman, 1971), French (Lewis, 1976), Czech (Pačesova, 1968), and Taiwanese (Linn, 1971).

Vocalization

Another process liquids undergo in final position is vocalization. In this case, the target liquid is produced as a vowel. This process also presents a case in which the result is more in line with the preferred CV syllable structure:

bawl	[bau]	*zipper*	[zɪpu]
table	[tebo]	*belt*	[bɛwt]

Assimilation Processes

The substitution processes observed in the previous section describe replacement of one phoneme by another one in a context-free fashion. For example, fricatives become stops in all instances, regardless of both the word position and other sounds that exist in that particular word. Assimilation processes are sound changes in which one sound becomes more like another sound in a specific context. In other words, the change is provoked by a preceding or a following sound. Following are the most commonly cited assimilatory patterns in the literature.

Consonant Harmony

This term refers to a noncontiguous assimilation process whereby one consonant becomes like another in terms of place or manner of articulation. The motive here is to favor the same or similar articulations in consonant productions. The assimilation can be progressive or regressive:

1. labial assimilation: child's use of a labial sound for a nonlabial (alveolar, velar) target due to a preceding or following labial consonant in the word:

       top   [pap] (regressive)   *boot*   [bup] (progressive)

2. alveolar assimilation: child' use of an alveolar sound for a nonalveolar (labial, velar) target due to a preceding or following alveolar consonant in the word:

       gate   [det] (regressive)   *dog*   [dɔd] (progressive)

3. velar assimilation: child's use of a velar sound for a nonvelar (labial, alveolar) target due to a preceding or following velar consonant in the word:

       dog   [gɔg] (regressive)   *coat*   [kok] (progressive)

Consonant harmony is also a very common process cross-linguistically. Vihman (1978) provides the best account to date. She compared the data from 13 children learning Chinese, Estonian, English, Czech, Slovenian, and Spanish and found that the majority (about two thirds) of assimilations were regressive. She also found that assimilations of place were much more common (45%) than manner (20%). (See Chapter 10 for more on this.)

Final Devoicing

The process whereby a child produces the voiceless counterpart of the target voiced obstruent in final position is termed final devoicing. As mentioned in Chapter 5, this can be considered an assimilation to voicelessness which occurs at the end of the word:

knob	[nap]	*bag*	[bæk]
bad	[bat]	*nose*	[nos]

Prevocalic Voicing

Prevocalic voicing is a process whereby the child produces a voiced obstruent in place of a voiceless target before a vowel. The voicing of the vowel influences the preceding consonant, and the adjacent sounds become more similar (same voicing):

toe	[do]	*pea*	[bi]
table	[debu]	*pie*	[ba]

Co-occurrence of Processes

The examples we have cited for the phonological processes mentioned above show only one process per word and do not necessarily represent the majority of utterances by children. Often children's productions contain more than one process, as exemplified in the following:

speak	[bi]	Consonant cluster reduction, Final consonant deletion, Prevocalic voicing.
sock	[gɔk]	Stopping, Velar assimilation, Prevocalic voicing.
cherry	[dɛwi]	Fronting, Stopping, Prevocalic voicing, Liquid gliding.

When the words have more than one simplification process, there might be cases in which we have to assume a particular ordering of the processes is in effect. For example, if the target *sick* is produced as [kɪ], it can be concluded that the child has applied the processes of stopping, velar assimilation, and final consonant deletion. The application of stopping and velar assimilation must come before the deletion of the final consonant, because the deletion of the final consonant would remove the necessary agent for velar assimilation. Also, only stops as obstruents are allowed in velar place of articulation. Thus, the following derivation is suggested:

Underlying form	/sɪk/
Stopping	tɪk
Velar assimilation	kɪk
Deletion of final consonant	kɪ
Phonetic representation	[kɪ]

In other instances, multiple processes may not be in a dependency relationship. For example, one of the common realizations of the word *black* is [bæ]. This shows the processes of consonant cluster reduction and final consonant deletion. However, these two processes do not need to apply in a specific order, as either order would account for the child's production.

Chronology of Processes

The simplification processes described above do not disappear in child speech at the same time. Different processes have varying permanence in developing phonologies. Although there are not many studies focusing on age norms, two investigations are worth mentioning. Stoel-Gammon and Dunn (1985) divided processes into two categories and give the following picture:

Processes Disappearing by 3 yrs	*Processes Persisting after 3 yrs*
Unstressed Syllable Deletion	Cluster Reduction
Final Consonant Deletion	Epenthesis
Velar Fronting	Gliding
Consonant Harmony	Vocalization
Reduplication	Stopping
Prevocalic Voicing	Depalatalization
	Final Devoicing

Another look at the chronology of processes is offered by Grunwell (1987), and is depicted in Table 6–4. In Table 6–4, the solid black line across an age band indicates that almost all children at this age will demonstrate use of the process. A broken line indicates that, at that age, an appreciable number of children will not be using the process or will be using it variably.

As might be observed, the two accounts, while differing in details, share many things. Stoel-Gammon and Dunn (1985) separate the two types of fronting, velar fronting and palatal fronting (depalatalization), whereas Grunwell (1987) differentiates between types of cluster reduction and stopping for individual fricatives and affricates. Additionally, there is a great deal of overlap in terms of the age at which a particular process disappears.

Bankson and Bernthal (1990), reporting on the processes most frequently found in a sample of 1,000 children between ages 3 and 9 years, place liquid gliding, stopping, cluster reduction, vocalization, and final conso-

Table 6–4. Chronology of phonological processes.

	2;0–2;6	2;6–3;0	3;0–3;6	3;6–4;0	4;0–4;6	4;6–5;0	5;0 →
Weak Syllable Detection							
Final Consonant Detection							
Reduplication							
Consonant Harmony							
Cluster Reduction (Initial) obstruent + approximant							
/s/ + consonant							
Stopping							
/f/							
/v/							
/θ/		/θ/ → [f]					
/ð/			/ð/ → [d] or [v]				
/s/							
/z/							
/ʃ/		Fronting "[s] type"					
/tʃ, dʒ/		Fronting [ts, dz]					
Fronting /k, g, ŋ/							
Gliding r/ → [w]							
Context-Sensitive Voicing							

Source: From *Clinical Phonology* (p. 229), by P. Grunwell, 1987 (2nd Edition). Batimore: Williams & Wilkins. Reprinted by permission.

nant deletion among the processes that persist longest in children's speech. Khan and Lewis (1986) reported similar results with an addition of velar fronting to this list.

The lists above characterize the situation in the development of English. However, as mentioned earlier during the discussion of the processes, these patterns are also observed in many other languages. There is not much information on the chronology of processes in different languages; however, the chronology provided for Portuguese by Yavas and Lamprecht (1988) and shown in Table 6–5, reveal certain similarities to the patterns found in English.

Although there are some language specific processes here, what concerns us are the processes that are shared by languages and the age at which they disappear. Cluster reduction is a late process in Portuguese, too, whereas processes such as assimilation, consonant harmony, and context sensitive voicing are early processes. Probably the most striking difference

Table 6–5. Chronology of phonological processes in normal development of Portugese.

	1;6–2;0	2;0–2;6	2;6–3;0	3;0–3;6	3;6–4;0	4;0–4;6	4;6–5;0
CC reduction							
Weak syllable del.							
Final fric. del.							
Final liq. del.							
Intervoc. liq. del.							
Initial liq. del.							
Obst. devoicing							
Fronting							
Liq. subst.							
Liq. gliding							
Stopping							
Assimilation							
Intervoc. voic.							

Source: From "Process and Intelligibility in Disordered Phonology," by M. Yavas and R. Lamprecht, 1988. *Clinical Linguistics and Phonetics*, 2(4), p. 334. Reprinted by permission.

A straight line indicates the ages during which the process is operative in the speech of the majority of the children. A broken line indicates the oldest age at which the process occurs.

observed between the English and the Portuguese data regards stopping. Whereas this process is classified as a late process in English, the Portuguese data reveal that it disappears quite early. This difference between the two languages is probably due to the fact that Portuguese does not have the two late acquired fricatives /θ/ and /ð/. If we exclude these two fricatives from the English data, the difference between the two languages, as can be computed from Grunwell's table, is not all that striking.

In closing this section, it should be remembered that these chronological accounts are merely broad generalizations, and many children show different patterns. There are also some patterns that are language specific, and the generalizations may apply in a different sequence. Substitutes for the targets /l/ and /r/ illustrate this point well. While English-speaking children reveal errors such as /r/ → [w] and /l/ → [w] or [j], the situation is different in Italian; /r/ is substituted by [l] or [n], and /l/ is substituted by [r] or [n] (Bortolini and Leonard, 1991). In Swedish, we see the substitutions /r/ → [h], and /l/ → [j] (Nettelbladt, 1983). Analyzing all of the above, Leonard (1995) gives a phonological explanation for each on the basis of the sensitivity to patterns of ambient languages. More specifically, the explanation for Italian stresses the very limited occurrences of /w/ and /j/ and the alveolar nature of the targets /l/ and /r/. Thus, the substitute is either the other alveolar liquid or another alveolar sound, /n/, which shares many of the same features. The unusual-looking glottal /h/ substitution in Swedish is accounted for by reference to /r/ which is uvular in this Southern Swedish dialect. Thus, what might appear as a highly unusual substitution may have a well-grounded explanation when the specific ambient language patterns and the nature of sounds are considered.

COMPLETION OF THE PHONETIC INVENTORY

During the previous stage, most basic phonological patterns are established, but the child's phonological system is far from being completed. A number of things still remain to be developed. During the stage between ages 4 and 7 years, certain contrasts such as fricatives and affricates are stabilized. At the end of this period, the child is capable of producing all of the English sounds. However, the child still has difficulty with longer words such as *thermometer* and *vegetable*, and they may not match adult targets. Morphophonemic development also begins in some structures. For example, /s/ and /z/ (not [əz]) for the plural morpheme are developed (Berko, 1958).

MORPHOPHONEMIC DEVELOPMENT

The final stage of phonological development relates to the acquisition of a system of rules for the combination of morphemes. In addition to completing the plural rule, there is evidence that vowel alternations, such as *sane - sanity* ([e] - [æ]), *succeed - success* ([i] - [ɛ]), *decide - decision* ([aj] - [ɪ]), *tone - tonic* ([o] - [a]), and *numeral - number* ([u] - [ʌ]), are productively used by older children. Also acquired are stress alterations regarding the compounds and phrases such as *hot dog* and *hot-dog*, *Redskin* and *red skin*, and the noun and verb pairs such as *an import* and *to import*, *an insult* and *to insult*.

CLINICAL RELEVANCE

Assessment

Phonological development has great relevance for the clinical population. To determine whether a child is phonologically disordered and needs professional help, we need a good understanding of normal phonological development. Among the stages of development we have reviewed above, the period of phonemic development that roughly corresponds to 1 year 6 months through 4 years is the most relevant, as this is the period in which the child establishes the basics of the system. At the end of this period, the child is expected to suppress most of the simplifying processes. Thus, by the time a child is 3 years 6 months to 4 years old, one can, with reasonable confidence determine whether any intervention is required.

Error patterns of segmental productions of children with phonological disorders are generally described in terms of distinctive features or phonological processes. The procedures and clinical applications of distinctive features were discussed in Chapter 4. In the following, the application of phonological processes to disordered data will be considered. The literature is quite rich on processes, and their impact is very significant in the investigation of disordered child phonology. In addition to numerous applications in several case studies of children with disordered phonology that have appeared in professional journals and textbooks, several assessment procedures are based on phonological process analysis. These are *Compton-Hutton Phonological Assessment* (Compton & Hutton, 1978), *Phonological Process Analysis* (Weiner, 1979), *Natural Process Analysis* (Shriberg & Kwiatkowski, 1980), *The Assessment of Phonological Processes* (Hodson, 1986), *Procedures for the Phonological Analysis of Chil-*

dren's Language (Ingram, 1981), *Phonological Assessment of Child Speech* (Grunwell, 1985), *Khan-Lewis Phonological Analysis* (Khan & Lewis, 1986), *Assessment Link Between Phonology and Articulation* (Lowe, 1986), and *Bankson-Bernthal Test of Phonology* (Bankson & Bernthal, 1990).

The number of processes used in these assessment procedures is vastly different. While Hodson (1986) has 40 processes, Weiner uses 16, and Shriberg and Kwiatkowski (1980) use only 8. This is due to the fact that some procedures separate the processes in greater detail while others treat them more generally. Another factor contributing to the discrepancy of the number of processes is the limitation of the definition of processes to natural phonological processes. Shriberg and Kwiatkowski(1980), for example, include only processes that are attested to in some phonological phenomenon other than normal phonological acquisition. Among these phenomena are historical changes, dialect variations, and slips of tongue.

Sample Process Analysis

In the following, the basic principles of process analysis will be shown by looking at the data from M that were examined earlier for distinctive features. This analysis does not necessarily follow the exact steps of any commercial manual; rather, the objective is to demonstrate general procedures for process analysis.

It was pointed out that, in this framework, the child is viewed as attempting to produce all targets of the ambient language, but, due to limited motor, cognitive, and linguistic capabilities, his or her productions show many simplifications of the adult models. Thus, the processes that describe the child's renditions reveal the errors relative to the adult productions.

A corollary of this is the view that the child's underlying representation is the same as the adult phonemic form, and the processes are explanations for the erroneous productions. As mentioned earlier, this is a very controversial presupposition and has been questioned by many scholars. Without going into a discussion of this issue, the following focuses on the procedures used in process analysis.

The first task is to go through the child's productions and identify the simplifications in the form of substitutions, omissions, or additions for each target item. This will be done with M's data, which were looked at earlier in Chapter 4:

1. brush   [bwʌs]   (r → w = LG), (ʃ → s = PF)

2. that   [dæt]   (ð → d = St.)

3. pencil   [bɛndəl]   (p → b = PV), (s → d = PV & St.)

4. sugar   [dʊgar]   (ʃ → d = PF, PV, St.)

5. dog   [dɔk]   (g → k = FCD)

6. dish   [dɪs]   (ʃ → s = PF)

7. speak   [bik]   (sp → b = CR, PV)

8. scratch   [kwæt]   (sk → k = CR), (r →w = LG), (tʃ → t = PF, St.)

9. ring   [wɪŋ]   (r → w = LG)

10. chair   [dɛr]   (tʃ → d = PF, St., PV)

11. window   [wɪndo]   -

12. bridge   [bwɪt]   (r → w = LG), (dʒ → t = PF, St., FCD)

13. five   [baɪf]   (f → b = St., PV), (v → f = FCD)

14. cow   [kaʊ]   -

15. soup   [tup]   (s → t = St.)

16. sick   [dɪk]   (s → d = St., PV)

17. talk   [dɔk]   (t → d = PV)

18. shoe   [du]   (ʃ → d = PF, St., PV)

19. zoo   [du]   (z → d = St.)

20. black   [bæk]   (bl → b = CR)

21. finger   [bɪŋgər]   (f → b = St., PV)

22. trees   [dwis]   (r → w = LG) , (z → s = FCD)

23. sheep   [dip]   (ʃ → d = PF, St., PV)

24. gun   [gʌn]   -

25. chicken   [dɪkən]   (tʃ → d = PF, St., PV)

26. car   [kar]   -

27. brown   [baʊn]   (br → b = CR)

28. flag   [bæk]   (fl → b = CR, St., PV), (g → k = FCD)

29. crash   [kwæs]   (r → w = LG) , (ʃ → s = PF)

30. fish   [bɪs]   (f → b = St., PV), (ʃ → s = PF)

31. rabbit   [wæbɪt]   (r → w = LG)

32. teeth   [dit]   (t → d = PV), (θ → t = St.)

33. they   [de]   (ð → d = St.)

34. sky   [kaɪ]   (sk → k = CR)

35. neck   [nɛk]   -

36. spoon   [bun]   (sp → b = CR, PV)

37. ball   [bol]   -

38. door   [dor]   -

39. bread   [bwɛt]   (r → w = LG), (d → t = FCD)

40. red   [wɛt]   (r → w = LG), (d → t = FCD)

CR = Cluster reduction, St. = Stopping of fricatives and affricates, PF = Palatal fronting, PV = Prevocalic voicing, LG = Liquid gliding, FCD = Final Consonant devoicing.

It is important to note that, in several cases, more than one process applies to the same target word, and it is indispensable that all processes should be identified. For example, target item number 28 *flag* is realized as [bæk]. The substitution of /fl/ → [b] is a result of four processes—cluster reduction, stopping, prevocalic voicing, and final consonant devoicing: /flæg/ cluster reduction /fæg/, stopping /pæg/, prevocalic voicing /bæg/, final consonant devoicing [bæk].

Once all of the processes that the child uses for the adult targets are identified, the next step is to figure out the percentage of occurrences of each process, as these will determine the planning of treatment. To do this, the targets are examined to make an inventory of the possibilities of occurrence for each process by putting a circle in the appropriate box. Finally, the processes observed in the child's speech are marked by an X in the circles wherever the simplification process takes place. These are needed to calculate the percentages of how many times a process applies among how many possibilities. Possibilities of occurrences are determined on the basis of a particular target's structure. For example, the beginning part of the target number 1, *brush* [brʌʃ], presents the opportunities for the processes cluster reduction, in which the initial cluster /br/ may be reduced to one sound, and the liquid gliding for a possible r → w replacement. The final sound of the same target, /ʃ/ may suffer palatal fronting (/ʃ/ → [s]) and stopping to [t]. It should be conceded that there are difficulties with this analysis. The main difficulty is to consider the same target equally vulnerable for the multiple processes in the same word position. In general, one process is more dominant in a particular position. The implications of this are discussed in the tabulation of the results below:

Target	Realization	CR	PF	St.	PV	FCD	LG
1. brush	[bwʌs]	○	(x)	○			(x)
2. that	[dæt]			(x)			
3. pencil	[bɛndəl]			(x)	(x)(x)		
4. sugar	[dʊgar]		(x)	(x)	(x)		
5. dog	[dɔk]					(x)	
6. dish	[dɪs]		(x)	○			
7. speak	[bik]	(x)			(x)		
8. scratch	[kwæt]	(x)	(x)	(x)	○		(x)

Target	*Realization*	CR	PF	St.	PV	FCD	LG
9. ring	[wɪŋ]						(x)
10. chair	[dɛr]		(x)	(x)	(x)		
11. window	[wɪndo]						
12. bridge	[bwɪt]	(○)	(x)	(x)		(x)	(x)
13. five	[baɪf]			(⊗)(○)	(x)	(x)	
14. cow	[kaʊ]				(○)		
15. soup	[tup]			(x)	(○)		
16. sick	[dɪk]			(x)	(x)		
17. talk	[dɔk]				(x)		
18. shoe	[du]		(x)	(x)	(x)		
19. zoo	[du]			(x)			
20. black	[bæk]	(x)					(○)
21. finger	[bɪŋgər]			(x)	(x)		
22. trees	[dwis]	(○)		(○)	(x)	(x)	(x)
23. sheep	[dip]		(x)	(x)	(x)		
24. gun	[gʌn]						
25. chicken	[dɪkən]		(x)	(x)	(x)		
26. car	[kar]						(○)
27. brown	[baʊn]	(x)					
28. flag	[bæk]	(x)		(x)	(x)	(x)	

(continued)

(continued)

Target	Realization	CR	PF	St.	PV	FCD	LG
29. crash	[kwæs]	◯	⊗	◯	◯		⊗
30. fish	[bɪs]		⊗	⊗	⊗		
31. rabbit	[wæbɪt]						⊗
32. teeth	[dit]			⊗	⊗		
33. they	[de]				⊗		
34. sky	[kaɪ]	⊗			◯		
35. neck	[nɛk]						
36. spoon	[bun]	⊗			⊗		
37. ball	[bol]						
38. door	[dor]						◯
39. bread	[bwɛt]	◯				⊗	⊗
40. red	[wɛt]					⊗	⊗

From the above data, the following results are obtained:

Consonant cluster reduction (CR):	7/12	58 %
Palatal fronting (PF):	11/11	100 %
Stopping (St.):	18/23	78 %
Prevocalic voicing (PV):	17/22	77 %
Final consonant devoicing (FCD):	7/7	100 %
Liquid gliding:	8/10	80 %

The prevalence of each process is relevant and the percentages are needed in treatment planning. However, we should also make the following observations: Whereas the groupings above correctly label the processes in M's productions, they are not specific enough. For example, although stopping applies in 78% of the possibilities, there seems to be a significantly different application of it depending on the position of the target in the word. Whereas all of the targets in initial position were stopped (15/15, 100%), in final position out of nine possibilities of occurrence only three (examples 8, 12, 32) were stopped (less than 35%); 6 targets (examples 1, 6, 13, 22, 29, 30) were not affected by this process. In fact, if we narrow the grouping a little more and separate the fricative targets from the affricate targets, the application of this process will be reduced to one out of seven, because two of the three targets which were stopped were affricates.

Consonant cluster reduction provides another opportunity to show the need to go beyond the general grouping and narrow the categorization of the targets. As the calculations show, cluster reduction applies in 7 cases out of 12 opportunities (58%). However, if the data are examined carefully, it will be realized that the application of this process is reduced to 17% (1/6) with respect to the clusters in which the second member is /r/. While example 27 undergoes cluster reduction, examples 1, 12, 22, 29, and 39 do not. This recategorization, of course, would raise the application of cluster reduction to 7/7 (100%) for the remaining clusters. These examples show that, sometimes, narrowing the groupings for processes is the only way to reveal significant generalizations. This is similar to what was concluded in Chapter 4 regarding data analysis through distinctive features.

CHARACTERISTICS OF DISORDERED PHONOLOGY

In what ways are children with phonological disorders different from normally developing ones? Grunwell (1985, 1987) tried to account for the differences through the use of the processes. According to this view, disordered children reveal **persisting normal processes**. In other words, these children employ the same processes that are observed during the normal development, but, unlike normal development in which they disappear at certain points, these processes continue. For example, consonant harmony and prevocalic voicing are early processes that normally disappear before 3 years of age. However, a child with phonological disorders might have these processes at age 4 years or even later. Another characteristic of the disordered system, suggested by Grunwell, is **chronological mismatch**. Here, some advanced patterns, such as consonant clusters, are seen co-occurring with consonant harmony or prevocalic voicing, which are normally considered early processes.

Yet another possible pattern that is unique to children with phonological disorders is **variable use of processes** in which more than one process operates with the same type of target structures. The result is unpredictable variability in the child's productions. For example, if the child is deleting final consonants in some cases but replacing them with [ʔ] in others, this results in totally unpredictable variability.

Systematic sound preference is also among the trademarks cited for disordered phonology (Grunwell, 1985; Stoel-Gammon & Dunn, 1985; Weiner, 1981). This is in evidence when a group of sounds with the same manner of articulation is represented by one or two sounds in the child's production. Because this process involves the loss of several contrasts when the child utilizes one sound for various targets, it implies a severe disorder because intelligibility becomes highly impaired. The following exemplifies this situation in which all voiceless fricatives are realized as [t]. The substitution results in a loss of multiple contrasts:

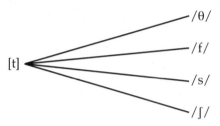

Targets such as *thin* [θɪn], *sin* [sɪn], *fin* [fɪn], and *shin* [ʃɪn] are all produced as [tɪn]. Weiner (1981) offers the following generalizations for systematic sound preference: (1) it affects a class of sounds with the same manner of articulation; (2) fricatives are affected more frequently than any other class of sounds; (3) it is limited to a single position in the word, more commonly word-initial position;[3] and (4) when only some members of a class of sounds are affected, voiceless and/or nonlabial sounds are more frequently affected.

The use of **unusual/idiosyncratic/atypical processes** is another characteristic of children with phonological disorders. Here simplifying processes that have been rarely attested in normal development are observed. Processes such as backing of alveolars (*pat* → [pæk]), gliding of fricatives (*fig* → [wɪg]), glottal insertion (*ladder* → [læʔər], frication of approximants (*lock* → [dɔk]), frication of stops (*ban* → [væn]), unusual cluster reduction (*train* → [ren]), and initial consonant deletion (*tape* → [ep], are not typically seen in normally developing children and are considered idiosyncratic.

The use of nondevelopmental processes is critical in Dodd's (1993) separation of **children with delays** versus **children with deviance**. Whereas the former are characterized as children who use normal developmental processes that are inappropriate for their chronological age, the latter are described as those who use some processes which do not occur among normally developing children.

The suggested distinction between delayed versus deviant is not something that is clearly established. Stoel-Gammon (1990) divided children beyond the first 50 word stage into three groups on the nature of the phonology-lexicon interface. According to this, Type A children are those with a small lexicon and a limited phonetic inventory for their chronological age. Type B children are those with an age-appropriate vocabulary, a small phonetic inventory, and many homonymous productions. And finally, Type C children are those with a large vocabulary, a small phonetic inventory, and the presence of atypical errors to make word contrasts. According to Stoel-Gammon, among these three groups, only group A qualifies for the label delayed, as they are the only children without mismatches between their sound repertoire and the size of their vocabulary. Although type B children also have the small phonetic inventory, the mismatch with age-appropriate vocabulary makes such systems deviant.

The use of unusual patterns is not unique to the disordered population and may also be seen in normally developing children. However, the significant difference between the two groups is that such patterns are exhibited more frequently and less systematically in children with disorders. Leonard et al. (1987) presented novel object names and their referents to normally developing and children with phonological disorders. After having sufficient exposure to these items, the children's use of the words was tested. There were three types of words. One type contained consonants that the child already used appropriately in the majority of instances (in phonology words). A second type of word contained consonants that the child attempted a number of times in the past but never produced accurately (attempted words). The last type of word contained consonants that the child had neither produced nor attempted in the past (out of phonology words). Normally developing children were more likely to show unusual productions for out of phonology words than for the other two types (17.9% for in phonology words, 20.2% for attempted words, and 45% for out of phonology words). This was expected because children did not have these words with consonants available to them. The results were quite different for children with phonological disorders. They did not produce significantly different unusual patterns in different word types (50.8% for in phonology words, 47.8% for attempted words, and 43.8% for out of phonology words). Although the percentage was understandable for the out of phonology words, the percentages for the other two types of words were surprisingly high.

Although they do not necessarily follow the patterns of the process framework, the following unusual errors are mentioned by Leonard

(1985) as being more likely with phonologically disordered children. One type of error involves the use of later developing sounds in place of earlier-developing sounds. Substitutions such as [l] for /k/, /t/, and /g/ (Weiner, 1981), [v] for /d/ and /g/ (Grunwell, 1981), and [θ] and [ð] in the initial position instead of other fricatives, affricates, liquids, and glides (Weiner, 1981) can be cited for this.

Another type of unusual error is characterized by productions whereby the child's form represents an addition to the adult form. Edwards and Bernhardt (1973) reported a child who inserted a homorganic nasal before an alveolar stop. Ingram (1976) reported a child who added nasals to the initial position of adult forms. Another child, reported by Leonard and Brown (1984) added [s] in the final position of all words that ended in a vowel in the adult target.

Use of sounds absent from the ambient language is another type of unusual error cited by researchers. The use of alveolar affricates (Fey, 1985), lateral fricatives (Edwards, 1980), and ingressive alveolar fricatives (Ingram & Terselic, 1983), all by English-speaking children, fall into this type of error.

Another difference cited concerns the feature [+strident]. As we saw earlier, this feature comes in late for both developmentally normal and children with phonological disorders. However, once this is integrated in the system of a normally developing child, it becomes rather firm. Children with phonological disorders, on the other hand, do not seem to retain [+strident] often.

Finally, there also seems to be a difference between the normally developing children and those with phonological disorders in terms of the order of certain distinctions. Whereas place distinctions appear before voice distinctions in normally developing children, the reverse seems to be true for children with phonological disorders (Ingram, 1990).

Looking at eight studies on children with disorders, Stoel-Gammon and Dunn (1985) compared the error patterns with normal children in the process framework. Although there were differences across the studies because of differences in age, methods of data collection, and other criteria, the authors were able to identify several common features among children with phonological disorders. Nine processes occurred most frequently among these children. These were cluster reduction, final consonant deletion, unstressed syllable deletion, stopping, velar fronting, palatal fronting, liquid simplification (gliding or vocalization), assimilations, and voicing processes.

It should be pointed out that there is great variability among different groups, and the percentage of occurrence of processes differs enormously among children in the same study. For example, Dunn and Davis (1983) reported that, among the nine subjects they looked at, the process of stopping revealed a variation between 3% and 61%; the percentage of liquid simplification was 7% in subject 4, whereas the same process was observed 92% of the time in subject 3.

It is quite obvious from our exposition that an overwhelming majority of studies in disordered phonology have focused on consonants, and vowel disorders largely have been ignored. The main reason behind this is the fact that there are far fewer vowel errors. For example, although many subjects with disorders produce only consonantal errors, there are no subjects who produce only vowel errors. Recently, however, there have been some studies that draw attention to the importance of disordered vowel systems (Penney, Fee, & Dowdle, 1994; Pollock & Hall, 1991; Reynolds, 1990; Stoel-Gammon & Herrington, 1990). Certain patterns, such as lowering of mid front vowels, /ɛ/ → [a], fronting of low back vowels to [a], and monophthongization of diphthongs /e/ → [a], emerge from this limited number of case studies. Pollock (1994) presented a framework for describing vowels and vowel misarticulations and offered several suggestions for collecting and analyzing data for assessment. To establish effective remediation processes for vowel misarticulations with confidence, however, many more studies are required.

ORGANICALLY BASED DISORDERS

The processes we have discussed so far relate to data that come from children with developmental disorders in that no known etiology is responsible for the erroneous productions. The dichotomous classification of developmental (functional) versus organic disorders has been common in the literature. Grunwell (1987) specified the following conditions to separate functional disorders from organic disorders: In order for a child to be classified as having a functional rather than an organic disorder, she or he should have normal physiological development, a normally functioning oral mechanism, and normal hearing. She or he should have no neurological problems relevant to speech production, and his or her comprehension of spoken language should be appropriate to mental age. The separation between functional and organic disorder is somewhat related to phonological and phonetic disability. Whereas functional disorders are phonologically based, organic disorders may be phonetically based. Although our focus in this book is on developmental phonological disorders, some of these organically based disorders will be mentioned briefly.

Dyspraxia, which is considered partially or totally synonymous with **apraxia,** is an impairment in the control of the motor system. This is a neurologically based motor speech disorder that interferes with the ability to execute normal speech movements. Developmental dyspraxia refers to children with articulation errors who have difficulty with volitional or imitative production of sounds. These children have normal intelligence, normal hearing, can understand spoken language, and have no muscle weakness. Children with apraxia exhibit more errors in consonants, especially for target fricatives and affricates and consonant clusters. The degree of error has a good correlation with the length, complexity, and frequency of the word. The speech of a child with apraxia has inconsistent substitutions, deletions, and additions. Reductions in the number of phonemes and distinctive features and a deletion of syllables are common.

Children with **cleft palate** also exhibit disordered productions resulting from organic damage. Because clefting of the soft palate impairs the child's ability to close the velopharyngeal port, the effect is the nasalization of his or her speech. This also impacts on the child's ability to have the necessary pressure in the oral cavity to produce stops, fricatives, and affricates. Children with cleft palate also have difficulties with consonant clusters and show inconsistencies in their articulations. Many of the processes cited earlier, such as consonant cluster reduction, stopping, glottal stop insertion, and liquid gliding, have been noted in these children (Hodson, Chin, Redmond, & Simpson, 1983).

Down syndrome is a well-known disorder resulting from a chromosomal abnormality. In general, the upper and lower jaws of these children are different in size and they are likely to show dental abnormalities. A smaller-than-normal oral cavity together with an unusually large tongue often results in a high level of unintelligibility. Children with Down syndrome are often hearing impaired (approximately 75%, Shipley & McAfee, 1992) and have some degree of mental retardation. The processes observed in children with Down syndrome are very similar to those in children with developmental disorders. Processes such as fronting, devoicing, stopping, gliding, weak syllable deletion, final consonant deletion, and cluster reduction are prevalent. In addition, these children reveal unusual processes and variable use of processes. Some researchers have claimed that the difference between normal children and children with Down syndrome is basically quantitative (Bodine, 1974; Smith & Stoel-Gammon, 1983). Dodd (1975), on the other hand, described the difference as qualitative because of the errors that cannot be formulated systematically, and inconsistent use of normal rules.

Children with **mental retardation** or children whose measured intelligence is below the expected level for their age also show common processes that occur in normally developing children. There is an inverse ratio between the number of errors in speech and Intelligence Quotient (IQ) (Wilson, 1966). The most common processes found in the speech of children with mental retardation are cluster reduction, stopping, depalatalization, fronting, gliding, deletion of final consonants, voicing processes, and assimilations (Ingram, 1976).

TREATMENT

In addition to providing a procedure for descriptive assessment, the phonological process approach also has been used to define treatment programs. A treatment approach based on phonological process analysis holds the premise that remediation of a process can influence all of the sounds that are similarly affected through generalization. Thus, instead of treating separate sound errors, facilitating the emergence of new sound patterns are accomplished through targeting only a few sounds that are representative of a process. For example, if a child has the process of fricative stopping, then by targeting only /f/ and /s/, we might expect the generalization to other fricatives without specific treatment. Once a clinician accepts the premise that suppression of the processes should be the target of the treatment, the next step is to establish the procedure for the selection of these targets.

Edwards and Bernhardt (1973) suggested the following three principles for the selection of processes for treatment. First, choose the processes that most interfere in intelligibility. Improvement of intelligibility is the main objective of the treatment. Second, if the decision cannot be made on the basis of the previous principle, choose the least stable processes. It is likely that optional processes are more susceptible to change than the ones that are stable in the child's system. Third, if neither principle above holds, choose the most common processes found in young children. In other words, the first processes that are chosen should be the ones that would produce the greatest change in intelligibility. If one cannot make a firm decision on the basis of these, then an optional process from the child's system should be chosen. If the first two principles are not sufficient to make a well-defined choice, then the order of acquisition in normal children should be followed. This will dictate the elimination of processes that end earlier in normally developing children.

Edwards (1983) added more details to these principles. According to her, it is not possible to give a specific order of processes in treatment because of the individual differences among children. However, the following considerations are important:

1. Choose processes that result in quick success. These may include processes that are optional in the child's system, processes that apply only in certain phonetic environments, and processes that affect sounds that are already in the child's phonetic inventory.

2. Choose processes that are crucial for each individual child. These would be the processes that affect the intelligibility of the child most by creating large numbers of homonyms and neutralizing contrastive features.

3. Choose early processes, or processes that affect the sounds acquired early.

4. Choose interacting processes that create substitutions based on more than one change in one rule.

It is obvious from the above considerations that the severity of errors and the intelligibility of the child's speech are among the most important concerns. In the process framework, intelligibility has also been dealt with by other scholars. Ingram (1976) and Grunwell (1981) have related unintelligibility to the processes that cause variability, whereas Grunwell (1985) points to the processes that are most deviant and to those that apply most frequently or result in greater homonymy. Nettelbladt (1983) proposes the differential effects of paradigmatic (substitution) and syntagmatic (sequential) processes. In her view, in children with moderate dysphonology (a term used by Nettelbladt for disordered phonology), paradigmatic substitution processes (e.g., stopping of fricatives, fronting of velars or palatals) dominate and only certain kinds of sequential syntagmatic processes, in particular, cluster reduction are found. In children with severe dysphonology there is a combination of paradigmatic (substitution) and strong syntagmatic (sequential) processes.

Hodson and Paden (1983) correlated a four-level intelligibility rating with the type and number of processes used by the child. The worst case of intelligibility *unintelligible except via gestures* is characterized by omission of stops, fricatives, and liquids. *Essentially unintelligible* is characterized by omission of syllables and initial and final obstruents, fronting, and backing. The third category, *sometimes intelligible* is distinguished by cluster reduction, strident deletion, stopping, and gliding. And finally, the *generally intelligible* group is characterized by nonphonemic distortions, affrication, and voicing or devoicing.

Hodson and Paden (1991) offer the following considerations when selecting potential targets for the initial cycles of phonological remediation for children with highly unintelligible speech, as these are thought to be the more important factors contributing to severity: (1) syllableness (whether the child's productions are matching the targets in number of syllables); (2) word-initial singleton consonants, that is, if any of the early developing phoneme classes—stops, nasals, glides—are lacking in CV utterances; (3) word final singleton consonants; (4) consonant sequences; (5) glides (if deficient by 70% or more); (6) alveolars (if the child is a backer). Other targets for remediation include nasals, stridents in /s/ clusters, velars, and liquids if their percentage of error occurrence exceeds 40%. Yavas and Lamprecht (1988), while recognizing the validity of all of the above, added that the number of words that contain more than one process may also be important. A similar concern is articulated by Edwards' (1992) Process density index. The idea here is to measure phonological severity by counting the average number of process applications per word. The average number of processes packed into each word, known as the Process density index, is found to be closely related to subjective judgments of intelligibility (Wolk, 1990).

Although it makes sense to suggest that words with one process have a higher chance of being more intelligible than words with three processes for the simple reason that the distancing effect of one process is smaller than that of three processes, even here we run into difficulties because the effects of the processes might vary in creating homophonous pairs or groups. A word that undergoes one process, yet results in a homophonous pair, might be more destructive for intelligibility than a word that undergoes more than one process without yielding such homonymy. The contribution of the type of process and its interaction with the process co-occurrence could be another crucial factor for intelligibility. For example, is it possible to determine the destructive effect on a word with three substitution processes in comparison to a word with two sequential processes?

Leinonen (1991) addressed the issue of communicative inadequacy by establishing a procedure for evaluating the functional loss (FLOSS) of a system by assessing the lack of lexical differentiation arising from the characteristics of the child's phonological system. In doing this, processes and combinations of processes are assessed as to the homophony they can

potentially lead to in the child's lexical system. Accordingly, three categories are established:

1. Processes that have no potential for homophony: These would be
   processes that do not conflate phonological contrasts and which operate as single processes (e.g., glottal replacement).

2. Processes that have no potential for multiple homophony: Here, for
   example, we can mention processes that are in counterfeeding relationship. This means that two processes that are observable in the
   child's system must be ordered in a certain way that is determined by
   the child's output. A counterfeeding relationship would imply that
   the second rule, if it were to apply before the first rule, would feed
   the first rule by increasing the number of forms to which it could
   apply. We will illustrate this with the following example. Consider
   the data from C (3;2):

tip	[dɪp]	*kip*	[tɪp]
dip	[dɪp]	*kick*	[tɪk]
tick	[dɪk]		

   From the data, we see two processes: voicing (t → d) and fronting
   (k → t). Because the child does not have voicing of the prevocalic
   /k/ in *kip* and *kick* (they do not become [dɪp] and [dɪk], respectively), but has it for *tip* and *tick*, we will have to order the two rules as
   (1) (t → d), and (2) (k → t). These two rules are in counterfeeding relationship, because if the second rule (k → t) were to apply before
   the first rule, it would feed it by increasing the number of forms to
   which it would apply. This would mean that the initial [t]s resulting from the fronting (k → t) in targets *kip* and *kick* would have un-
   dergone voicing.

3. Processes that have potential for multiple homophony: These would
   be created either by feeding processes (reverse ordering of the
   fronting and voicing in the above case where *kip* would be realized as
   [dɪp], too), or by the co-existence of non-interacting processes. For example, stopping (s → t), fronting (k → t), and devoicing (d → t) for the
   following targets will create multiple homophony:

sip	
kip	[tɪp]
dip	

The assessment of the functional adequacy of the child's phonological system has direct implications for the planning of treatment goals. Because homophony should be kept to a minimum for communicative adequacy, elimination of the processes which have greatest potential for homophony is a reasonable goal. To this end, processes which have potential for homophony, including multiple homophony, are suggested to have priority over processes which cannot produce homophony. Further, processes which have potential for multiple homophony will have priority over processes which have no potential for multiple homophony.

Word position seems to be an important variable in determining the order of processes for therapeutic purposes. Leinonen (1991) proposed that processes operating in the syllable-final-word-final (SFWF) position merit priority over processes operating in the syllable-initial-word-initial (SIWI) position, and processes operating in the SFWF and SIWI positions merit priority over processes operating in the syllable-final-within-word (SFWW) and syllable-initial-within-word (SIWW) positions. Because the potential for creating homophony are different in different word positions, the following order of priority was suggested: (1) SIWI: fronting, gliding, prevocalic voicing, stopping, WI cluster deletion; (2) SFWF: final C deletion, fronting, WF devoicing, stopping, gliding.

Whereas these principles are useful as general guidelines, many details contributing to the communicative inadequacy of a child's speech remain to be worked out, and the elusive concept of intelligibility is far from being understood completely. However, the search goes on, and this is one of the key questions for principled therapy.

Tyler, Edwards, and Saxman (1987) provided a detailed application of phonological process-based treatment procedures and their efficacy. Using two procedures (minimal pair and modified cyles) based on phonological process analysis of their four subjects' speech, the authors showed that dramatic improvements took place in the phonological systems of the children in 2½ months. The results were the same regardless of which phonological process-based procedure was applied; there was generalization of the target patterns to sounds affected by the phonological process but that were not trained. For example, subject B in the study was trained with targets /f, and s/ and generalization was observed to the untrained targets /z, v, ʃ, θ, and ð/. The authors noted, however, that the correct production of untrained sounds lagged behind that of the trained sounds. Similar results were obtained by Weiner (1981).

SUMMARY

In this chapter, we examined the stages of phonological development. The period of phonemic development that roughly corresponds to 1 year 6 months to 4 years of age was identified as the most active and most relevant for the clinical population. It was pointed out that there are several cross-linguistic developmental patterns and, in a general fashion, it is possible to establish chronologies for developmental simplifications of child productions of the adult targets. Natural phonology, which has been used extensively to describe erroneous productions, was explained and a sample data analysis in this framework was offered. Certain patterns of disordered phonology that are not found in normal development were identified and therapeutic implications derived from Natural phonology were discussed. The more recent views on phonological development and their implications for the clinical population will be given in the chapters on syllable (Chapter 9) and on feature geometry and underspecification (Chapter 10).

NOTES

1. Brazilian Portuguese permits only /l, r, s/ in syllable final position.

2. Palatal fronting is named "depalatalization" in some publications (e.g., Stoel-Gammon & Dunn 1985).

3. Yavas and Hernandorena (1991) illustrate that sound preference may occur in more than one position. Their 7-year-old Portuguese-speaking subject had this process in syllable initial-within-word position as well as in syllable-initial word-initial position.

EXERCISES

1. Identify the phonological process(es) in the following words.

meat	[mi]	_____
this	[di]	_____
feather	[fɛdə]	_____

dog	[dɔ]	_____
put	[bu]	_____
sip	[di]	_____
pig	[bi]	_____
sock	[tɔt]	_____
pretty	[bɪdi]	_____
gas	[dæt]	_____
dig	[tɪt]	_____
bad	[dæt]	_____
save	[sæs]	_____
boat	[dot]	_____
soup	[pup]	_____
feet	[pip]	_____
come	[mʌm]	_____
glass	[gæt]	_____
stop	[pap]	_____
drink	[dɪk]	_____
cheese	[tit]	_____
bottle	[batu]	_____
kiss	[tɪt]	_____

2. The following substitutions are found both in normally developing and in children with phonological disorders:

a. z → s   b. r → w   c. v → b   d. θ → t

e. ð → d   f. p → b   g. f → p   h. l → w

i. dʒ → tʃ   j. ʃ → s   k. θ → f   l. ð → θ

m. v → f   n. k → t   o. θ → s   p. l → j

Match these substitutions with the following:

fricative stopping_____

fricative substitution   _____

liquid gliding   _____

velar fronting   _____

devoicing   _____

palatal fronting   _____

3. First, give two examples in words of each of the following processes, and then state which of these are seen mostly in children with phonological disorders (i.e., not commonly found in normally developing children).

 a. gliding of fricatives

 b. velar assimilation

 c. frication of stops

 d. stopping of fricatives

 e. alveolar assimilation

 f. frication of approximants

 g. liquid gliding

 h. backing of alveolars

4. Predict the child realizations of the following targets based on the application of the particular processes specified for each item:

peep	Prevocalic voicing, FC deletion	[	]
fell	Stopping, vocalization	[	]
bread	CC reduction, FC devoicing	[	]
grass	Liquid gliding, stopping	[	]
coat	Progressive velar assim.	[	]
zip	Regressive labial assim.	[	]
trick	CC reduction, alveolar assim.	[	]

beside	Weak syl. deletion, stopping	[	]
rabbit	Liquid gliding, FC deletion	[	]
please	CC reduction, stopping	[	]

5. The existence of devoicing, stopping, palatal and velar fronting, and final consonant deletion can result in a homophonous production [taɪ] for targets that have initial /θ, s, ʃ, t, k, d, g, tr, kr, gl/. Find examples that will illustrate this 10-way homophony.

Chapter 7

NATURALNESS AND MARKEDNESS

$\mathbf{T}$he phonological changes mentioned in previous chapters are not, for the most part, arbitrary. The same processes are repeated in many different situations. These processes end up producing certain types of segments and sequences that are more favored than others. During the descriptions of many phonological phenomena, the terms marked and unmarked were used for the expected (natural) and unexpected (not natural), respectively. In this chapter, these phenomena will be looked at in a more systematic manner.

NATURAL SEGMENTS AND SYSTEMS

Scholars have long observed that certain segments are more frequently attested in languages than others. Thus, for example, the front unrounded vowels /i/ and /e/ are more frequent and, hence, considered more natural than the front rounded vowels /y/ and /ø/, which are marked. The phonologists' view of marked and unmarked is not based solely on the inventories of languages. Phonological acquisition, phonological disorders, slips of the tongue, and historical changes are also considered to be important and are used as evidence. Consequently, we expect that children acquiring German or Turkish, languages that have all four vowels mentioned above, will acquire /i/ and /e/ earlier than /y/ and /ø/, a prediction that has been confirmed. Also, in historical changes and slips of tongue, unrounding of rounded front vowels is found more frequently than the reverse. For these reasons, the vowels /i/ and /e/ are considered unmarked, as opposed to /y/ and /ø/, which are treated as marked.

Before examining individual classes of sounds in terms of naturalness, we should point out that the generalizations we will give are not absolute. These tendencies form a continuum that identifies cases in terms of degrees of markedness or naturalness. In many cases, what appears as natural or unmarked has explanations in terms of articulatory ease, acoustic power, duration, and the like and phonetic motivation is evoked. However, such principles should not be treated as strongly predictive, as no good explanations will be found for the failures of predictions based on markedness.

Consonants

Obstruents

Stops: Stops are the most common consonants found in all known languages. They are reported in 100% of languages by Ruhlen (1976), who covered 693 languages from different families. Maddieson (1984), who reported on the 317 language UCLA Phonological Segment Inventory Database (UPSID), also confirmed the 100% existence of stops. Some common patterns that are observed regarding stops in languages are as follows: Almost all languages (over 99%) have stops in three places of articulation: bilabial, dental/alveolar, and velar. Some notable exceptions are Tahitian and Chavante for lack of velar stops, Hawaiian for lack of dental/alveolar stops, and Aleut, Cherokee, Oneida, and Tlingit for lack of bilabial stops.

Another significant patterning refers to voicing. The most basic type of stop is the voiceless unaspirated (e.g., /t/). This is followed by voiced stops (e.g., /d/). A language with only one stop series almost invariably has unaspirated voiceless stops, and a language which contrasts only two series typically has a voiceless/voiced contrast (Maddieson, 1984).[1] This is commonly expressed in the implicational tendency that "the existence of voiced stops presupposes the existence of voiceless stops in a language" (p. 27). Although this is true as a strong tendency, it may be also influenced by another dimension, place of articulation. For example, whereas this tendency of the existence of the voiced member presupposing the voiceless member is exceptionless for velars (if a language has a /g/, it always has a /k/), it is not so for bilabial stops (a language can have a /b/ without necessarily having a /p/).[2] As stated succinctly by

Gamkrelidze (1978), "voicing is best combined with labiality, and voicelessness with velarity" (p. 17). As a consequence, it would not be very unusual to find a system like the following, which has /b/ and /k/ and lacks the voiceless bilabial /p/ and the voiced velar /g/:

	t	k
b	d	

It is, on the other hand, very difficult to find a language with the reverse trend, having /p/ and /g/ without the voiceless velar /k/ and the voiced bilabial /b/:

p	t	
	d	g

The implicational tendency, then, is that /g/ implies /d/, which implies /b/.

If we look at the languages that have a voice contrast in the stop series with one stop missing, we see that the missing element is typically /p/ or /g/. If a language is missing two stops, these are typically /p/ and /g/.

Apart from the three popular places of articulation—bilabial, dental/alveolar, and velar—stops are also found in retroflex, palatal, uvular, and glottal places of articulation. These latter are not as common, and whenever they are found in a system they presuppose the existence of stops in the common three places of articulation. The abrupt release that is required for a stop articulation is not easy in the palatal/palato-alveolar place of articulation. This is due to the dome-shaped configuration of the upper surface of the palate and, as a result, languages more commonly have affricates, instead of stops, in this place of articulation.

In child language acquisition, stops are among the earliest sounds acquired by children. Prather et al. (1975) showed that the normally developing 36-month-olds' correct production of stops is over 90% for all stops. Data from some clinical populations also indicate high correct production of stops. In adults with cerebral palsy, the percentage is higher than 80% (the only exception is /g/ with 78%) (Platt, Andrews, Young, & Quinn, 1980).

Fricatives: Whereas fricatives are found in almost all of the world's languages, they are not as common as stops. More than 90% of languages have at least one fricative (almost all exceptions are Australian languages). The voiceless dental/alveolar sibilant, /s/, is by far the most common fricative sound found in languages of the world, followed by /f/ and /ʃ/. Thus, languages with fewer fricatives are likely to have these three voiceless fricatives, which are articulated in the front part of the mouth. The voiced/voiceless contrast in fricatives is likely to be seen in systems with four or more fricatives. A system with four fricatives would likely include /f, v, s, and z/.

Although, in general, voiceless fricatives are more common than voiced fricatives, there seem to be some exceptions related to place of articulation and sibilance. Whereas voiceless fricatives dominate the scene in general, bilabial and dental nonsibilant fricatives favor voicing. Looking at the ratio of unpaired voiced fricatives in total voiced fricatives, Maddieson (1984) found no language with /z/ but lacking /s/, and very few with /z/ but lacking /ʃ/(2 in 51 languages, 3.9%). The situation was very different with regard to bilabial and interdental fricatives: 24 in 32 languages (75%) had /β/ without /ɸ/, and 12 in 21 languages (57.1%) had /ð/ without /θ /.

Several factors may help to explain the preference for certain fricatives. Table 7–1 incorporates some of them.

In Table 7–1, acoustic description refers to energy concentration in frequencies for each individual fricative. For the saliency of a sound, the

Table 7–1. Characteristics of fricatives that are thought to be influential on their frequency.

Fricative	Acoustic Description	Acoustic Power (dB)	Duration (ms)	Perceptual Data
/f/	low to mid	6.9	122	1.92
/v/	low to mid	8.4	78	6.03
/θ /	low	1.0	119	9.86
/ð/	low	10.1	119	9.43
/s/	mid to high	9.2	129	0.43
/z/	mid to high	9.8	85	0.87
/ʃ/	mid to high	18.1	118	0.87
/ʒ/	mid to high	13.0	85	2.62

higher the better. Acoustic power in decibels (Edwards, 1992) relates to the loudness of a sound. Here, too, the higher the number the more salient the sound becomes. Another dimension, duration of the sound (in milliseconds), is given in the third column. Once again, the higher number is a plus for saliency. The final column, the perceptual data, refers to the relative difficulty of recognizing the sound in question. Here, contrary to the previous examples, the higher numbers are an indication of the sound's difficulty in recognition, a decrease in saliency (Edwards, 1992).

Analyzing the data here, it is clear why /s/ is the most common fricative; its saliency is confirmed in all dimensions. It has energy concentration in the mid to high frequencies, considerable acoustic power (9.2 dB), the longest duration, and the least amount of difficulty in recognition. With the exception of the interdentals, for all pairs of fricatives, the voiceless member has more favorable ratings for duration and perceptual data. Thus, the preference for /f/, /s/, and /ʃ/ mentioned earlier is explained. The reverse trend for interdentals (57% of languages had /ð/ without having /θ/) can be made understandable through an imbalance of acoustic power in decibels: Although the more common /ð/ has considerable acoustic power (10.1 dB), the voiceless counterpart, /θ/ is much weaker (1.0 dB). This seems to be the determining factor regarding the frequency of /ð/, as the two sounds are very much alike with respect to other variables.

Fricatives are not acquired early by children and, as mentioned earlier, they undergo the process of stopping in early stages. When that tendency is suppressed and fricatives start coming into the child's system, correct productions are observed more for the labio-dental /f/ than for /s/. This is somewhat different from what we have observed in the inventories of the languages of the world in which dental/alveolar was the favorite place of articulation.

In summary, with certain notable exceptions, voiceless obstruents are more common than their voiced counterparts, and the existence of the voiced obstruents implies the existence of its voiceless counterpart. As for the preferences for place of articulation, there are differences. The following list gives the preferences, in descending order, on the basis of frequencies found in languages:

Stops	*Fricatives*	*Affricates*
Dental/Alveolar	Dental/Alveolar	Palatal
Labial	Labial	Dental/Alveolar
Velar	Palatal	Labial

Palatal   Velar   Velar
Uvular   Uvular

With this information in mind, let us examine the following obstruent systems, and analyze them in terms of the universal preferences discussed thus far:

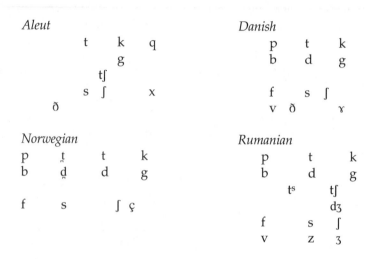

Aleut

	t	k	q
		g	
	tʃ		
s	ʃ		x
ð			

Danish

p	t	k
b	d	g
f	s	ʃ
v	ð		ɣ

Norwegian

p	t̪	t	k
b	d̪	d	g
f	s		ʃ ç

Rumanian

p		t		k
b		d		g
	tˢ		tʃ	
			dʒ	
f		s		ʃ
v		z		ʒ

Of the four languages, Rumanian is the only one that reveals the most common pattern and, therefore, is not remarkable for its obstruents. The reasons are that six stops are distributed in three most favored place of articulation. Also, they are matched pairwise in voicing. Two of the three affricates are expectedly in the palatal region (one voiceless, one voiced) and the third one is alveolar. Finally, its six fricatives occupy the three most favored places of articulation (alveolar, labial, and velar) with voiced-voiceless pairs.

Danish and Norwegian are also quite unremarkable for their stops. The retroflex stops of Norwegian are in addition to the basic three places of articulation and, thus, are not unexpected. The fricatives in these two languages merit some comment. The six fricatives of Danish, although made up of three voiceless and three voiced, have a rather unexpected distribution. With the exception of the labio-dentals /f/ and /v/, the remaining fricatives are unpaired with respect to voicing. Although /ð/ seems to be rather natural without its voiceless counterpart /θ/ (a pattern found in 57% of languages in UPSID), /ɣ/ without /x/ is not as common. Although the alveolar and palatal sibilants are voiceless and, thus, natural, the lack of their voiced counterparts in a six-fricative system is remarkable.

Norwegian fricatives also demonstrate a discrepancy of voiced-voiceless pairs. As mentioned earlier, a more typical four-fricative system generally utilizes two places of articulation with pairings in voicing. For example, the following are quite typical for such systems:

f	s		s	ʃ
v	z		z	ʒ

The comments on Danish and Norwegian are related to rather mild deviations from the expected patterns. In Aleut, however, some extremely unusual patterns become obvious. The stops are probably the most significant. The lack of bilabial stops is made even more unusual because of the existence of uvular and voiced velar stops, contrary to implicational principles. As for the fricatives, the pattern also is not what is expected from a four-fricative system. Probably the most unusual aspect is the lack of the generally more common bilabial /β/, and the existence of the infrequent uvular /ɣ/.

In summary, it can be said that, although voiceless generally typifies obstruents, the marked/unmarked (unexpected/expected, respectively) nature of a sound is greatly determined by the context in which it occurs. For example, voicing of an obstruent in intervocalic or postnasal position is absolutely natural (unmarked). Such cases are frequently seen in child language and are attested in the phonologies of many languages.

Sonorants

Nasals: Languages normally have at least one nasal consonant in their inventories. A few counterexamples are considered oddities which are not explainable by areal or genetic groupings. Although lacking nasal consonants is unexpected, having only one nasal in the system is equally, if not more, strange. The UPSID data reveal that two nasals (31.9% of languages), three nasals (30% of languages), and four nasals (26.2% of languages) are the most popular patterns in languages. Together, they constitute more than 88% of languages.

In terms of place of articulation, dental/alveolar is the most preferred, which is followed by bilabial. Although velars and palatals are ranked third and fourth, respectively, retroflex and uvular nasals are less frequent. Finally, typical of sonorants, nasals are unmarkedly voiced.

Liquids: Similar to the pattern observed for nasals, languages tend to have at least one liquid, and most languages have more than one. Unlike nasals, which form a rather homogeneous group, liquids include laterals (approximant or fricative) and nonlateral r-sounds (trill, tap/flap, approximant).[3]

Depending on the type of liquid, certain tendencies with respect to voicing are revealed. Although a lateral will most likely be a voiced approximant (in approximately 80% of languages), a fricative lateral is most likely to be voiceless. On the other hand, all types of nonlaterals, r-sounds, favor voicing.

As for the place of articulation, the following tendencies are observed: Laterals typically are produced at dental/alveolar place (87%). Nonlaterals, however, show an interesting place and manner interaction. Although interrupted nonlaterals (trills, taps/flaps) generally are produced at the dental/alveolar region, the continuant nonlaterals (approximant r-sounds, e.g., American English) show a preference for retroflex place of articulation.

Glides. Maddieson (1984) stated that more than 90% of languages have one or more glides. /w/ and /j/ are the most commonly occurring glides. As noted in Chapter 2, these glides are the nonsyllabic versions of the high vowels /u/ and /i/, respectively. Whenever the two glides appear in a phonological system, they imply the existence of the respective vowels in that language. In UPSID data, the existence of /w/ is associated with the occurrence of /j/. Because /i/ is more common than /u/ in languages, /w/ implying /j/ is not surprising. Other than the two most common palatal and labio-velar glides, labio-palatal /ɥ/ and velar /ɯ/ varieties are found in some languages.

Summarizing the patterns of sonorants, we can say that they are unmarkedly voiced. Nasals and liquids (with the exception of approximant r-sounds) show a strong preference for dental/alveolar place of articulation, whereas glides are common in bilabial and palatal areas. As for the naturalness of sonorants with respect to language acquisition, nasals and glides are unmarked early sounds, whereas liquids are problematic and marked.

The following sonorant systems reveal some unusual patterns. Let us examine how they differ from the expected patterns:

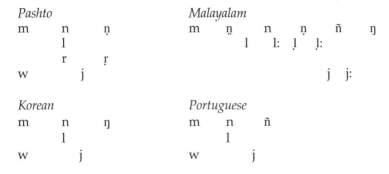

The points that are worthy of comment vary from language to language. For Portuguese, the remark will be on the lack of velar in a three-nasal system in which the most common dental/alveolar and bilabials are followed by the palatal nasal rather than the expected velar. The only remark for Korean is the lack of a nonlateral liquid. Pashto deserves a comment for the retroflex nasal instead of the expected unmarked velar nasal.

Malayalam is the only language among the four for which the comments will be lengthier. To start with, it has an unusually large nasal system in which a record number, six, places of articulation are used. In some accounts, contrasts are increased even to 12 because of length at each of these places of articulation. Liquids are also rather marked because of the unusually heavy lateral bias. Finally, the only glide, /j/, while not very unusual, deserves a mention for the lack of /w/.

Summarizing what has been said about consonants in languages of the world and the patterns of acquisition, with certain exceptions, the two fields of data share many commonalities. This is demonstrated in Table 7–2. Apart from the discrepancies related to sibilants (higher incidence in languages versus lower accuracy in children's production) and affricates (lower incidence in languages versus higher production accuracy), the two columns agree closely. If affricates are considered as the combination of a stop and a fricative and calculated as such, they do not come out as discrepant.

Vowels

Vowel systems are generally examined according to their size and patterning. The most common small system is generally a three-vowel system with /i, a, and u/ (e.g., Arabic). In such a system, only two degrees of height are observed. When the number of vowels in a system increas-

Table 7–2. Phonological universals and children's production accuracy.

	Percentage of Languages having[a]	Percentage of Correct Production[b]
Stops	100.0	98.5
Nasals	99.6	96.0
Sibilants	90.6	80.2
Laterals	81.7	93.4
Vibrants[d]	77.3	88.4
Fricatives	73.0	73.2
Affricates	69.8	86.6

Source: From *Phonological Acquisition and Change*, by J. L. Locke, 1983, p. 111. New York: Academic Press. Reprinted with permission.

[a] Based on 693 languages listed in Ruhlen.

[b] Based on 438 English-speaking children tested by Snow (1963)

es, it is almost always the case that the third degree of height, mid, is introduced. Although there are some languages with four vowels, the five-vowel system is the most common. The prototypical five-vowel system is /i, e, a, o, u/ (e.g., Spanish). In a vowel system in which there are four degrees of height, the minimum number of vowels increases to seven. In such a system, the most common is /i, e, ɛ, a, ɔ, o, u/ (e.g., Italian, Portuguese).

In all of these typical systems, we see that front vowels are generally unrounded and non-low back vowels are generally rounded. This tendency is explained with reference to the maximal distance principle. Because rounding makes a vowel more back than the unrounded counterpart, a front vowel such as /i/ would be more front than /j/. Similarly, /u/, as a rounded vowel, would be more back than its unrounded counterpart /ɯ/. Thus, having the maximally front /i/ and the maximally back /u/ creates maximum perceptual separation and is the unmarked pattern.

Systems with more than eight or nine vowels are not very common and do not yield themselves neatly to easy classifications in terms of patterning. The above-mentioned number of vowels all refer to the basic types and do not include contrasts created by length, nasalization, or other additional features. A vowel system may also include a set of nasal or long vowels that correspond to the basic set. With reference to vowel length and nasalization, another generalization can be made: Contrast in long or nasal vowels implies a contrast in short/oral vowels.

Looking at common/uncommon segments and considering different sizes of phoneme inventories in languages, it may seem that smaller inventories would contain the most frequent segments, and that, as the size of the inventory increases, less common segments (in descending order of frequency of occurrence) would be added. Maddieson (1986) rejects such a formulation as extreme. The reasons for this are: (a) no single segment is found in all languages and (b) there does not seem to exist a single hierarchy for segmental naturalness that would coincide with the increasing number of segments in a system. Instead, he suggests a more relaxed, universal tendency that "a smaller inventory has a greater probability of including a given common segment than a larger one, and a larger inventory has a greater probability of including an unusual segment type than a smaller one" (p. 110). Thus, it is possible to predict which segments are more likely to occur in a small or large inventory, but not to predict absolutely which segments would occur in a given inventory.

Examining the distribution of 13 of the most frequent consonants in smaller inventories (57 languages with 20–24 segments) and relatively large inventories (54 languages with over 40 segments), the situation depicted in Table 7–3 emerges.

Before ending this section, the following point should be emphasized. Although certain statistical tendencies are revealed by the inventories of the languages of the world, the oddities resulting from these generalizations may actually be normal (common) if certain areal and genetic groupings are considered. For example, the lack of fricatives is limited almost exclusively to languages of Oceania. Pharyngeals are generally rare, but are commonly found in Semitic and Caucasian languages. Implosives are an areal characteristic of Sub-Saharan Africa, Southeast Asia, and Southern Mexico, and are rarely, if at all, found elsewhere. Finally, clicks are found only in Southern Africa, primarily in the Khoisan family.

MARKEDNESS IN GENERATIVE PHONOLOGY

In Chapter 4, we saw that segments undergoing a phonological rule form a natural class in which certain features are shared by all members of the

Table 7–3. Inventory size and frequency of selected segments.

Segment	Small Inventory Languages (in %)	All Languages (in %)	Large Inventory Languages (in %)
More likely in small inventories			
/p/	89.5	82.6	77.8
/k/	93.0	89.3	79.3
/ŋ/	59.6	52.7	51.9
Equally likely in large or small inventories			
/m/	94.7	94.3	92.6
/w/	75.4	75.1	77.3
More likely in large inventories			
/b/	45.6	62.8	77.8
/g/	42.1	55.2	75.9
/ʔ/	33.3	30.3	55.6
/tʃ/	22.8	44.5	64.8
/f/	15.8	42.6	51.8
/ʃ/	17.5	46.1	70.4
/j/	78.9	85.5	94.4
/ñ/	22.8	33.8	37.0

Source: From "The Size and Structure of Phonological Inventories," by I. Maddieson, 1986, p. 111. In *Experimental Phonology*, by J. Ohala and J. J. Jaeger, Orlando, FL: Academic Press. Reprinted by permission.

group. It was also pointed out that fewer features are required to specify a natural class of sounds than to specify any one member of that class. For example, the class of voiced fricatives of English, /v, ð, z, ʒ/, can be specified as [–sonorant, +continuant, +voiced], whereas the description of any one member of this class would require more features because the place of articulation needs to be specified. Consequently, it may be assumed that feature counting could lead to an evaluation of naturalness. That this is not so simple can readily be discovered. For example, although the following class of voiceless stops /p, t, k/ is described as [–sonorant, –continuant, –delayed release, –voiced], (i.e., with four features), a much less natural group of the sounds /m, r, l, j, d, z, b, v, a, o/ can be described with one feature, [+voiced]. If feature counting revealed the relative naturalness/markedness, then the latter group should appear in more phonological rules than the former. Not only is the former group more commonly found in phonological rules of languages, it is rather difficult, if not inconceivable, to find any rule or process having the second group that groups vowels, nasals, liquids, glides, and voiced obstruents as its input.

To give another example, this time from the same group of sounds, vowels, let us look at the following:

a. /i, e, o, u/　　　　　b. /e, ø, u, ɨ/

Although these two groups require the same number of features in their specifications,

a. $\begin{bmatrix} \alpha \text{ back} \\ \alpha \text{ round} \\ - \text{ low} \\ - \text{ cons} \\ + \text{ syl.} \end{bmatrix}$　　　　b. $\begin{bmatrix} \alpha \text{ back} \\ \alpha \text{ high} \\ - \text{ low} \\ - \text{ cons} \\ + \text{ syl.} \end{bmatrix}$

it is clear that the first group of sounds is natural and can be found together in a phonological rule, whereas the second group is highly unnatural, and it is quite inconceivable that these sounds would behave together in a phonological rule. Nevertheless, the number of features needed to specify either group is the same and feature counting cannot discriminate the natural (unmarked) from the unnatural (marked). Thus, the attempt to quantify the notion of naturalness through counting distinctive features fails.

To remedy this situation, generative phonology introduces a number of marking conventions that are designed to evaluate the intrinsic content of the features. The details of these conventions are highly complex, but the following example shows how they are used to differentiate the expected (unmarked) from the unexpected (marked). Referring to the case of the two groups of vowels just seen, the following marking convention is relevant:

[u round]　　→　　[α round]　/　_____
　　　　　　　　　　　　　　　　$\begin{bmatrix} \alpha \text{ back} \\ - \text{ low} \end{bmatrix}$

This convention states that the unmarked value of the feature [round] is identical to the feature specification for [back] for non-low vowels (where '_____' inside a segment indicates a simultaneous context). This way, only the (a) vowels, /i, e, o, u/, would be treated as unmarked (natural), as group (b), /e, ø, u, ɨ/, has the vowels /ø, ɨ/ in which the rounding and the backness have the opposite values.

Each segment is evaluated with respect to individual features that are pertinent, and marked value for a feature (*m* below) has a cost of 1, and the unmarked value (*u* below) is cost free. Pluses and minuses have a cost of 1 for complexity. This way, the complexity (thus, naturalness or markedness) of each segment is calculated. The following shows the relative markedness of a select group of obstruents:

	p	*b*	*t*	*d*	*k*	*g*	*f*	*v*	*s*	*z*
anterior	u	u	u	u	m	m	u	u	u	u
coronal	–	–	+	+	u	u	m	m	u	u
continuant	u	u	u	u	u	u	m	m	m	m
voiced	u	m	u	m	u	m	u	m	u	m
Complexity	1	2	1	2	1	2	2	3	2	3

Here, the following relations hold: [+anterior] is treated as unmarked, as frontal articulations are favored for obstruents. The + and – values for [coronal] are assigned for bilabial and dental/alveolar stops because no decision is made regarding the relative markedness of these places of articulation for stops. [–continuant] is unmarked because stops are more common than fricatives. And finally, [–voiced] is unmarked, as voiceless obstruents are more common than voiced obstruents.

Although these relations may seem rather reasonable in terms of individual segments, among different systems, we realize there is no solid base for determining markedness. The values derived from the above example will show that the following two systems, which have the same number of segments, will be assigned equal degrees of complexity:

a.	p	t	k		b.		t	k
		d	g			b	d	g
							s	
	v	z					z	

Although both systems will have the identical complexity (12), it is not very difficult to see that (b) is much more expected than (a). The reasons are as follows: Although both systems have five stops each, the missing element in (a) is highly unusual. If a language has /g/ and /d/, then it is very much expected that it will also have /b/. System (b), on the other hand, lacks /p/ which is not all that unusual. As for the fricatives, system (b) has the most basic /s/ and its voiced counterpart, whereas system (a) has two voiced fricatives without any voiceless members. Although a typical two-fricative system would more likely have two voiceless fricatives, /s and f/, the /s, z/ set given in language (b) is definitely less marked than the two voiced fricatives, /v and z/, in language (a). Thus, while certain segments are more or less natural than others, this does not mean that, by adding the complexities of individual segments, we can directly arrive at the naturalness of a system.

NATURALNESS OF SYLLABLES

Like segments and phonological systems, syllables can be put on a continuum of naturalness or markedness. CV is the most preferred (unmarked) syllable type, and it is not missing in any language. It also is the syllable type acquired first by children. All other syllable types are marked. The degree of markedness of a syllable increases as we put more consonants in a row. For example, CVC is more marked than CV, but less marked than CCV, CCVC, CVCC, and so on.

It has been stated by generations of scholars that there is a principled relationship between the intrinsic content of the sounds and their respective distribution throughout syllabic structure. The center (nucleus) of the syllable normally is occupied by either a vowel or a diphthong, and the surrounding segments (onset and codas) are composed of segments with lower sonority. Sonority of a sound is its relative loudness compared to other sounds with the same length, stress, and pitch. Two factors that are directly related to the sonority index of a sound are (a) the degree of opening (stricture) of the articulation, and (b) its propensity for voicing. The more open articulation a sound has, the greater its sonority level will be. Also, if two sounds have the same degree of opening, the voiced one will have a greater degree of sonority than the voiceless counterpart. Although scales of sonority used by different phoneticians and phonologists vary in detail, they all agree on the relative sonority of different groups of sounds. The 10-point sonority scale in Table 7–4 is from Hogg and McCully (1987). Glides and affricates are not included in Table 7–4, but it is not difficult to place them here. Glides are assigned the same sonority value as the high vowels, as they are the nonsyllabic versions of them. Affricates, by definition, should be placed between the stops and the fricatives.

Table 7–4. Sonority scale.

Sounds	Sonority Values	Examples
Low vowels	10	/a, æ/
Mid vowels	9	/e, o/
High vowels	8	/i, u/
Flaps	7	/r/
Laterals	6	/l/
Nasals	5	/m, n, ŋ/
Voiced fricatives	4	/v, ð, z/
Voiceless fricatives	3	/f, θ , s/
Voiced stops	2	/b, d, g/
Voiceless stops	1	/p, t, k/

Source: From *Metrical Phonology: A Coursebook*, by R. Hogg and C. Mc-Cully, 1987, p. 33. Boston, MA: Cambridge University Press. Reprinted with permission.

As we see, obstruents are the lower sonority items and vowels are the higher ones. In between, we see liquids and nasals in descending sonority levels. Across languages, there seems to be an optimal ordering of elements with respect to a syllable peak, which is well-articulated by the Sonority Sequencing Principle (Selkirk, 1984, p. 116)

> In any syllable, there is a segment constituting
> a sonority peak that is preceded and/or followed
> by a sequence of segments with progressively
> decreasing sonority values.

Schematically, this relationship is shown in the following manner:

Onset   *Nucleus*   *Coda*
stop > fric. > nasal > liq. > vowel < liq. < nasal < fric. < stop

Because the co-occurrence of consonants within the onset and coda is governed by principles of sonority, languages frequently permit onset clusters of the form /pl/, /dr/, and /kl/, but the reverse sequencing is rare or not seen at all. Similarly, there is an undeniable preference in languages for coda clusters to put the lower sonority item at the end of the syllable. For example, /mp/ and /nd/ are much more common than /pm/ and /dn/ as codas. Consequently, between the following two hypothetical monosyllabic words with onset and coda clusters, *prant* and *rpant*, the former is the natural, and the latter is highly marked.

The appeal to sonority is not only to separate what is natural from unnatural but also to show the relative degrees of naturalness. When languages allow clusters of two consonants in onset and codas, certain patterns are followed with respect to sonority distance between the two elements. Here, we find that, the greater the sonority distance is between the members of the cluster, the more natural the sequence is. Although none of the following onset clusters violates the sonority sequencing principle because C1 always has lower sonority value than C2 in all, clusters /pr/ or /kr/ are more natural than clusters such as /bl/ or /fr/. The reason for this is that /pr/ or /kr/ gives us the sequence of a voiceless stop with /r/, which is a transition in sonority values from 1 to 7. On the other hand, a /bl/ cluster reveals a transition from a voiced stop to a lateral (from 2 to 6), and /fr/ is a transition from a voiceless fricative to an /r/ (from 3 to 7).

The mirror image of this tendency is observed in codas. Among the codas /nd, ld, rt/, none of which is in violation of the sonority sequencing principle, the following relative naturalness emerges: The least marked cluster will be /rt/, which has the greatest sonority distance between its members, 7 to 1, followed by /ld/ with 6 to 2. The most marked in the group is /nd/, which has the minimum sonority distance of 3 (the result of the transition from 5 to 2). The obvious implication from these is that, if a language permits the sequencing of two consonants with a smaller sonority distance, then it will also allow clusters with greater sonority distances, a prediction that is borne out in languages.

NATURAL PROCESSES

When the preferred types of segments and sequences that are brought about through tendencies in acquisition or phonological events from languages of the world are examined, it becomes apparent that most of them share a common goal called *ease of articulation*. In Chapter 5, several phonetically motivated processes that are found in the phonologies of languages were discussed. The following looks at the motivation for some common patterns that are seen in phonological acquisition.

Cluster reduction and final consonant deletion both have the objective of creating more preferred syllable types. Cluster reduction sequences segments as CV(C); final consonant deletion creates open syllables. In the former, different clusters are reduced in different ways. For example, it is very common to see initial /bl/ → /b/, /pr/ → /p/, and /kl/ → /k/, in which the second member of the cluster is deleted. On the other hand, initial clusters such as /st/ and /sk/, are reduced by deleting the first member. In each case, the more marked member of the cluster is deleted. In final consonant deletion, the motivation is to have the universally unmarked CV open-syllable type.

The process of stopping, which applies to fricatives and affricates, is another testimonial for the naturalness of stops. This cross-linguistically very common process in child phonology can be explained with reference to the complexity of the fricative target in which a relatively long period of narrowed approximation of the articulators demands great muscular control. As opposed to this, stops involve very straightforward and simpler contact of the articulators. The process of stopping applies more frequently to voiced fricatives than to voiceless ones (the ratio seems to be 6 to 1) (Olmsted, 1971). Here again, it is important to remember that different word positions reveal different degrees of stopping. For example, /ð/ → [d] is far more common word-initially than word-finally.

Stopping of fricatives and affricates also is observed in phonologies of languages of the world as regular processes. This, however, generally is limited to certain word positions or before or after certain segments. For example, in Albanian, /f/ becomes [p] and /v/ becomes [b] word-finally and before consonants. In Quechua, /β/ becomes [b] and /ɣ/ becomes [g] initially and after nasals. Because these cases generally are limited to certain environments, this stopping cannot be equated with what happens in child language in which the process generally operates in a context-free fashion. Final consonant devoicing is also a common process that is seen in phonological acquisition as well as in phonological rules of languages. As mentioned in Chapter 5, it is phonetically motivated and considered an assimilatory process whereby the voicing of the final obstruent is assimilated to the end of the word silence. In English, there is a tendency to devoice final obstruents in adult speech. This, however, does not mean that former lexical contrasts such as *back* versus *bag* are being lost. They are clearly indicated by a contrast in vowel length whereby the vowel has greater duration before the voiced obstruent.

As far as stops are concerned, there seems to be a clear relationship between the place of articulation and devoicing. Devoicing is observed more commonly with velars than alveolars. Bilabials are most resistant to devoicing. In other words, as the place of articulation moves further back, the propensity for devoicing becomes greater. The motivation for these differential effects based on the place of articulation of the target stop is due to speech aerodynamics. The larger the supraglottal area is for a stop, the better it can accommodate glottal flow for some time before oral pressure exceeds subglottal pressure and stops the vocal cord vibration. Because the cavity size is increasingly smaller as we go from bilabial to alveolar and then to velar, velars have the least chance of maintaining the glottal flow and, thus, are more quickly devoiced.

Fronting of velars and palatals creates favored front articulations. As seen earlier, generative phonology markedness assigns an unmarked value to [+anterior]. The fronting process results in segments that have this specification. Thus, /k/ → [t], /g/ → [d], and /ʃ/ → [s] result in more unmarked (less marked) segments. It is important to note that while palatal fronting (/ʃ/ → [s]) is common in child phonology and also in adult slips (Shattuck-Hufnagel, 1975), the reverse, /s/ → [ʃ] palatalization contextually before high front vowels or palatal glides, is also natural.

Finally, processes that seem to be restricted mainly to child phonology, such as liquid gliding, also result in unmarked segments.[5]

Although it is customary to see explanations for these phenomena in articulatory terms, acoustic explanations for them cannot and should not be ignored. In Chapter 4, Stevens and Keyser's (1989) enhancement model was shown to be quite effective in explaining child substitution processes such as fronting and stopping. Other processes such as liquid gliding and devoicing also lend themselves to this model's enhancement relationships. In fact, Stevens and Keyser's primary objective was to provide an explanation for the most commonly found 10 consonants among 500 cited by Maddieson (1984), whose work is based on 317 languages. As such, the enhancement model provides a metric for markedness.

In analyzing child substitutions, we saw that the substitutes revealed more preferred feature combinations than the targets based on the enhancement relationships. This way, the directionality of substitutions was accounted for, thus enabling us to distinguish normal (unmarked) substitutions from unusual (marked) ones. This account, in addition to separating marked from unmarked, brings in the rather neglected, but welcomed, acoustic dimension.

In this chapter, we have looked at several topics that are related to naturalness in phonology. Finding a principled way to distinguish unmarked segments, syllables, and processes from marked ones has been of longtime concern to phonologists, as these have reflections in several areas of applied phonology as well as in its implications to phonological theory.

The topic of markedness also will be of considerable interest in the acquisition of the phonology of another language, which will be dealt with in the next chapter. The latest developments on markedness in phonological theory will be discussed in Chapter 10 in relation to the theory of underspecification.

NOTES

1. "Series" is defined in terms of sets of stops that share the same manner (same phonation type, i.e., voiceless, voiced, breathy voiced, laryngealized), same airstream, same relative timing (aspirated versus unaspirated), and same relative timing of velic closure (nasal, oral).

2. This is explainable with reference to the aerodynamics of voicing which is given later in this chapter.

3. Whether a fricative counts as an obstruent or a liquid is a matter of phonological analysis. For example, /x/ and /ʁ/ of Portuguese (phonetically, fricative) function as liquids in the phonological system.

4. A cover term for taps and trills.

5. There are some processes that are observed in developmental phonology in which the opposite tendency is observed. For example, in consonant harmony, alveolars seem to assimilate to velars or to labials more often than the reverse. See Chapter 10 for an explanation of this phenomenon.

EXERCISES

1. Comment on the marked/unmarked nature of the following systems:

CHEROKEE (Macro-Siouan, W North Carolina; 10,000 speakers)

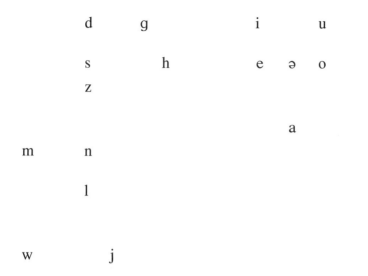

HAWAIIAN (Austro-Tai, Hawaii; 250 speakers)

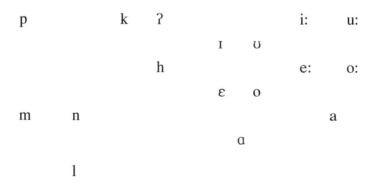

GUARANI (Andean-Equatorial, Paraguay; 2.5 million speakers)

p   t   k   kʷ   ʔ   i   i   u   i: i: u:

    s   ʃ   x   e   o   e: o:

v   ɣ   ɣʷ   a   a:

m   n   ŋ   ŋʷ

w   j

2. Consider the following list of hypothetical words with initial or final consonant clusters and comment on their naturalness:

Initial Clusters	*Final Clusters*
[ploz]	[tipm]
[mbet]	[θɛsr]
[rpum]	[ŋond]
[snot]	[getl]
[kluð]	[ðims]
[vdon]	[zuls]
[zkir]	[murt]
[zret]	[hertʃ]

3. First, give the consonant and the vowel inventory of English. Then evaluate them with respect to expected/unexpected patterns.

Chapter 8

BILINGUAL PHONOLOGY

To many people living in a monolingual environment, bilingualism may seem a little exotic. It may be regarded as a phenomenon restricted to a few countries such as India, Canada, Switzerland, and Paraguay. The facts, however, speak rather differently: Bilingualism is present practically everywhere to a greater or lesser degree. Because bilingualism exists across all social classes and in every age group, no segment of the society is immune to it.

Before we examine aspects of bilingual phonology, we must decide who qualifies as bilingual. For decades, scholars have struggled with this question because bilingualism defies delimitation and is open to a variety of descriptions and interpretations. For example, Bloomfield (1933) required nativelike control of two languages, and Weinreich (1968) and Mackey (1970) considered a bilingual as an individual who alternately uses two languages.

The following situations, among many others, are all examples of bilingualism:

- A 4-year-old whose home language is Haitian Creole and who has been attending an English-speaking preschool in South Florida

- A Brazilian child from a German- or Italian-speaking family in the southern state of Rio Grande do Sul who is going to school where all subjects are taught through the medium of Portuguese

- A schoolchild from a Mexican family living in the southern United States who increasingly uses English both at home and outside, but whose grandparents address him in Spanish only.

These and many other comparable situations have led scholars to take a more flexible stand on the definition of bilingualism, which is well-characterized in the following quote by Beatens-Beardsmore (1982): "Bilingualism as a concept has open-ended semantics" (p. 1) In other words, it is not possible to label bilingualism with only one neat definition because it is a concept with a wide range of variation.

BILINGUALS LEARNING PHONOLOGY

One of the controversial aspects of bilingualism concerns the question of the number of systems the speaker uses. This question is intimately tied to the type of bilingualism considered here. Bilinguals can be divided into two groups: simultaneous bilinguals and successive bilinguals.

In simultaneous bilingualism, in which the two languages are acquired simultaneously, the initial question is to what extent the bilingual child develops two separate linguistic systems, in this case, phonologies. There seems to be some controversy over this matter. Ingram (1981) looked at a 2-year-old English/Italian bilingual child and claimed that his subject showed evidence of two separate phonological systems with different characteristics that were traceable to the two languages involved. Based on this, Ingram suggested that these different preferences were proof of two systems.

Duchar and Clark (1992) stated that their subject, a Spanish/English bilingual child, who was studied between the ages 1 year 7 months and 2 years 3 months, developed separate voicing systems for the two languages.

On the other hand, several other researchers (Burling, 1959; Imedadze, 1967; Leopold, 1949; Major, 1977; Vogel, 1975; Vihman, 1985; Yavas, 1995) have suggested an initial undifferentiated system. Yavas (1995), studying the first 50 word period of his Portuguese/Turkish bilingual son, found avoidance patterns that were clearly language independent. For example, regardless of the language, words with initial fricatives or initial liquids were avoided. Such examples support an undifferentiated system that prefers less marked phonological patterning at that stage of development regardless of the language.

The controversy is probably due to the stage(s) studied in each case mentioned above. Those who defend two separate systems have dealt with subjects beyond the first 50 word period who had multiword utterances, whereas the defenders of an undifferentiated system have concentrated on an earlier stage. Accordingly, it seems that the separation of the two systems is generally accomplished around age 2, when the child is out of the first 50 word period.

Once the child starts separating the systems, patterns become subject to a dominance relationship. In a great majority of cases, unequal exposure to the languages, contexts in which each language is used, and so on, blur the picture, and one of the languages becomes more dominant. Because perfectly balanced bilinguals are very rare, competencies in two languages should be treated as a continuum. Watson (1991) discussed the following three possibilities regarding the two language systems of a balanced bilingual after the initial stage of one mixed system. It is possible: (1) to have two completely independent phonological and phonetic systems, each identical in all ways to those of monolinguals; (2) to have a degree of integration between the two systems; (3) to have two systems that differ in some way from those of monolinguals.

It is argued that studies on balanced bilinguals support the last possibility with respect to production. This means that these individuals achieve nativelike competence at the phonemic level, matching the monolinguals in both languages, while having some differences at the phonetic level. These phonetic differences, although they can be captured clearly by acoustic measurements, are not distinguishable from the productions of monolinguals, because there is phonetic variation among monolinguals as well. Thus, it appears that the balanced bilingual functions, for all practical purposes, like a monolingual in the two languages, although without perfectly matching their phonetic productions. Watson suggested that the bilingual reaches a compromise between the need to sound sufficiently like a native speaker of the two languages and, at the same time, the need to reduce the processing load of phonetic details in the two systems.

In successive bilingualism, the person normally acquires one language (the home language) and starts acquiring the other language when she or he starts (pre)school or later in life. In such situations, the influence of one language over the other will be more evident.

CRITICAL AGE HYPOTHESIS

Before dealing with the interference patterns in bilinguals, an issue that seems to be very important in the determination of a bilingual's capability of acquiring nativelike phonology must be considered. This is the age factor.

The question to be discussed is why certain individuals can manage to acquire the phonology of the second language in a nativelike manner, whereas others fail to do so. This issue is especially intriguing because many bilinguals have apparent native control over all aspects of the second language except phonology. It is rather common to meet an individual who is very fluent in syntax but has obvious non-native pronunciation. Former Secretary of State Henry Kissinger and former National Security Advisor Zbigniev Brezinski are good examples of such bilinguals. It is, on the other hand, rather difficult to find individuals who have perfect native phonology, but faulty syntax or morphology. These observations suggest that phonology is a special case in second language acquisition.

In answering the question of why certain people can acquire all aspects of a second language in a nativelike manner except phonology, one factor, age of learning, stands out. Many other variables can affect the language-learning situation in naturalistic settings. These include input conditions, personality, motivation, and other such factors. Although these factors are influential, there is no clear correlation between them and success in pronunciation per se.

A point that is made frequently relates to the comparison of individuals who live in similar situations but show different (native/non-native) phonological patterns in the second language. As seen in many immigrant families, although the parents become very fluent in English, their phonologies are always non-native. Children, on the other hand, can and usually do, acquire native phonology if their age of learning is prepuberty. These facts led researchers to suggest a critical age for learning pronunciation.

Simply put, it is suggested that there is a sensitive period from birth to puberty in which it is possible to acquire second language phonology in a nativelike manner. This capacity seems to deteriorate after puberty and, consequently, the other factors (environmental and personal), however favorable, will not be sufficient to make the L2 (second language) pronunciation of the learner accent-free. Thus, a person who acquires a second language before the end of this critical period will have a marked phonological advantage over a later learner.

Oyama's (1976) study is probably one of the best demonstrations of this point. She looked at the pronunciation ability of 60 Italian immigrants with different lengths of residence and different ages of arrival in the United States. The results showed that, although length of residence bore no relationship to the foreign accent, there was a strong correlation between accent and the subjects' age of arrival.

Thompson (1991) examined a wide range of independent variables including age of arrival (age of learning), length of residence, degree of English language usage, sex, and self-reported characteristics such as ability to mimic, motivation, and extraversion, and found that the age of arrival (age of learning) was the best predictor of accent.

The idea that the relationship between the capacity to acquire L2 phonology and age of learning is one of progressive decline is also supported by Scovel (1988); Asher and Garcia (1969); Tahta, Wood, and Loewenthal (1981); and Patkowski (1994).

Although the majority of researchers agree on around the time of puberty (roughly 12–15 years of age) as the critical age for L2 phonology, there are some who set the ceiling for this period at a younger age. Long (1990), for example, stated that "exposure needs to occur before age six to guarantee that an L2 phonology can become native like" (p. 274). Flege and Fletcher (1992) suggested that accented speech is highly unusual in individuals whose age of learning is not older than 6. However, it becomes increasingly evident after that age.

Among the topics in interlingual phonology that have dealt with the age of learning, voice onset time (VOT) has been a popular focus of attention for Spanish-English bilinguals. The relevance of studying VOT comes from the fact that its values have been claimed to be closely correlated with overall degree of authentic nativelike speech or global foreign accent (Flege & Eefting, 1986, 1987; Major, 1987).

Spanish and English differ in their VOT values for stop consonants. English voiceless stops /p, t, k/ at the beginning of a stressed syllable have long lag VOT (aspirated), whereas Spanish voiceless stops have coincident and short lag VOT (unaspirated). It has been observed that late Spanish-English bilinguals produce English voiceless stops either with VOT values identical to their L1 (first language) or with compromise values—significantly shorter VOT values than monolingual English speakers produce (Flege, 1987, 1991; Flege & Port, 1981; Lowie, 1988; Nathan et al., 1987).

There is, on the other hand, evidence that early L2 learners may keep the two languages separate and produce stops in an authentic manner in the two languages involved. Williams (1977) reported that subjects who learned both English and Spanish by age 6 were equal to monolingual English and Spanish speakers in VOT values. Mack (1989) reported subjects who learned French (a language similar to Spanish with respect to VOT) and English by the age of 7 and who showed VOT values for stops identical to those of monolinguals in English and French. Flege (1991), examining the production of English /t/, found that most early L2 learners (age of learning 5 or 6 years) produced the targets with mean VOT values that fell within or exceeded the range of values observed for native speakers of English.

To examine whether the ceiling of the sensitive period requires the age of learning to be as low as 6 years or could go as high as 12 or so, Yavas (1996) studied two groups of Spanish-English bilinguals in relation to VOT values of English voiceless stops. Early bilinguals, who learned Spanish as their first language and added English when they started school or preschool, and later bilinguals, who learned English around 12 years of age, were compared. Results showed that, although early bilinguals' VOT values were significantly different (greater) than those of later bilinguals and were closer to the prototypical monolingual English speakers, the later group's VOTs were still within the possible limits of the native range. These results suggest that our ability to acquire the aspects of L2 pronunciation in a nativelike manner diminishes with the increase of age but is not lost fully at the age of 12.

It is important to add the following caveat before concluding this section: Although there is unanimous agreement that a sensitive period for acquisition of a second language phonology exists, this does not mean that accent-free speech is guaranteed for learners before puberty. It only states that the potential to acquire nativelike phonology continues until the end of this period, and is not available thereafter. However, in order to realize this potential, all other relevant conditions—cognitive, socio-effective, input, and so on—must be optimal.

INTERFERENCE PATTERNS

When successive bilinguals are considered, it is commonly observed that, depending on the dominance patterns, the first language of the learner exerts influence over the later language. In a classic study, Weinreich (1953) suggested that a speaker identifies a phoneme of the secondary system with one in the primary system and, in reproducing it, subjects it to the phonetic rules of the primary system. Weinreich described interference in the following four ways:

Under-Differentiation of Phonemes

This occurs when two sounds of the secondary system for which counterparts are not distinguished in the primary system are confused. The examples cited from Spanish and English in Chapter 3 illustrate this well. In Spanish, /d/ is a phoneme with two conditioned variants: [d] occurs in word-initial position and after [n], [ð] occurs in intervocalic position. In English /d/ and /ð/ are separate phonemes. A speaker whose primary system is Spanish might treat English /d/ and /ð/ as allophones of one phoneme, failing to note and produce the contrast in words like *day* and *they* when dealing with English as the secondary system.

Over-Differentiation of Phonemes

This involves the imposition of phonemic distinctions from the primary system on the sounds of the secondary system, in which they are not required. For example, a speaker whose primary system is English may interpret Spanish [b] and [β] as allophones of two phonemes /b/ and /v/.

Reinterpretation of Distinctions

This occurs when the speaker distinguishes phonemes of the secondary system by features that are merely redundant in that system, but are relevant in the primary system. For example, Finnish has distinctive vowel length; a speaker whose primary system is Finnish may disregard the vowel quality difference in English words like *sit* and *seat* and distinguish between them on the basis of the difference in the duration of the two-syllable nuclei.

Phone Substitution

This applies to phonemes that are defined identically in two languages but for which pronunciation differs. For example, Portuguese /t/ is dental and unaspirated, and English /t/ is alveolar and contextually aspirated; yet, both are classified as [+coronal, +anterior, –voiced, –continuant].

Sounds of the dominant language are not the only things that are transferred in the acquisition of another language; there is evidence that learners attempt to maintain their native language syllable structure. When the target language allows syllable structures that are not permitted in the native (dominant) language, learners modify them according to what is allowed in their language. As cited earlier, Spanish does not allow the sequence of /sC/ (where C = any consonant) in word-initial position. Thus, the target English words with such structures are modified according to the structures permitted in Spanish. Words such as *school*, *speak* are realized as [ɛskul], [ɛspik] respectively.

In addition to these segmental and sequential concerns, we can observe rhythmic differences between the two languages involving stress and intonation. Tiffin (1974) suggested that intelligibility of Yoruba and Hausa speakers' productions of Nigerian English was closely related to the stress patterns of the native languages. Between the two, the Hausa suprasegmental system more closely resembles that of English. Consequently, the Hausa speakers' English was more intelligible than that of Yoruba speakers.

To give some other examples, we can look at the following conflict between Arabic and English: Although Arabic sentence stress is similar to English (content words are usually stressed and function words are unstressed), function words keep their full forms without any of the vowel reduction that is typical for English in unstressed position. This may create problems for Arabic speakers learning English.

Certain suffixes in Italian have English counterparts. For example, *-ta* corresponds to English *-ty* and *-zione* corresponds to English *-tion*:

abilita	ability	relazione	relation
carita	charit	nazione	nation

In Italian words with these suffixes, the suffixes are stressed. This is different from English; therefore, Italian speakers learning English may transfer these habits into new situations and make stress errors.

Mismatches between native and target language were held responsible for foreign accent in Adams' (1979) study of Vietnamese and Cambodian learners of English. Native language influence on intonation of L2 was also cited by Purschel (1975), Willems (1982), and Van Els and DeBot (1987).

HIERARCHIES OF DIFFICULTY

In the 1950s and 1960s, the hey-day of structural linguistics, it was thought that everything that appeared in a bilingual's speech could be explained on the basis of the contrasts involving the structures of the two languages. A huge industry was created to establish contrastive phonologies between the source language (L1) and the target language (L2), and several books were written comparing systems such as Spanish-English, German-English, and Italian-English contrastive phonologies.

The discrepancies between the two languages involved also gave scholars many opportunities to observe different degrees of difficulty experienced by learners. Hierarchies of difficulty were attempted on the basis of whether certain categories were present or absent in the native and target languages and, if they are present, whether they are obligatory or optional. The following hierarchy is from one of the most well-known studies in this respect (Stockwell & Bowen, 1983):

Difficulty

Magnitude	*Order*	*Native language*	*Target language*
	1	∅	Obligatory
I	2	∅	Optional
	3	Optional	Obligatory
	4	Obligatory	Optional
II	5	Obligatory	∅
	6	Optional	∅
III	7	Optional	Optional
	8	Obligatory	Obligatory

Optional categories are phonemes that may or may not occur in a particular phonological context. Obligatory categories are allophones that must be used in a given phonological context. Finally, zero, or null, categories are cases of the complete absence of a sound in the language. The degree of difficulty is shown in descending order; whereas Magnitude I Order 1 represents the most difficult learning situation, Magnitude III Order 8 is the easiest.

However, scholars dealing with the acquisition of L2 phonology soon realized that the predictions based on such a hierarchy were not solid. For example, the palato-alveolar fricative /ʃ/ is a phoneme of English, but does not occur in Spanish. This discrepancy qualifies as Magnitude I Order 2 and, thus, should create considerable difficulty. Although the difficulty is real and can easily be observed, there are problems encountered in this explanation. Not all sounds that are lacking in L1 will be equally difficult. It appears that some relationship exists between the frequency of a sound in languages and its difficulty in L2 learning. A sound like /ʃ/, which appears in many languages, should not be as difficult as a rare sound like /ħ/, which is rare in languages. Thus, the relative markedness of the sound could determine its relative ease or difficulty in L2 acquisition.

Also, through a series of experiments, Flege (1987) demonstrated that sounds that are similar to those in L1 are more difficult to learn than sounds that are novel. If the two languages have the same sounds, then no difficulty is observed. However, when we compare totally new sounds with phonetically similar sounds, it was found that the new sounds were successfully produced in a nativelike manner by learners, whereas there were problems with phonetically similar ones. The explanation for why such sounds create greater difficulty comes from the idea that the representation of a sound in the native language guides the learning of a sound in the second language. Because a phonetically similar, but not identical, sound in L1 already has a representation, it makes the creation of a representation for a similar but different sound in L2 difficult.

In addition to the difficulty of similar sounds in languages, the hierarchy runs into problems regarding situations that are characterized identically but, in fact, reveal different degrees of difficulty. A well-known example comes from obstruent voicing and devoicing. Let us now compare the following two L2 learning situations:

Both English and German have the stop phonemes /p, t, k, b, d, g/ and both languages have contrasts between the voiced and voiceless stops in initial and medial positions. In final position, however, the situation is different; whereas English allows the contrast (e.g., *bag* vs. *back*), German neutralizes the opposition in favor of the voiceless members. Thus, only /p, t, k/ are allowed in final position in German. As a result of this discrepancy, we can predict that a speaker of German would have problems with target-final voiced stops in English. That this prediction is correct can be seen in examples in which English final voiced stops are realized with the voiceless counterparts (e.g., *bag* → [bæk], *bed* → [bɛt]).

The second case to be considered comes from an English-French contact situation. This time, we look at the voicing contrast for another obstruent. Both English and French have /ʃ/ and /ʒ/ contrast in medial and final positions, but only French extends this contrast to initial position. That is, English does not have this contrast initially, and allows only /ʃ/ in the initial position. As a result of this discrepancy, an English speaker who is learning French is expected to have difficulties for French words that have initial /ʒ/ targets.

The two situations discussed (German–English and English–French) are descriptively identical in that phonemes in both L1 and L2 show the voicing contrasts in obstruents in all word positions only in the L2s; the L1s are defective in this respect and the situation can be illustrated in the following manner:

	/ʒ/				/b, d, g/		
	initial	*medial*	*final*		*initial*	*medial*	*final*
L1(Eng.)	–	+	+	L1(Ger.)	+	+	–
L2(Fre.)	+	+	+	L2(Eng.)	+	+	+

Any person who has had contact with learners in the two situations described above must have witnessed that the difficulties experienced by the German speaker learning English final voiced stops are far greater than the English speaker attempting initial /ʒ/ sounds in French. This results in a situation in which two descriptively identical conflicts between L1 and L2 result in two very different degrees of difficulty. Such cases led scholars to modify their positions with respect to degrees of difficulty. Whereas predictions given earlier were made solely on the basis of matches and mismatches between L1 and L2, researchers turned their attention more to markedness. Eckman (1977, 1985) suggested a principle which states that the areas of the target language that are different from and relatively more marked in the native language will be difficult. Eckman defines the concept marked in the following way: "A structure X in some language is relatively more marked than some other structure Y if cross-linguistically the presence of X in a language implies the presence of Y, but the presence of Y does not imply the presence of X" (p. 290).

As far as voicing of obstruents is concerned, we see the following patterns in languages: Contrast in final position implies a contrast medially, which, in turn, implies a contrast initially. The reverse, however, does not hold. Consequently, the final position is the unmarked position for the voiceless and the marked position for the voiced obstruents. Because the

German speaker acquiring English is dealing with marked segments (final voiced stops) and the English speaker acquiring French is not, the greater difficulty of the former can be accounted for.

DISTINCTIVE FEATURES IN INTERLANGUAGE PHONOLOGY

Weinreich's (1953) model of sound substitutions and interference patterns is not the only approach to account for interference phenomena. In a model proposed by Ritchie (1968) and Michaels (1973), sound substitutions are analyzed on the basis of phonological features. This model is based on Halle's (1959) condition imposed on the underlying segments in which the maximum number of feature specifications in underlying segments is rendered predictable by phonological rules. Decision trees are drawn in which each node represents a feature and each branch from a node represents a value (+ or –) of the feature (see Figures 8–1, 8–2, and 8–3). The first node divides all segments into two classes, the second node further divides each of these into two classes, and so on. Each path through the tree represents a distinct segment. Each segment is identified by asking a sequence of questions to categorize it according to its phonological features, for example, is it sonorant, is it coronal, and so on for each feature in each level of the model.

According to the model, an L2 learner screens the sounds in such a manner when confronted with a foreign segment. The learner asks feature questions of the foreign segment and assigns to it the various subsets of the native language inventory. Ritchie (1968) did not mention the possibility of a strict order, or hierarchy, in which questions must be asked, because it is believed that the identification of any one segment is more efficient for a given language if the questions are asked in one order than if they are asked in another. Once feature prominences are determined for a given L1, the substitution for incoming foreign segments is predicted.

The substitutions for English interdental fricatives, /θ / and /ð/ have been a very popular topic for this approach, and different replacements of these targets by speakers of various languages in the form of [s, z] or [t, d] were explained by different prominence patterns in different systems. In Figure 8–1, we will look at the analysis of the Spanish substitution of [t] for English / θ/ via distinctive feature decision trees. As seen in Figure 8–1, this analysis will not yield the desired result; /θ /, having [+continuant] specification, will not reach the actual rendition [t], which is [–continuant].

Another attempt to explain L2 sound substitutions within the framework of distinctive features was proposed by Carter (reported by Holden, 1972). Unlike the earlier attempts at predicting substitutions, Carter stated two well-defined principles that govern the order of questions to be asked. These are: (1) parsimony, which dictates that the most economical or symmetrical feature system should be employed, and (2) hierarchy, which states that certain features must (universally) be ordered before others. In reviewing the models above, Figure 8–1 will not be acceptable, because it does not follow the requirement of parsimony, as the [continuant] feature gives a 7 to 3 division for the [–sonorant] group. If we want to have a more parsimonious division, we can modify the picture by placing the feature [continuant] lower in the tree. This is given in Figure 8–2. Although this modified diagram gives a more parsimonious picture (at least for 5 to 5 coronal), it still cannot predict the actual rendition [t], because the last branching in the tree favors [s]. The only course we can take to remedy this situation, and reach the actual rendition [t] by a distinctive feature tree is to replace [continuant] with the feature [strident]. This is given in Figure 8–3. Although the tree in Figure 8–3 correctly finds the actual rendition, [t], it is not acceptable for the following reasons: First, the feature [strident] is totally unnecessary in the differentiation of Spanish phonemes. Second, the purpose of [strident] is used for contrasts between certain pairs of fricatives and affricates with the same or similar places of articulation. Yet, in Figure 8–3, [strident] is used to differentiate stops from fricatives and affricates. Feature systems normally utilize [continuant] for this function. Finally, the picture obtained violates the principle of parsimony by yielding a 7 to 3 division of the [–sonorant] group for the feature [strident].

The above concepts seem to show that the prediction of the Spanish rendition of English /θ/ cannot be accomplished in a nonarbitrary fashion via distinctive feature decision trees. This does not mean that the attempt to account for the foreign sound substitutions is useless and should be abandoned. Rather, the model needs to be rethought and revised. New approaches via more current phonological models such as feature geometry and radical underspecification are at work, and will be dealt with in Chapter 10.

UNIVERSAL PATTERNS

Although phonological interference is still considered very influential (and longer lasting than morphological or syntactic interference) and contrastive phonological information is indispensable, we have come to

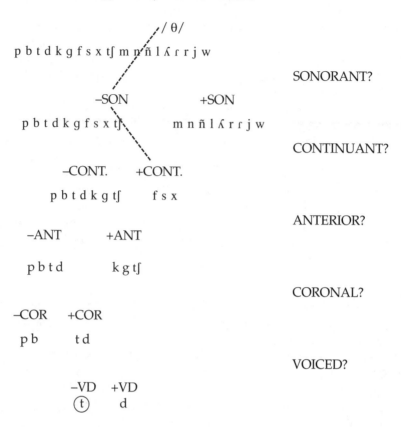

Figure 8–1. Prediction of the rendition of English / T/ by Spanish speakers (continuant after sonorant).

realize that interference does not account for everything in the speech patterns of our subjects. What bilingual speakers do in their phonological patterns is not due solely to the effects of L1 interference. There are universal markedness constraints with respect to phonological acquisition that can explain specific patterns in the speech of our clients or students. Recent years have been fairly productive in giving us convincing evidence regarding the effects of universal markedness constraints. Following are some examples of studies that point in this direction.

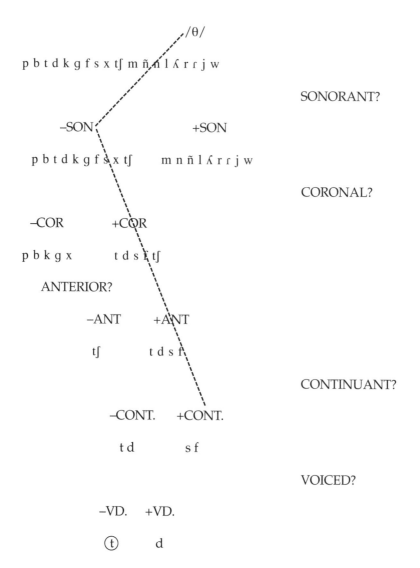

Figure 8–2. Prediction of the rendition of English /T/ by Spanish speakers (coronal after sonorant).

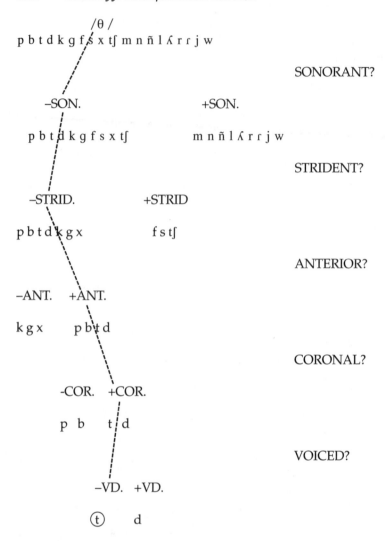

Figure 8–3. Prediction of the rendition of English / θ /, by Spanish speakers (strident after sonorant).

Coda Consonants

Eckman and Iverson (1994) analyzed consonant pronunciation errors in syllable codas in English made by native speakers of Cantonese, Korean, and Japanese. The objective of their study was to find out whether the errors made by the subjects were explainable through markedness constraints based on universals. It was hypothesized that the success of the subjects could be predicted on the basis of the sonority of the coda consonant. Specifically, low sonority codas, such as stops and fricatives (obstruents, would cause more difficulty than high sonority codas, such as liquids and nasals (sonorants). The explanation for this comes from the fact that, universally, obstruents are more marked (less expected) in coda position relative to sonorants. When a language has CVC syllables, the coda positions are most commonly occupied by sonorants. There are two patterns that are observed in languages that allow CVC syllables: (a) obstruent and sonorant codas and (b) only sonorant codas. That is, there is no language that has obstruent codas but lacks sonorant codas. This indicates that sonorants are more natural as codas than obstruents. Table 8–1 shows percentages of mistakes on the English coda targets in the Eckman and Iverson (1994) study.

In all three groups, obstruents constituted the greatest number of errors. As seen in Table 8–1, native language interference cannot be taken as the deciding factor, because what is permitted or not permitted does not nec-

Table 8–1 Percentage of errors in English coda targets by Cantonese, Korean, and Japanese-speaking learners.

% Error	Target	L–1 Features
Cantonese		
77%	Obstruents	(/p,t,k/ permitted in L1)
20%	Liquids	
3%	Nasals	(permitted in L1)
0.5%	Glides	(permitted in L1)
Korean		
84%	Obstruents	(permitted in L1)
13%	Liquids	(/l/ permitted in L1)
2%	Nasals	(permitted in L1)
1%	Glides	
Japanese		
59%	Obstruents	
21%	Liquids	
19%	Nasals	(/n/ permitted in L1)
1%	Glides	

essarily agree with the percentage of errors. For example, both Korean and Cantonese permit obstruents in coda positions, but the subjects committed more errors in that category than in that of consonants that are not allowed in coda position (liquids in the case of Cantonese and glides in the case of Korean). The conclusion from the results is that pronunciation problems of codas cannot be predicted simply on the basis of comparison between the native language and the target language. Rather, explanations for the difficulties of the learners must incorporate universal markedness of particular types of segments in particular positions. The fact that obstruents cause more difficulty than sonorants in coda positions, regardless of the native language background of the learners, is a function of low sonority segments being more marked than high sonority segments in this position.

Onset Clusters

Another issue that shows the importance of markedness relates to different degrees of difficulty encountered in the acquisition of onset clusters of English. In several studies, Carlisle (1988, 1991a, 1991b, 1994) examined the difficulties of Spanish speakers in their acquisition of English onset clusters /sl/, /sN/ (where N = /m/ or /n/), and /sT/ (where T =/p/, /t/, or /k/). As mentioned earlier, Spanish does not allow any word initial /sC/ clusters (where C = consonant) and, expectedly, these clusters create problems for Spanish speakers acquiring English. However, it has been noted that different /sC/ clusters pose different degrees of difficulty, and these different degrees cannot be explained with reference to the native language patterns. Specifically, Carlisle found that /sl/ clusters are the easiest, followed by /sN/ targets. /sT/ onsets are found to be the most difficult. The explanation for this phenomenon comes from universal markedness based on the sonority sequencing generalization which dictates that the sonority values should rise as we move from the margin of the syllable to the peak. (Selkirk, 1982). Among the three targets in question, one of them, /sT/, violates this principle, because the first member of the onset, /s/ (which is a voiceless fricative), has a higher sonority rating, 3, than the second member of the onset cluster /p, t, or k/, which are voiceless stops with a sonority ranking of 1. Thus, as we move from the first to the second member of the onset cluster, a fall in sonority is created. Because this is unexpected according to universal tendencies, it is understandably the most difficult target for the learners. The remaining two targets, /sl/ and /sN/, both satisfy the sonority sequencing generalization because, as we move from the first member (voiceless fricative) to the second member (lateral or nasal), there is an increase in sonority. Further, the fact that /sl/ is found easier than /sN/ targets is still explainable through sonority ranking. Laterals are higher in sonority than nasals (6 vs. 5), and a move from /s/ to a lateral shows a greater amount of increase in sonority than a move from /s/ to a nasal. Thus, a greater change in sonority seems to be easier for the learner.

The suggestion that errors regarding clusters follow universal principles is supported by examples from different language groups. In several languages, unmarked obstruent + sonorant clusters are treated one way, while marked s + stop clusters are treated another way. Broselow (1993) examined the error patterns of Egyptian Arabic, Sindhi, and Bengali speakers during contact with English, and stated that their behavior is entirely congruent with the above pattern. In none of these languages are onset clusters permitted. Consequently, speakers modify target English clusters. However, as the following examples demonstrate, the treatment given to the marked s + stop clusters is clearly different from the treatment of the unmarked obstruent + sonorant clusters:

Egyptian Arabic

street	→	[istirit]	sweater	→	[siwetar]
splendid	→	[izbilendid]	slide	→	[silajd]
study	→	[istadi]			

Sindhi

school	→	[ɪskul]	please	→	[piliz]
spelling	→	[ɪspɛlɪŋ]	slipper	→	[silipər]

Bengali

stamp	→	[istamp]	glass	→	[gelas]
school	→	[iskul]	slate	→	[shelet]

The acquisition of coda consonants and onset clusters reveals processes that interlanguage learners go through when there is mismatch between their first and the second languages. In these cases, the effort is to modify the marked targets into unmarked structures. It was shown in Chapter 6 that children acquiring English as their first language also deal with the same marked targets. Although the marked targets are the same for these two populations, the solutions preferred by adult second language learners are different from those that are utilized by first language learners. For example, when children encounter a CVC target, they typically delete the final consonant, as in *dog* → [dɔ]. The solutions preferred by second language learners is typically to add a vowel after the last consonant, *dog* → [dɔgə]. These different processes—deletion versus epenthesis—also are manifested in dealing with another marked structure, onset clusters. Whereas children typically use deletion as in *play* → [pe], second language learners prefer epenthesis, *play* → [pəle]. Although the ways the two populations choose to deal with the marked targets are different, the effect is the same, namely, to get rid of the marked structures by replacing them with unmarked open syllables.

The question that immediately comes to mind is why the two populations prefer different processes to attack the same marked targets. Weinberger (1994) suggested that these differences are explainable with reference to the recoverability principle which states that "recoverable representations take precedence over unrecoverable ones" (p. 293). According to Weinberger, recoverability is one of the components of grammar that is not available in early childhood and develops gradually. If we compare the resulting forms in child language and adult interlanguage learning, the adult forms resulting from epenthesis are recoverable, whereas the child forms resulting from deletion are not. The following examples illustrate this difference (Weinberger 1994):

	Target	*Epenthesis* (recoverable target)
adult	*seed*	[sidə] "seed, cedar"
		deletion (nonrecoverable target)
child	*seed*	[si] "seed, seat, seep, seek, seize, siege, . . ."

When the last consonant is deleted and the target is nonrecoverable, this creates considerable ambiguity in the resulting form. The adult form undergoing epenthesis, on the other hand, creates very limited ambiguity. Because adults have the recoverability principle available to them, they avoid multiple ambiguity by retaining the last consonant through epenthesis. First language learners, on the other hand, do not have recoverability available to them and, thus, have no reason to retain the final consonant, so they delete it.

Acquisition of English Liquids

Acquisition of English /l/ and /r/ by speakers of other languages is yet another topic that demonstrates the relevance of markedness in interlanguage phonology. Paolillo (1995) studied the acquisition of English liquids by speakers of Mandarin, a language that has different patterns in liquids than English. Contrary to the contrast of /l/ and /r/ in English, which is in any position of the syllable (onset, nucleus, and coda), Mandarin has the contrast only in syllable initial position; there are no syllabic liquids in Mandarin, and only /r/ is found in syllable-final position.

From this contrastive information, it is reasonable to expect that Mandarin speakers should be able to differentiate the two liquids in English only in onset position. English contrasts found in other positions would be problematic for them.

Paolillo (1995) examined the rendition of liquids in the following five environments: postconsonantal (e.g., *from, plenty*), word-initial (e.g., *republic, lesson*), intervocalic (e.g., *parent, family*), syllable nucleus (e.g., *razor, able*), and postvocalic (e.g., *years, ball*), and found four different substitution patterns. These were complete neutralization, in which the two sets of phones are completely neutralized; subset neutralization, in which one set of phones has a broader range of variation than the other (/r/ is represented by [l] and /l/ is represented by [l], [ɨ], and [əl]); overlap neutralization, in which the two sets of phones are largely distinct, but with some overlap (/r/ is represented by [l], [w], and [j], and /l/ is represented by [l]); and no neutralization, which represents a nativelike pattern. Subset and overlap neutralizations may seem similar because the phone [l] is shared between the two categories, but this is less so in subset neutralization than in overlap neutralization.

Looking at the results of his investigation, Paolillo found a sequence of acquisition moving from complete neutralization to a weak distinction (subset neutralization), to greater distinction (overlap neutralization), to no neutralization (complete contrast). It also was found that there was a hierarchy of environments in which neutralization occurred. This was #___ < Ç < V__V < C___ < ___C/# (word-initial < syllabic < intervocalic < postconsonantal < and postvocalic). If learners neutralize the target English liquid contrast in one environment, they usually neutralize it in all the environments to the right. This means that, if there is a neutralization in an intervocalic target, then there will be a neutralization in postconsonantal and postvocalic environments. The explanation for this hierarchy comes from the relative acoustic salience of the sounds in each of these environments. Relative salience is higher in initial or syllabic positions than in other transitory positions or in clusters. Most overlap neutralizations occur in the least favorable (most marked) postvo-calic environment, and stronger contrasts are found in initial (most unmarked) position for which the relative salience is higher. The order of acquisition, which is in accordance with the relative salience of different environments, indicates that more marked structures are more difficult to learn. Thus, the patterns of acquisition of English liquid contrasts reconfirm the principle that the difficulties encountered by the learners cannot solely be explained via native language transfer, and that the universal markedness of sounds in a given environment must be considered.

Final Devoicing

Finally, we will deal with another common process in the speech patterns of L2 learners, final devoicing. This process generally affects voiced obstruents in final position but, in some cases, it is restricted to stops only. It is a common process in developmental phonology in which the final voiced targets in words like *dog* and *bed* are realized by native English-speaking children with voiceless versions [dɔk] and [bɛt]. As mentioned earlier in Chapter 5, many languages, such as German, Russian, Basque, Turkish, Bulgarian, and Polish, allow only voiceless stops in final position. When English is learned as a second language, the same tendency is observed in the speech of the learners. If this happens in the learning patterns of subjects whose native language is German, Russian, Polish, or Turkish, we might suggest first or dominant language interference. But the process is not restricted to these learners and is observed in the speech of people whose native languages are Portuguese, Mandarin, and Japanese, which do not allow any stops, voiced or voiceless, in final position. It was mentioned earlier that, for obstruents, final position is the unmarked position for voiceless and the marked position for voiced. This means that, when speakers of languages that have no final stops show a tendency to devoice the English final voiced targets, this must be due to universal markedness rather than any native language interference. Thus, although a simple contrastive analysis cannot predict this, an accurate prediction can be made on the basis of markedness.

There are some considerations that make certain targets more prone to devoicing than others. In Chapter 7, it was mentioned that there is a correlation between the place of articulation of the target-final voiced stop and its propensity for devoicing, and as we move the place of articulation farther back, the chances for devoicing increase. As a result, velars devoice most easily, and alveolars devoice easier than bilabials.

Another factor contributing to final devoicing comes from the height of the vowel preceding the final voiced stop. Increasing the height of the vowel creates a more favorable environment for devoicing of the stop targets. The reason for this is that high vowels, by raising the tongue and creating more constriction than other vowels, cause higher supraglottal pressure, and are more prone to devoicing (Jaeger, 1978). This vulnerability to devoicing seems to be carried over to the following final voiced stops (Parucci, 1983; Plevyak, 1982).

Yavas (1997b) studied these factors with data from 19 subjects whose native languages were Mandarin Chinese, Japanese, and Portuguese and found support for the above hypotheses. Subjects revealed more devoicing as the place of articulation of the final voiced stop moved from bilabial to alveolar and from alveolar to velar. Also, as shown in Figure 8–4, changing the vowel preceding the final voiced stop made a significant difference for alveolar and velar stops.

To sum up these studies, several problems in the acquisition of L2 phonology do not seem to lend themselves to explanations based in the first language of the learners. Because these tendencies are found in learners from diverse languages as well as in developmental phonologies in monolingual children, the native languages of the learners (L1 interference) cannot be held responsible, and universal constraints must be brought into the discussion.

The relationship between L1 interference and universal constraints is a complicated one. Major (1987) offered a strictly hierarchical interrelationship between language-specific transfer errors and universal developmental errors. In his Ontogeny Model, the claim made is that transfer effects (L1 interference) decrease over time, whereas universal developmental errors are infrequent initially, then increase, and finally decrease.

Major suggested that the same pattern occurs in relation to style; as style becomes more formal, interference errors decrease while universal developmental errors increase. Supporting evidence is cited from Wode (1981), Dickerson (1977), and Major (1986).

Developing bilingual phonology is a very complex matter and requires more information regarding its different aspects; for example, the importance of the age factor, first language phonology, how those patterns are acquired, and the contrastive information between the structure of the first and the second language that is being learned. This vitally important information will need to be complemented by universal markedness conditions that are observed in second language acquisition. In addition to these data, information about the degree of dominance between two languages in the bilingual is needed to complete the whole picture, as this will inevitably affect the interaction of the first language interference and the universal constraints in shaping his or her speech patterns.

CLINICAL RELEVANCE

When we look at children growing up with more than one language, we observe that their production of the ambient language may show certain patterns that are erroneous with reference to the monolingual speakers of

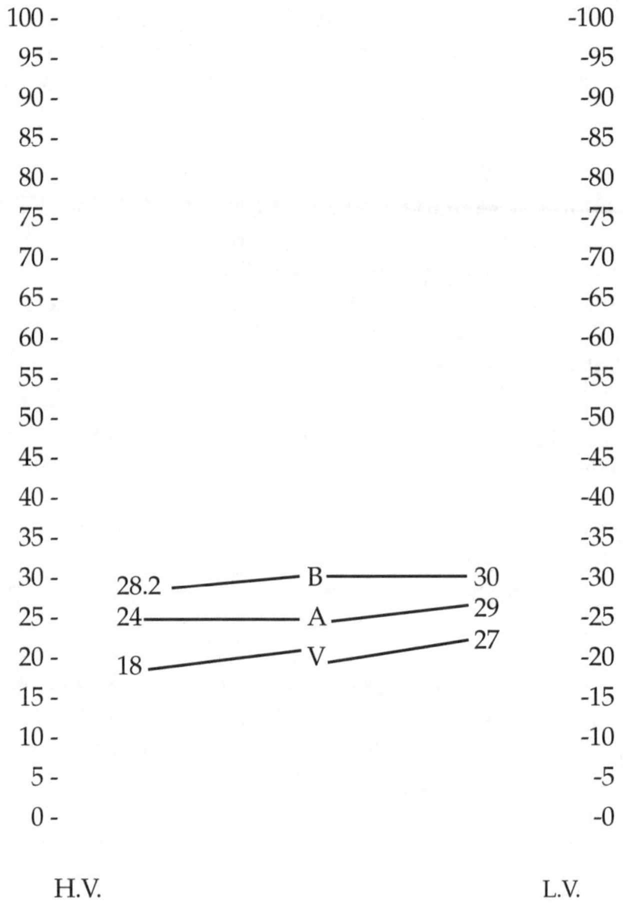

100 -		-100
95 -		-95
90 -		-90
85 -		-85
80 -		-80
75 -		-75
70 -		-70
65 -		-65
60 -		-60
55 -		-55
50 -		-50
45 -		-45
40 -		-40
35 -		-35
30 -	28.2 ——— B ——— 30	-30
25 -	24——— A ——— 29	-25
20 -	18 ——— V ——— 27	-20
15 -		-15
10 -		-10
5 -		-5
0 -		-0

H.V.   L.V.

B = Bilabial, A = Alveolar, V = Velar, H.V. = High vowel,
L.V. = Low vowel

Figure 8–4. Percentage of the voicing of final stops according to the place of articulation of the target stop and the height of the preceding vowel.

that language. In these circumstances, we would like to find out whether these nonconforming patterns are due to the influence of the child's other language(s), or if this is an indication of some kind of language disorder. In other words, close attention must be paid to possible interference patterns as being a phenomenon distinct from phonological disorders. Researchers have been aware of this rather complex situation for some time, and therapists are at a loss in many cases, as developmental norms need to be defined in order to analyze and treat the disorders meaningfully. This author's personal experience with Hindi-, Urdu-, and Bengali-speaking children with English as their secondary system in the United Kingdom, Italian or German speaking children with Portuguese as their secondary system in Southern Brazil, and Spanish or Haitian Creole speaking children with English as their secondary system in Florida point to the same problem. Thus, the question that arises is whether phonological patterns that do not conform to the target language are due to first language interference or these children are speech disordered.

In all three situations of bilingual acquisition cited above, which seem representative of many more situations from around the world, children grow up in the home environment with their first dominant language and start acquiring the target community language when they begin schooling around age 5 or 6 years. When children learn one language, we know that they simplify the adult targets, and we looked at these patterns in Chapter 6. For convenience, Table 8–2, which represents some of the most common simplification patterns, is provided.

As stated earlier, the number of simplification processes can be multiplied if we want to further differentiate them. In addition to being very common in normal phonological development, these processes also are observed frequently in children with phonological disorders. In addition, as seen in Table 8–3, their employment is not restricted to English, and they have been attested in several languages.

The seven languages cited in Table 8–3 come from four different language families: English and Swedish are Germanic; Spanish, Portuguese, and Italian are Romance; Turkish is Altaic; and Cantonese is Sino-Tibetan. This is significant because the similarities among languages should not be attempted via a genetic (language family) link.

A simple look at Table 8–3 shows that there are many shared elements across languages. In all languages, children reduce consonant clusters, delete and/or devoice final consonants, stop fricatives, front velars and palatals, glide liquids, delete unstressed syllables, and reveal assimilatory changes. These are observed with normally developing children as well as those with phonological disorders. The difference between the two groups is that normally developing children suppress these tendencies at certain points in their development, whereas the clinical population continues to employ these patterns long after the processes should be suppressed according to the developmental time-table. There are some places in the table that are marked "NA," which stands for "not applicable." For example, consonant cluster reduction is not applicable to

Table 8–2. Common simplification processes in developmental phonology.

Simplification Process	Target	Child's Realization
Cluster reduction	bread	[bɛd]
	stop	[tap]
Final consonant deletion	bean	[bi]
	mouse	[mau]
Final consonant devoicing	dog	[dak]
	nose	[nos]
Stopping	van	[bæn]
	that	[dæt]
Velar fronting	key	[ti]
	go	[do]
Palatal fronting	ship	[sɪp]
	fish	[fɪs]
Liquid gliding	rabbit	[wæbɪt]
	line	[jain]
Assimilation	boot	[bup] (labial)
	dog	[gag] (velar)
	bunny	[mani] (nasal)
Weak syllable deletion	beside	[said]
	pajama	[dʒamə]

Turkish because there are no targets in the language that would provoke this simplification. Consequently, the child is not challenged for this process. In terms of final consonant devoicing, we see NA for Portuguese, Italian, Cantonese, and Spanish, with a question mark for Spanish. Because this process focuses on obstruents and these languages do not allow any voiced obstruent in final position, the NA label is justified. That is, there is nothing to devoice in final position in these languages. The only possible exception is Spanish with the existence of final /ð/, as in *universidad*. However, this is rather marginal and, in many varieties, such words are not pronounced with a final /ð/. The reason that Cantonese has NA for the weak syllable deletion is that most words in this language are monosyllabic and some are disyllabic. Because this process generally applies to targets longer than disyllabic, it is irrelevant for Cantonese.

Table 8–3. Common simplification processes in normally developing children and children with phonological disorders in different languages.[1]

Simplification Process	English		Portuguese		Spanish		Italian		Turkish		Swedish		Cantonese	
	N	PD	N	PD	N	PD	N	PD	N	PD	N	PD	N	PD
Cluster reduction	X	X	X	X	X	X	X	X	NA		X	X	X	X
Final consonant deletion	X	X	X	X	X	X	X	X	X	X	X	X	X	X
Final consonant devoicing	X	X	NA		NA?		NA		X	X	X	X	NA	
Stopping	X	X	X	X	X	X	X	X	X	X	X	X	X	X
Fronting	X	X	X	X	X	X	X	X	X	X	X	X	X	X
Liquid														
Gliding	X	X	X	X	X	X	X	X	X	X	X	X	X	X
Assimilation	X	X	X	X	X	X	X	X	X	X	X	X	X	X
Weak syllable deletion	X	X	X	X	X	X	X	X	X	X	X	X	NA	

Note: N = normally developing; PD = phonologically disordered; X = phonological process exhibited in that language; NA = not applicable.

Table 8–4. Unusual phonological processes.

Process	Target	Child's Realization
Unusual cluster reduction	train	[ren]
	stick	[sɪk]
Initial consonant deletion	tape	[ep]
	sit	[ɪt]
Liquid nasalization	[kadera]	[katena] "chair"
(Portuguese)	[elis]	[emis] "they"
Fricative gliding	fig	[wɪg]
Stopping of glide	will	[bɪl]
Frication of approximant	lock	[ðak]
Frication of stops	ban	[væn]
Backing	pat	[pæk]
Nasal gliding (Portuguese)	[ə̃nus]	[əju] "years"
Delabialization (Swedish)	[foːgel]	[toːgel] "bird"

If such patterns are common in different languages both in normally developing children and those with phonological disorders, then how do we differentiate these two populations? In Chapter 6, it was stated that both Grunwell (1985, 1987) and Dodd (1993) emphasized the use of unusual processes as a yardstick to separate the disordered population from normal children. Table 8–4 shows some of the most commonly cited patterns that are found in the clinical population and are not generally found in normally developing children. If there were examples from English-speaking children, these were provided in the table. In the case of unavailability of English data, another language is cited.

These processes are considered unusual or idiosyncratic because they are exactly the opposite of the common processes that are observed in normally developing children. For example, the targets *train* and *stick* are simplified as [ren] and [sɪk], respectively, instead of the expected [ten] and [tɪk]. What is unusual here is the deletion of the unmarked member of the clusters, /t/, instead of the marked members, /r/ and /s/. Therefore, although normally developing children delete these marked consonants and come up with realizations like [ten] and [tɪk], exactly the opposite occurs in the unusual reduction.

Another example, which was dealt with in Chapter 4 in relation to distinctive features, relates to the frication of stops exemplified by *ban* becoming [væn]. In normal development, stops are acquired much earlier than fricatives, and fricative targets are realized with stop substitutes. In other words, it is extremely common to see fricative stopping and, as mentioned earlier, this was due to the fact that stops are much more manageable articulations with their complete contact of the articulators, whereas fricatives require much more muscular control as the articulators do not touch each other but only approximate to create the necessary friction. In the example cited above, *ban* → [væn], we see the reverse (frication of a stop). That is why the label unusual is used. If we consider the data from the seven languages mentioned earlier, we see that some of these unusual patterns are found in many of them whereas others are encountered only in a restricted group of languages. For example, unusual cluster deletion, initial consonant deletion, and backing are observed in all seven languages.[2] The processes that are found only in some of these languages reconfirm the earlier conclusion that the similarities between languages defy any genetic grouping. For example, Spanish (Romance) and Swedish (Germanic) share delabialization, while Turkish (Altaic) and English (Germanic) show frication of approximants. Liquid nasalization is reported in Portuguese (Romance) and Swedish (Germanic), and Spanish (Romance) and English (Germanic) share frication of stops.

It is important to remember, however, that the data from the seven languages cited above do not come from an equal number of sources, and that there is a problem of imbalance in the data. The situation is one of a continuum. English is the most widely studied language and reliability of the data from this language is greatest. Spanish is probably the next most reliable, as we see many more publications on Spanish than on the other languages. Turkish stands alone at the other extreme. Other than some unpublished theses and dissertations, there is not much existing information on normally developing Turkish-speaking children or those with phonological disorders.

If a child is acquiring one language, certain patterns will be observed. If, on the other hand, two languages are involved, some kind of interference from the dominant language is expected. Because a perfect bilingual is the exception rather than the rule, interference from the dominant language becomes a very important issue. Weinreich's (1953) criteria showed that interference patterns follow certain principles. In addition, rhythmic interferences may occur resulting from the stress versus syllable-timed character of the two languages.

An important issue to be discussed here relates to bilinguals' productions that may reveal erroneous patterns with reference to the ambient language. Because a bilingual individual, like his or her monolingual counterpart, may suffer developmental difficulties in the patterns of his or her language, we must make sure that we are capable of separating language interference from disorder.

Using information from the languages previously mentioned, the following simplification processes are probable results of interference when the secondary system of the bilingual is English:

1. More final devoicing is expected if the primary system of the subject is Turkish. This language has the rule of final stop devoicing. Thus, the natural tendency of final devoicing is emphasized more from the rule of the primary system.

2. More weak syllable deletion is expected from speakers whose primary system is Portuguese or Swedish. These two languages, like English, are stress-timed. Although the process of weak syllable deletion is primarily a function of the number of syllables in the target word, vowel reductions in the unstressed syllables of the stressed-timed languages facilitate the deletion.

3. More final consonant deletion is expected from the speakers whose primary system is Italian, Spanish, or Portuguese. These three languages are striving for an open syllable pattern that is diametrically opposed to a syllable-final consonant.

4. More initial consonant cluster reduction is expected by subjects whose primary system is Turkish. As mentioned earlier, all of the languages mentioned here reveal initial consonant cluster reduction. However, Turkish is the only language among them that does not present a challenge for the acquisition of an initial consonant cluster. For this reason, subjects whose primary system is Turkish should take a longer period to be able to suppress the tendency to reduce consonant clusters.

5. More consonant harmony assimilations are expected from the speakers whose primary systems allow more closed syllables. Because assimilations are more commonly available when there is a consonant

at the beginning and end of a syllable, this process will not be very common for speakers of mostly open syllable languages such as Spanish, Italian, or Portuguese.

6. More prevocalic devoicing and less aspiration are expected if the primary system of the speaker is a Romance language such as like Spanish, Portuguese, or Italian. In Romance languages, voiceless stops are unaspirated, that is, the situation more closely approaches simultaneity in terms of the moment of release and the voice onset time. These voiceless unaspirated stops are easier to produce than the voiced stops of English, which require glottal pulsing prior to the moment of release (voice lead). Thus, prevocalic devoicing is an easier substitute. This configuration is also easier than aspirated productions, which require a considerable period of voicelessness between the moment of release and the voicing for the following segment (voice lag). Speakers with primary systems in Turkish or Swedish are not likely to err in aspiration, as their systems are similar to English.

7. More problems regarding the differences between English stressed and unstressed syllables are expected if the primary system of the speaker is one of the syllable-timed languages (i.e., Spanish, Italian, or Turkish). English stressed syllables, typical of a stress-timed language, are considerably longer than unstressed syllables. Also, there is significant vowel reduction in unstressed syllables. Such characteristics are diametrically opposed to what syllable-timed languages do. In such languages, the lack of vowel reduction and only slight differences in duration between stressed and unstressed syllables are the trademarks. For example, stressed syllables in Spanish are typically about 1.3 times longer than unstressed syllables, whereas English stressed syllables are characteristically about 1.5 times longer (Delattre, 1965). The differential effects are especially significant in utterance-medial open syllables in which Spanish stressed syllables are only 1.1 times longer than unstressed syllables as opposed to the 1.6 times difference found in English (Dauer, 1983). Also, vowels in 92% of the unstressed CV English syllables are realized phonetically as relatively short central vowels, whereas the nuclei of 90% of the unstressed CV syllables in Spanish are manifested by longer peripheral vowels (Dauer, 1983).

8. Fricative stopping, at least for some specific targets, is expected to last longer if the primary system of the speaker is Spanish. This is because Spanish does not have a /v/, and the natural substitute is a /b/. Stopping of the two interdental fricatives of English, /θ/ and /ð/, is expected in all five languages, as none of them, with the exception of Spanish allophonically, has these sounds.

9. Another Spanish-specific substitution refers to the replacement of the voiceless palato-alveolar fricative /ʃ/ with the affricate /tʃ/ which shares voicing and place of articulation. Stops becoming fricatives are normally considered unusual (deviant), but this process may happen with subjects whose primary system is Spanish. In Spanish, /d/ is contextually realized as /ð/. Thus, the English target *adore* may be realized [əðor].

10. Many languages, including Spanish, Portuguese, and Cantonese, do not make the distinction between high front vowels /i/ and /ɪ/ that contrast in English (e.g., *beat-bit*). Thus, longer lasting confusion is expected between pairs such as *peach-pitch*, and *leave-live* by speakers of these languages.

Finally, to the above processes and implications that are related to the patterns of language contact situation, we need to add the implications from markedness constraints. For example, we have said that more final devoicing will be expected from subjects whose primary system is Turkish in their contact with English. To this general statement, we must add the specifics that come from the markedness of individual targets. Considerations such as the place of articulation and the height of the preceding vowel will help to determine different degrees of difficulty.

Similarly, the prediction that the subjects whose primary system is Turkish will have greater difficulty with initial consonant clusters must be supplemented with information about different clusters. For example, less marked clusters, such as /stop + liquid/, will be expected to be in the system of the learner earlier than marked clusters, such as /s + stop/.

Italian, Spanish, and Portuguese speakers are expected to show more final consonant deletions, as these languages basically do not, with certain exceptions, have final obstruents. However, among the closed syllable targets in English, it would not be surprising if the ones ending in fricatives appeared in the learners' system before the more marked syllables ending in stops.

The above list and considerations are by no means exhaustive, and many more implications can be derived from it. The goal of this section has been to show the possible interactions of native language patterns with natural processes that might be observed in the acquisition of second language phonology. The important message is that detailed information is needed on the two languages involved in order to be able to account for what goes on in the productions of bilinguals. The urgent need for data on the developmental patterns of the languages involved is key for our understanding the speech patterns of our clients.

Studies that have examined phonological patterns in normally developing bilingual children (Gildersleeve, Davis, & Stubbe, 1996) and bilingual children with suspected speech disorders (Dodd, Holm, & Wei, 1997) indicate that children in both bilingual groups exhibit patterns that are different from matched monolingual peers revealing more errors. Within the bilingual group, we generally observe a greater number and a higher percentage of occurrence of all patterns in children with disorders in comparison to normally developing children. For example, if we consider the difference between a normally developing bilingual child and a bilingual child with phonological disorders whose first language is Portuguese and is in the process of acquiring English as the second language, the following picture may emerge: Around the age of 4 years, the normally developing bilingual child will reveal cluster reduction, a low percentage of final liquid deletion, and perhaps weak syllable deletion. She or he might show a low percentage of a less common process such as backing. Due to interference from Portuguese, English productions for targets /t/ and /d/ before /i/ will be realized as [tʃ] and [dʒ], respectively. For the same reason, word initial /r/ may turn into [x]. Exhibition of patterns that are atypical in one of the languages may be manifested because of interference from the other language. For example, stopping, which is very unusual for this age in Portuguese (see Table 6–5), and context-free obstruent devoicing, which is normally not seen in English (see Table 6–4), may be present. If the same child were to have a phonological disorder she or he would manifest higher percentages of the same patterns and would exhibit other patterns that are not present in the normally developing child.

Finally, some remarks are in order regarding the assessment of bilingual children. In assessing the phonological development of a bilingual child, both languages should be the focus of attention and each should be examined in detail even if the child seems to be a dominant speaker of one of the languages. In doing this, all phonemes of the languages should be assessed in different word positions, and phonotactic patterns should be evaluated. Assessment tools that are designed for English, no matter how perfect they are, will not be appropriate for the other language and may be the cause of over- or underdiagnosis. Unfortunately, assessment tools designed for languages other than English are limited to a few languages. Among them are Spanish (Carrow, 1974; Hodson, 1986; Mason, Smith, & Hinshaw, 1976; Toronto, 1977), Cantonese (So, 1992), Vietnamese (Cheng, 1987), and Portuguese (Yavas, Hernandorena, & Lamprecht, 1991). Thus, many speech-language pathologists may have to employ assessment alternatives in dealing with a language for which a reliable assessment tool is lacking.[3]

Another issue that confronts the professional who deals with bilingual children is the dialect of the first language. Just as there are several varieties of English in different countries (British, American, Australian, South African, Canadian, Indian, etc.), and even within one country (New England variety, Southern variety, General American, and African American vernacular in the United States), other languages have dialectal variations. Because none of the varieties or dialects of a given language is or can be considered a disordered form of that language, the child's dialect information is essential. Any assessment of the child's speech will must be made according to the norm of the particular variety she or he is learning. For example, in Cuban Spanish, which is similar to the Puerto Rican variety, the colloquial productions generally delete the syllable final /s/ and, consequently, the target *pescado* [peskaðo] "fish" is pronounced as [pekao]. If the child's production lacks the syllable final /s/, this should not constitute a disorder labeled "syllable-final stridency deletion."

To give another example, consider the following: In Brazilian Portuguese, one finds the target *estar* "to be" pronounced as [eʃtax] (variety spoken in Rio de Janeiro) and [estaɾ] (variety spoken in the Southern state of Rio Grande do Sul. If the professional who is dealing with a Portuguese-English bilingual child does not have the dialectal information, focusing on the final consonant of the first syllable, the change (ʃ → s) might be erroneously classified as palatal fronting (or depalatalization). Mislabeling the child as phonologically disordered would result in sending him or her inappropriately to intervention. Goldstein and Igleasias (in preparation) looked at 54 normally developing Spanish speaking preschoolers and found that 25 of their subjects (46%) were labeled as phonologically disordered due to dialectal variation. Thus, it is imperative for the speech-language pathologist to have accurate information regarding the variety of the first language of the child and have access to the normative data on this variety.

SUMMARY

In this chapter we have looked at different aspects of bilingual phonology. Different types of bilingualism were considered. The critical age hypothesis, which has a strong claim about a bilinguals' capability of acquiring nativelike phonology, was reviewed. We saw that interference patterns are important in understanding bilingual phonology, but they cannot account for all production errors. To be able to explain what interference from the dominant language cannot, universal patterns were referred to. We saw that normally developing and children with phonological disorders children from very different languages exhibit many common patterns in normal as well as idiosyncratic processes. Several cross-linguistic situations were discussed and predictions regarding the dominant language were offered. Finally, some considerations for assessment of bilingual phonology were given.

We conclude that the normative data from a bilingual child's two languages are extremely important for any reliable assessment, but we should reemphasize that data on the normal development of the two languages separately, although necessary, will not be adequate, and the important information will come from further data on the normal development of the bilingual children.

NOTES

1. Sources for Table 8–3 are as follows: English data come from various published sources. For Spanish, in addition to the author's own files, Goldstein (1988), Goldstein (1996), and Goldstein and Iglesias (1996a, 1996b) were consulted. Nettelbladt (1983) and Magnusson (1983) are the sources for Swedish, while Bortolini and Leonard (1991) was used for Italian. Cantonese patterns are derived from So and Dodd (1994, 1995) and Dodd, Holm, and Wei (1997). Data on Portuguese are from Yavas and Lamprecht (1988), Yavas (1990), Yavas and Hernandorena (1991), and Yavas (1994). Turkish data are from Topbas (1988) and the author's own files.

2. The status of these two processes is rather questionable, as they have been noted in some normally developing children too.

3. For assessment alternatives and intervention strategies, see Yavas and Goldstein (in press).

EXERCISES

1. Spanish does not have /z/, /v/, and /ʃ/. English words that have these target sounds receive the replacements [s],

[b], and [tʃ], respectively. Consider the following words and determine the homophones that will be created by the neutralization of the distinctions because of these substitutions in the speech of a Spanish speaker who is learning English.

Example: *peas* [piz] → [pis]

Result: Both *peas* and *piece* will be pronounced [pis]

a. *very* _____

b. *phase* _____

c. *zip* _____

d. *rays* _____

e. *shop* _____

f. *vowel* _____

g. *shore* _____

h. *eyes* _____

2. Vowel length: English vs. Italian

English

- Stressed vowels are longer in final position.
- Stressed vowels are longer before voiced consonants than before voiceless consonants.

Italian

- Stressed vowels are shorter at the end of a word.
- Vowels are short if there is a following consonant.

On the basis of these facts, what problems do you expect to find when the primary language is Italian and the secondary language is English regarding the following targets:

true _____

cab _____

sooner _____

Pete   _____

see   _____

mad   _____

cause   _____

jam   _____

3. Alveolar stops: English versus German, Spanish, and Portuguese.

   Alveolar stops /t, d/, behave differently in these four languages. The following rules will be relevant for the comparison.

   English

   - Both stops occur can occur in all word positions.
   - /t/ is aspirated at the beginning of a stressed syllable.

   German

   - Both stops occur at the initial and medial positions, but only /t/ can be found in final position.
   - /t/ is aspirated similarly to English.

   Spanish

   - Both stops occur at the initial and medial positions, but only /d/ (marginally ?) occur in final position.
   - /d/ becomes [ð] in intervocalic position.
   - /t/ is unaspirated.

   Portuguese

   - Both stops occur only in initial and medial positions.
   - /t/ becomes [tʃ] and /d/ becomes [dʒ] before /i/.
   - /t/ is unaspirated.

   On the basis of these patterns, what (if any) problems do you expect for German, Spanish, and Portuguese speakers regarding the alveolar stops in the following English targets:

(Note: When English targets have final alveolar stops, Portuguese speakers tend to insert an epenthetic /i/ after the stop, whereas Spanish speakers tend to delete the stop.)

	German	Spanish	Portuguese
time	_____	_____	_____
bed	_____	_____	_____
renter	_____	_____	_____
adore	_____	_____	_____
meat	_____	_____	_____
teacher	_____	_____	_____
need	_____	_____	_____

4. Front vowels: English versus Spanish

   English has five front vowels, /i, ɪ, e, ɛ, æ/, whereas Spanish has only two, /i, ɛ/. Consequently, several difficulties result when the speaker's primary system is Spanish and the secondary system is English. On the basis of these, state which of the following English contrasts will be difficult:

   ages - edges _____

   beat - bit _____

   beat - bet _____

   bit - bet _____

   bait - bat _____

   bet - bat _____

5. Although contrastive phonological information is indispensable for the prediction of learners' difficulties, it is not sufficient in many cases because, for certain phenomena, constraints based on universal markedness have been shown very influential in explaining the degree of difficulty of targets. Order the following targets in terms of degree of difficulty and state the rationale:

a. *Single coda consonants*

beer _____

beat _____

beam _____

beach _____

deal _____

b. */s + C/ onsets*

speak _____

sleep _____

smear _____

c. *liquids*

ball _____

Florida _____

elect _____

_____

d. *Final voiced stops*

food _____

pig _____

tub _____

rib _____

dog _____

bad _____

Chapter 9

SYLLABLES AND FEET

Although the syllable was mentioned as far back as the ancient grammars of Greek and Latin, Standard Generative Phonology ignored it and took the morpheme as the basic unit of phonology. One of the most important reasons for this was the difficulty encountered in defining the syllable. As we observed in Chapter 2, there is no agreed-upon phonetic definition of syllable and, consequently, it was thought that a unit that has no solid definition could not and should not be taken as the basic unit of phonology. The avoidance of such a clearly phonological unit has lead to rather embarrassing results. Many phonological generalizations were expressed in a strange fashion because the syllable was not used. For example, vowel nasalization in French was expressed in the following way (Schane, 1968):

$$V \rightarrow [\text{nasal}] / \underline{\hspace{2cm}} C \quad \begin{cases} C \\ \# \end{cases}$$
$$[\text{nasal}]$$

(The brace notation is used to indicate either possibility in the set of options in the rule.)

This rule states that vowels are nasalized when followed by a consonant that is followed by another consonant or word boundary. The common environment, C and #, does not form a natural class. However, this environment is not unique to the above rule and seems to occur in various other generalizations. For example, the r-less dialects of English are said to drop the *r* in that same environment

$$\underline{\hspace{2cm}} \quad \left\{ \begin{array}{l} C \\ \\ \# \end{array} \right.$$

park the car   [paːk ðə kaː]

Many English dialects have a velarized /l/ (raising the back of the tongue) under certain conditions. In *pole* and *spalding*, /l/ is velar, but in *polar* it is not. The context for velarization is again the same.

$$[+\text{lateral}] \rightarrow \left[\begin{array}{l} +\text{high} \\ \\ +\text{back} \end{array} \right] \;/\; \underline{\hspace{2cm}} \quad \left\{ \begin{array}{l} C \\ \\ \# \end{array} \right.$$

The obstruent devoicing rule we have seen in languages such as German, Russian, Polish, and Turkish is another one that refers to the same environment:

$$[-\text{sonorant}] \rightarrow [-\text{voice}] \;/\; \underline{\hspace{2cm}} \quad \left\{ \begin{array}{l} C \\ \\ \# \end{array} \right.$$

Three separate rules of degemination, epenthesis, and vowel shortening in Turkish all take place in the same environment (Clements & Keyser, 1983). Finally, this very same environment also is needed for an epenthesis rule in Yawelmani (Kenstowicz & Kisseberth, 1979).

If such an environment is commonly found in languages for a variety of phonological rules, then one would expect that the two elements (consonant and word boundary) form a natural class. Because they do not, one wonders about the motivation of putting these unrelated things together as the environment in which the processes occur. If, however, the syllable is accepted as a legitimate unit in our phonological description, then it becomes clear that these processes are all referring to the same environment, namely, syllable final (coda) position.

The relevance of the syllable for the expression of significant phonological generalizations has numerous supporting examples in diverse languages. Several phonological events target a specific syllable. In Turkish, voiceless velar stops are deleted intervocalically in non-initial syllables. In Japanese, high vowels are deleted before velar stops in non-initial syllables. In Swahili, nasal prefixes of a certain class of nouns are syllabic if they are attached to monosyllabic roots, but are not syllabic if they are attached to longer roots. In Turkish, non-high rounded vowels, /o, ø/, can occur only in initial syllables. In Spanish, the shape of the diminutive suffix is regulated by the number of syllables: After disyllabics, we find -sita/-sito, and after trisyllabics, we have -ita/-ito. To express such significant generalizations using a unit other than the syllable would necessarily result in extremely cumbersome descriptions.

Another significant role played by the syllable concerns phonotactic constraints in languages. This term refers to the system of arrangement of sounds and sound sequences. Speakers of English can easily judge which of two non-occurring words, [blɪk] and [bmɪk], could be a possible word in their language. They tacitly know that, although English words can start with the sequence [bl], the sequence [bm] is not a possible sequence in that position. This is not to say that the sequence of [b] plus [m] is not at all allowed in English. For example, the words such as *submit* and *submarine* have this sequence. The difference between these words and the disallowed *bmik* is not one of position, that is, word initial versus word medial. Rather, it is a matter of syllable structure; the sequence [bm] in *submit* and *submarine* belongs to two separate syllables, whereas it belongs to the same syllable in *bmik*. Thus, the restriction is that [bm] cannot occur syllable initially.

Similarly, speakers are aware of the fact that English words can start with a sequence of [tr] but not with [tl]. However, again the restriction is for more than just the word-initial position, and the reference should be made to syllable-initial position. This knowledge reveals itself for the different behavior with respect to the following words:

attraction	Atlantic
attrition	atlas
atrocity	Atlanta

The words in the left column all begin with a schwa [ə] followed by an aspirated alveolar stop, whereas the words on the right begin with, most commonly, a non-reduced vowel followed by an unaspirated stop. Actually, the expected rendition of the consonant following the initial vowel on the right would be the glottal stop [ʔ].[1]

The reasons for the different renditions of the first vowel and the immediately following consonant in the two groups of words are the different sequencing of sounds in syllables and, consequently, the sensitivity of the phonological rules to these sequencing. The words in the left column put the syllable boundary between the initial vowel and the following consonant because the cluster [tr] is a possible cluster ([ə.træk.ʃən], [ə.trɪ.ʃən], [ə.tra.sə.ti]). On the other hand, the words in the right column have a consonant ending the first syllable ([æʔ.læn.tɪk], [æʔ.ləs], and [æʔ.læn.tə]), as [tl] or [ʔl] is not a possible syllable-initial sequence.

As for the application of the three rules, aspiration, glottalization, and vowel reduction, we can note the following: The aspiration rule applies in the initial position of a stressed syllable; only the words in the left column satisfy this condition and, thus, have aspirated alveolar stops following the initial vowel. The glottalization rule requires the consonant, /t/, to be in syllable-final position, and the words in the right column have exactly that condition satisfied. As for the difference between the reduced and unreduced vowels of the initial syllable, the above syllabification would be relevant. Because open syllables universally have a greater tendency to reduce, we would expect the words in the left column to do just that. In summary, the sequential restrictions among sounds, once considered within the perspective of the syllable, become much more explanatory.

STRUCTURE OF THE SYLLABLE

Although the relevance of the syllable has been established as an undeniable unit in the phonological structure, there does not seem to be unanimous agreement regarding the constituent structure of this unit. Kahn (1980) suggested that the syllable node (α) dominates the constituents immediately, as exemplified in the following:

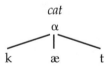

A similar, but more detailed, position was taken by Clements and Keyser (1983), suggesting that the relation between syllable and segments is mediated by the CV tier (a timing tier) and the syllable is breakable as onset + nucleus + coda:

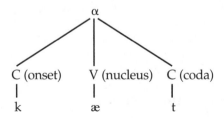

However, a more widespread view (Anderson, 1986; Durand, 1990; Selkirk,1982; Vincent, 1986) proposes a major break between the onset of the syllable and the rest of the syllable, called the rhyme. The rhyme, in turn, is breakable into its constituents, the nucleus and the coda. In this hierarchical view of the syllable, there are units intermediate in size (onset-rhyme) between the syllable and the phoneme. The onset is the initial consonant or consonant clusters of the syllable; for example, the onset of the word *strap* is /str/, the onset of *trap* is /tr/, and the onset of *rap* is /r/. The onset is not obligatory in English in that a well-formed syllable may not have one (e.g., *at, in, out*). The rhyme is the remaining part of the syllable following the onset. In the above examples, /æp/ is the rhyme of all three words *rap, trap,* and *strap*. A rhyme may have a short or diphthongized vowel and a consonant or consonant cluster (*sit, seat, tent, taint*) or a diphthongized vowel without anything following it (*say*). Within the internal structure of the rhyme, the vowel or the diphthong is the nucleus (or peak), and the consonant or consonants following make up the coda.[2]

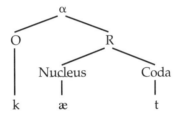

In addition to the above, as agreed by many, the CV tier may be added to this representation.

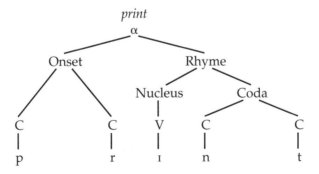

There are advantages of positing an intermediary CV tier between the segments and the suprasegmental structure. The treatment of affricates, for example, has always been problematic. On the one hand, they are recognized as being a sequence of a stop and a fricative; on the other hand, they are treated as single units in phonological terms. The phonological one-unit treatment is justifiable because, although affricates can appear in initial position before a vowel, no stop + fricative sequences are allowed in initial position in English. Also, historically, English affricates developed from single stops. If a CV tier is employed in the representation, then this apparent discrepancy of one phonological unit with a phonetic sequence of two sounds phonetically can be accounted for.

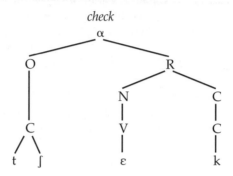

Here, the first C position is associated with two segments, indicating that a single phonological unit is made up of two articulatory events.

The CV tier is also useful in dealing with long vowels and diphthongs where they will be assigned to two units of timing, as opposed to short vowels. Thus, *sit*, *seat*, and *site* will be represented as follows:

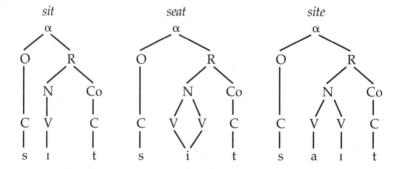

SONORITY

In Chapter 2, it was stated that there is no agreed-upon phonetic definition of the syllable. Although defining this unit is not easy, speakers normally have little difficulty in deciding how many syllables a given word has. There are, of course, some words that show variable pronunciation and, thus, create disagreement among speakers. For example *settling*

could be said to have two or three syllables, and *realistic* could be debated to have either three or four. However, the overwhelming majority of cases have rather straightforward answers. *Book* and *this* have one
syllable, *pencil* and *phoneme* have two, and *aroma* and *December* have
three syllables.

In Chapter 7, a principled relationship between the intrinsic content of
the sounds and their respective distribution throughout syllabic structure was seen. Specifically, the nucleus of the syllable is normally taken
by a vowel or a diphthong and, moving from the center to the margins,
a progressive decrease of segments in their sonority values is observed.
Thus, the naturalness of a word, *print*, with its initial and final clusters,
and the markedness and the rarity of the word, *rpitn*, can be explained
with reference to the Sonority Sequencing principle.

Because the nucleus of the syllable is occupied by higher sonority elements, it has been suggested that the number of peaks of sonority in a
word should be equal to the number of syllables. This principle can be
seen at work in the following examples:

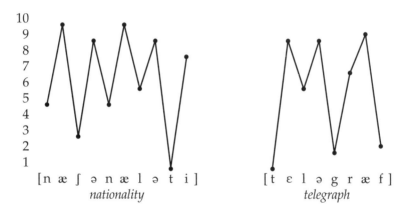

[n æ ʃ ə n æ l ə t i]
nationality

[t ɛ l ə g r æ f]
telegraph

In the first word, we have 5 peaks of sonority and 5 syllables, and in the
second word we have 3 and 3 respectively.

Although this principle holds in thousands of English words, it does not
mean that there are no exceptions to it. English onset clusters that start
with /s/ followed by a stop create a problem for sonority sequencing.
Examples such as *space*, *stick*, and *skin* illustrate this well. The problem is
created because there is a lowering of the sonority value from the first to
the second member of the onset. In these cases, /s/, with a sonority index
of 3, precedes the stops /p, t, k/, which have a sonority value of 1. That
the problem is created solely by /s/ is easy to show, because its removal

from these words would leave us with *pace, tick,* and *kin,* which are harmonious with the sonority sequencing.

A similar problem is encountered for certain final clusters that are exemplified by the members of the codas in *lapse* [læps] and *axe* [æks]. Here, instead of the expected lowering of sonority at the edge of the syllable, these coda clusters reveal the opposite tendency by increasing the sonority values, thereby violating the sonority sequencing. These examples are all from words with one morpheme. If we look at monosyllabic words with more than one morpheme, the number of cases involving the violations of the sonority sequencing is multiplied. The simple addition of the plural suffix, for example, is sufficient to create numerous additional violations (e.g., *texts, winds*).[3] As a result of these violations, these words also create discrepancies between the number of syllables and the number of peaks of sonority. For example, *stick* and *lapse* will have the following appearances:

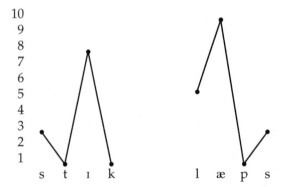

Despite their monosyllabicity, both of these words show two peaks of sonority and, thus, violate the general principle that the number of peaks of sonority is indicative of the number of syllables.

SYLLABIFICATION

The sonority hierarchy, in spite of some problems, has aided us in determining the number of syllables in a word by counting the peaks of sonority. Thus, the words *nationality* and *telegraph* were shown to have five and three syllables, respectively, resulting from the number of peaks of sonority in them. Although the count generally gives the number of syllables accurately, it does not indicate exactly where the syllable divisions lie in these words. For example, is [ʃ] in *nationality* the coda of the first syllable or the onset of the second syllable? What about the [g] in *telegraph*? Is it the coda of the second syllable or the onset of the third?

In cases such as (C)VCV(C) in which the vowels constitute the syllable peaks and the consonants are at the margins of the syllables, the division will be such that the C between vowels constitutes the onset of the second syllable, rather than the coda of the previous syllable. This principle comes from the fact that all languages have CV (open) syllables, whereas many languages lack VC (closed) syllables. This consideration favors the following syllabification for *nationality*: [næ.ʃə.næ.lə.ti]. In cases in which we have two consonants between two vowels, VCCV, the decision will require other considerations. The two consonants must be analyzed in terms of the well-formedness condition in that language. If the two consonants do not form an acceptable onset, then the syllable division will be between the two consonants. Words such as *balsam* [balsəm] and *artery* [artəri] illustrate this point well. The two consonants between the vowels in these words are [ls] and [rt], respectively; because these sequences do not conform to the well-formedness condition in English, they will not be the onsets of the second syllables. Note that these sequences also violate the expected sonority sequencing in that there is no increase in sonority from the first consonant to the second; actually, there is lowering. The first consonant in each case is assigned to the coda of the first syllable: [bal.səm] and [ar.tə.ri].

If, however, the sequence of two consonants is in accordance with the well-formedness condition, then the two consonants are placed in the onset of the same syllable. Thus, the syllabification of the word *telegraph* is [tɛ.lə.græf]. This is because [gr] is a possible onset in English. It also happens that the expected sonority sequencing by increasing it from 2 (a voiced stop) to 7 ([r]) is followed here.

It is important to emphasize the phonotactic rules (well-formedness conditions) of the language. For example, the words *Atlanta* and *atlas* seen earlier were syllabified as *at.lan.ta* and *at.las*, respectively. The consonantal sequence [tl] was divided and the two consonants were placed in different syllables. Similarly, *subway* is divided as *sub.way*. The reasons for these divisions do not come from sonority sequencing but rather from the well-formedness condition of the language. As far as sonority sequencing is concerned, both /tl/ and /bw/ conform with the rise in sonority (from [t] to [l] is a rise from 1 to 6; from /b/ to /w/ is a rise from 2 to 8). Thus, the syllable divisions were made on the basis of an English-specific condition. It is interesting to note that English allows onsets such as /dw/ and /bl/ while prohibiting /bw/ and /tl/ or /dl/. Because the sonority changes from the first member to the second member of the onset are identical in the disallowed /bw/ and /tl/ as well as the allowed /dw/ and /bl/, the sonority scale cannot be an explanation. The restriction seems to come from the place of articulation in that the two segments cannot both be the members of the same place of articulation.

Because /dw/ and /bl/ do not share the same place of articulation, they are allowed.

Similarly, the words *submarine* [sʌbmərin] and *admit* [ədmɪt] have the sequences of consonants [bm] and [dm], respectively, and these sequences of voiced stops followed by nasals show an increase in sonority from the first consonant to the second. This fact, however, is not enough to qualify them as onsets in English. As observed, the syllabifications of these words split these consonantal sequences as in the following : [sʌb.mə.rin], [əd.mɪt]. The separation of [bm] and [dm] result from a language-specific constraint that does not allow such sequences in English. This does not mean that other languages follow suit and, in fact, such sequences can be found in some languages. For example, stop plus a nasal is an acceptable onset in Norwegian (proper name *Knut*). Czech allows both /tn/ and /tl/ as onsets, /tnout/ "to hit," /tlit/ "to rot." In Hebrew /pn/, /bn/, /gm/, /gn/, /dm/, /tn/, /tm/, and /kn/ are all possible (/pnimi/ "interior," /bniya/ "construction," and /gmisut/ "flexibility").

The fact that language-specific constraints override general rules also can cause the same or similar sequences to be parsed differently in different languages. For example, a word such as *livro* [livru] "book" in Portuguese is syllabified as [li.vru], as [vr] is a possible onset in Portuguese. The same sequence of [vr] appears in Turkish *avrat* [avrat], but the syllabification is [av.rat], because Turkish does not allow any consonant clusters as syllable onsets. Similarly, English speakers typically syllabify the word *asleep* as [ə.slip], because the sequence [sl] is in accordance with the phonotactic rules of English. The same word, however, will be attempted as [əs.lip] by Spanish speakers, because Spanish does not allow [sl] as an onset.

What has been said so far can be summarized by the following maximal-onset principle: We place the syllable boundaries in such a way that onsets are maximized without violating the syllable structure conditions of the language. If a consonant or a sequence of consonants cannot be part of the onset, they are placed in the coda of the previous syllable. We will illustrate this step by step with the word *temptation* [tɛmp.te.ʃən]. The vowels [ɛ], [e], and [ə] are the sonority peaks and form the nuclei of the three syllables. Starting from the end of the word, we have the sound [n]. This sound necessarily goes to the coda position of the third syllable, because there is nothing else to follow. The next consonant to the left is [ʃ]; this can precede the nucleus [ə] and, thus, will be the onset of the third syllable. The nucleus of the second syllable [e] is preceded by [t]. This is an acceptable sequence as the onset of the second syllable. The sound,

[p], which stands before [t], must go to the coda of the previous syllable, because [pt] cannot form a possible onset in English. [m] standing before [p] is also part of the coda of the first syllable because this combination is allowed. It is interesting to note that the three consonants in the middle of this word, [mpt], are split as [mp.t] in *temptation*. This, however, should not give the impression that they cannot be together in the same syllable. For example, as the word *tempt* shows, these three sounds together form the coda of this monosyllabic word. The reason that they split in the word [tɛmp.te.ʃən] is due to the maximum onset principle, which assigns [t] to the syllable onset position.

In the same connection, the two previously mentioned words, *balsam* and *artery*, are divided as [bal.səm] and [ar.tə.ri]. Although both could carry potential codas of [ls] and [rt] (e.g., as in *pulse*, and *art*), they are nevertheless divided between the consonants. Again the reason is the maximum onset principle. Because [səm] and [tə] are possible syllables with these onsets, these splits have the priority.

AMBISYLLABICITY

The cases we have looked at so far are rather straightforward, and the conventions of syllabification have accommodated them comfortably. There are, however, several other words for which it cannot easily be determined where the boundary of each syllable lies. Consider the following:

honest	*Africa*	*Canada*	*ticket*
ugly	*origin*	*apple*	*metric*

Although the divisions suggested by the maximum onset principle would syllabify these words as *ho.nest, A.fri.ca, Ca.na.da*, and so on, speakers of English cannot be so sure about these divisions. Although many speakers may follow this division, several others give answers such as *hon.est, Af.ri.ca, Can.a.da*. Yet, there are several others who do not feel comfortable with either way and, at times, give fluctuating answers. Situations like these are clear indications that the consonant in question cannot clearly be assigned either to the coda of the preceding syllable or to the onset of the following syllable. Consonants that are felt to be ambiguously syllabified as, in the above words, are called **ambisyllabic** and treated as belonging to both syllables. The regularities governing ambisyllabic consonants always point to the coda position of a stressed syllable and the onset of the following unstressed syllable. The quality of the vowel in the stressed syllable also matters. For example, although words such as *digest* [daɪdʒɛst], *rival* [raɪvəl], *legal* [ligəl],and *shooting* [ʃutɪŋ] have

consonants between a stressed and an unstressed position, these segments are unambiguously assigned to the onsets of the second syllable in
each case. Thus, the syllabifications of [li.gəl], [daɪ.dʒɛst], [raɪ.vəl], and
[ʃu.tɪŋ] are agreed on by all native speakers of English. The difference between these words and the earlier group is that the nucleus of the
stressed syllable in the last group is either a long tense vowel or a diphthong. In other words, as mentioned earlier in relation to CV tiers, they
have two units of timing. Thus, we represent *rival* in the following way:

rival

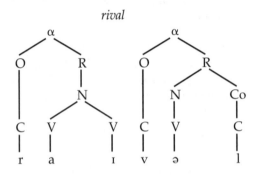

In the cases in which there were doubts due to ambisyllabicity, the nucleus of the stressed syllable has a short vowel (one unit of timing), as exemplified by the word *ticket*:

ticket

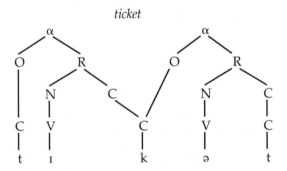

It will be shown later in this chapter that syllables that attract stress for
nouns in English have two units of timing in the nucleus (branching nucleus). When a disyllabic word does not have syllables with a branching
nucleus, then the stress goes to the first syllable, as in *ticket* and *apple*. By
stressing the syllable with a short vowel (one unit of timing), its timing
increases phonetically but does not reach to two units of timing as in the
case of the branching nucleus. This gives the feeling that the following
consonant is the coda of this syllable. This fact, however, creates a conflict
with the maximum onset principle, which would normally assign the

consonant to the onset of the following syllable. The result is the formation of the apparently undetermined, ambisyllabic consonants.

Before leaving the topic of syllabification, some comments are in order regarding the syllabification conventions of written language. This is not a trivial matter, as this is the system that is taught to elementary school students, and it follows certain principles that are not identical to the principles of spoken syllabification. The first principle concerns the sounds represented by the five vowel letters (*a, e, i, o, u*) and the letter *y*, which stands for vowels in certain words. If one of these letters represents one of the tense vowels [i, e, a, ɔ, o, u] or diphthongs [aɪ, aʊ, ɔɪ], the next letter representing the consonant goes in the following syllable. However, if the vowel represented by these letters is a lax vowel [ɪ, ɛ, æ, ʊ, ʌ], then the next letter goes with the preceding syllable. Thus, the following dictionary syllabifications are given:

ri.val	*fin.ish*
pu.ni.tive	*stud.y*
le.gal	*med.i.cine*
la.bor	*rad.i.cal*

Although native speakers' spoken syllabifications are in complete agreement with the dictionary (written language) syllabifications for words in the left column, this is not the case for the words in the right column. The reason that the dictionary syllabification differs from the spoken is that the vowel letters (*i, u, e, a*) in the first syllables of these words represent lax vowels. When this is the case, the consonant following the lax vowel goes with the preceding, rather than the following, syllable in the conventional dictionary representation, which is contrary to spoken syllabification. The vowel letters in the first syllables (*i, u, e, a*) of the words in the left column all represent tense vowels or diphthongs [aɪ, u, i, e, o], whereas the same letters in the words in the right column represent lax vowels [ɪ, ɛ, æ, ʌ]. That is why the dictionary representations are given as shown. Although native speakers' spoken syllabifications agree with the dictionary syllabifications of the words in the left column, there is a clear discrepancy for the words in the right column. Many speakers, unlike the dictionary representations, tend to syllabify these words as [fɪ.nɪʃ], [stʌ.di], [mɛ.də.sən], and [ræ.də.kəl] in the spoken language without much controversy.

Another principle that guides the conventions of written syllabification is related to prefixes and suffixes, which are not divided. As a result, the dictionary representations of *un.able* and *sleep.ing* are contrary to the spoken syllabifications of [ʌ.ne.bəl] and [sli.pɪŋ]. The latter word is especially significant, because it demonstrates the fact that the second principle, which states that prefixes and suffixes cannot be divided, takes precedence over the first. In *sleeping*, there is a long tense vowel in the first syllable and, according to the first principle, the following consonantal letter should go to the onset position of the next syllable. However, because *-ing* is a suffix, and the second principle requires the independence of suffixes, *p* remains in the first syllable.

STRESS ASSIGNMENT AND SYLLABLE WEIGHT

As seen earlier in this chapter, the segment is not the ultimate unit for phonological generalizations, and the syllable is crucial for the expression of several phonological phenomena. The question now arises whether there are larger units above the level of the syllable that are relevant for phonological generalizations.

In looking at languages of the world in terms of the word stress assignment, two patterns emerge. On the one hand, there are languages with fixed stress in that the location of the main stress in polysyllabic words is quite straightforward. For example, stress falls on the last (ultimate) syllable in French, and on the next to the last (penultimate) syllable in Polish. On the other hand, the stress assignment in many languages is not as straightforward and the determinant is the syllable structure. In languages where word stress assignment is sensitive to syllable structure, the weight of the syllable must be considered. Syllable weight essentially refers to the weight of the rhyme, as the onset plays no role in such rules. A syllable is **light** if it contains no branching rhyme, V (e.g., [ta]):

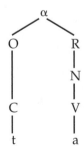

A syllable is generally **heavy** if it has a branching rhyme:

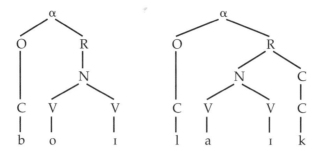

Although the above cases are clear, there remains a questionable rhyme structure, namely VC, that behaves differently in different languages. In some languages (Type A), such as Latin and Turkish, VC syllables count as heavy, whereas in others (Type B), such as Huatesco and Mongolian, they count as light. For example, the following sequence [tæp] will have the assignment of heavy in type A languages, as it has a branching rhyme:

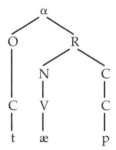

However, the same sequence will have the assignment of light in type B languages in which heavy requires a branching nucleus, and the coda is irrelevant for the weight of the syllable. Different assignments of the same sequence in different types of languages are illustrated in the following diagram:

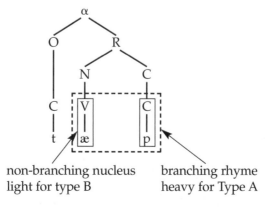

non-branching nucleus
light for type B

branching rhyme
heavy for Type A

Although the above statements represent the facts accurately, sometimes they need to be appended by language-specific conditions. For example, although Cayapa, an Amerindian language spoken in Ecuador, is a Type A language with closed syllables generally counting as heavy, syllables closed by glottal stop are treated as light. In Mongolian, which was given as an example of a Type B language, closed syllables, expectedly, count as light unless they are closed by [ŋ]. Chuvash, a type A language, does not count closed syllables as heavy if the vowel is [ə].

The significance of syllable weight is seen in the stress rules of languages, because heavy syllables are the ones that generally receive the main stress.[4] For example, in Latin, polysyllabic stress falls on a heavy penultimate syllable; if the penultimate syllable is light (no branching rhyme), the stress is placed on the antepenultimate syllable.

When stress rules refer to the weight of the syllable (weight of the rhyme), they are said to be quantity-sensitive. In languages that have such rules, it is generally the case that one syllable or a segment at word edges does not count. Such segments or syllables are called **extrametrical**. In the following, we will illustrate the concept of extrametricality by looking at the rules of stress in English. First, consider the following list of disyllabic verbs:

a. *cóver*   *cárry*   *cópy*
b. *combíne*   *digést*   *deláy*

In (a) the primary stress falls on the first syllable, whereas in (b), it falls on the second syllable. The rule governing this can be stated in the following way: Stress the first heavy syllable from the right end of the word. If the word does not have any heavy syllables (branching rhyme), then, by default, stress falls on the first syllable. The last consonant is extrametrical. Because the last consonant is extrametrical, *cover* does not have any heavy syllables and the stress falls on the first syllable. Words in (b) all have heavy second syllables: *combine* and *delay* have branching nucleus, and *digest* has a branching rhyme after the extrametrical final /t/.[5, 6]

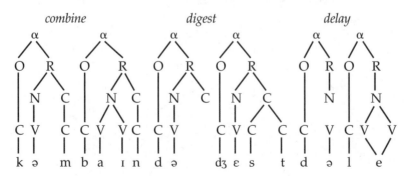

Now, consider the following disyllabic nouns:

a. *tícket*   *fócus*   *cávern*
  ríver   *túlip*   *pócket*
b. *políce*   *brigáde*   *arcáde*

In (a), the primary stress falls on the first syllable, whereas in (b), it falls on the second syllable. The rule governing this is the same as that stated for the verbs: Stress the first heavy syllable from the right end of the word. If the word does not have any heavy syllables then, by default, stress falls on the first syllable. There is a difference, however, and it pertains to the definition of heavy syllable. Although a heavy syllable for the verb rule demands a branching rhyme, for nouns it is defined as a syllable with a branching nucleus, and the coda consonants are extrametrical. The words in (a) do not have heavy second syllables, and are stressed on the first syllables. Although the second syllables of these words have branching rhymes (i.e., have coda consonants), these consonants are extrametrical and do not contribute to the weight of these syllables. Words in (b), however, have heavy second syllables (branching nucleus) and are stressed on the second syllable.

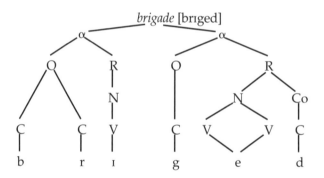

Let us look at longer words now. Consider the following:

a. *horízon* *tomáto* *affidávit* *aróma*
b. *intéstine* *uténsil* *agénda* *memorándum*
c. *díscipline* *América* *cítizen* *déficit*

Ignoring the last consonant, which is extrametrical, we can state the rule as follows: Stress falls on the penultimate syllable if it is heavy, but, if the penultimate syllable is not heavy, stress falls on the antepenultimate syllable. A heavy syllable requires a branching rhyme (long vowel, diphthong, or closed syllable). Words in (a) and (b) are stressed on their penultimate syllables. The first group has diphthongs or long vowels, and the second group has closed syllables in the penultimate syllable. Words in

(c) are stressed on the antepenultimate syllable, because they all have light penultimate syllables.

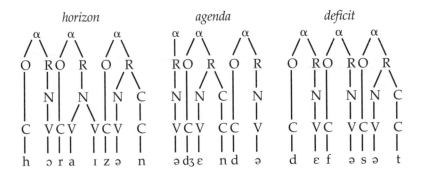

The discussion about English stress so far should be taken as general statements, but the complete picture is much more complex, and non-phonological factors interfere. For example, the same sequences are stressed differently because of noun-verb oppositions (an *import* versus to *import*; an *insult* versus to *insult*).

Also, the addition of affixes reveals interesting patterns regarding stress in English. Although the addition of prefixes does not change word stress, the suffixes may have varying affects on the word stress.

One group of suffixes, like prefixes, has no effect on the primary stress of the word:(*-ing, -er, -less, -able, -ment, -ness, -ful, -some,* and *-hood*). Examples include work*ing*, small*er*, child*less*, read*able*, measure*ment*, good*ness*, law*ful*, lone*some*, and boy*hood*.

Among the groups of suffixes that affect the main stress, one type attracts stress to themselves. Suffixes such as *-ette, -esque, -ee, -ese,*and *-ique* are stressed. *cigarette, grotesque, refugee, Portuguese,* and *technique* are examples of this group.[7]

Another group of suffixes have the effect of moving the stress to the syllable immediately before them. These include *-ic, -ity, -ial, -cial, -tial, -ify, -itude,* and *-tion*. Words such as *fantastic, humidity, trivial, financial, essential, terrify, attitude, definition* exemplify this pattern.[8]

Finally, there is a group of suffixes that put the stress on the syllable immediately preceding if it is heavy (branching rhyme). Examples include *refusal* (long vowel), *recital* (diphthong), and *accidental* (closed syllable). However, if the preceding syllable is not heavy, the stress moves one more syllable to the left, as in *seasonal* and *practical*.

FEET

Sequences of syllables consisting of a stressed syllable plus one or more unstressed syllables form a timing unit called **a foot**. Stress is a relational concept in that one syllable in a word is more prominent than the other(s). For example, in the word *able*, the first syllable is more prominent than the second syllable, whereas in *urbane* the opposite holds. This relative prominence is expressed via branching binary trees according to the strength relationship. S stands for the strong syllable, and W stands for the weak syllable:

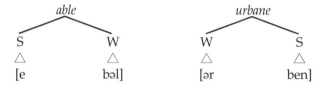

Syllables join for foot formation. The dominant syllable is called the **head**, and it governs its neighbor(s) to the right or left. S and W are interpreted relationally: S means stronger than W and W means weaker than S. Feet consisting of more than two syllables must be broken into binary branching where prominence relations are shown:

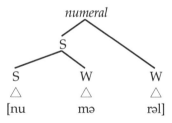

Putting together what has been said so far, the internal structure of different words with one foot can be shown:

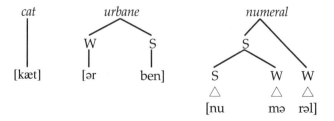

Many words, of course, have more than one foot in their structure. These may include disyllabic as well as polysyllabic words. Consider the following:

hotel	[hòtél]
textile	[tékstàɪl]
collateral	[kəlǽtərəl]
automatic	[ɔtəmǽtɪk]
authenticity	[ɔθəntísəti]

The first two words are disyllabics with different stress patterns than the earlier-mentioned *able* and *urbane*. Whereas in *able* and *urbane*, one syllable is stressed and the other is unstressed, in *hotel* and *textile*, both syllables have stress, one with a greater prominence than the other. The significance of this is that the latter pair of words have two feet in their structure, as opposed to the one-foot structure of *able* and *urbane*. Compare the trees with different structures:

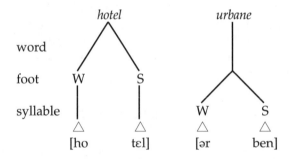

Just as disyllabic does not mean one foot in the structure, polysyllabics do not necessarily include more than one foot, as shown in the following:

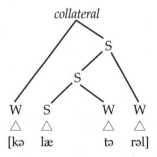

The word *automatic* is an example of a polysyllabic word with more than one foot:

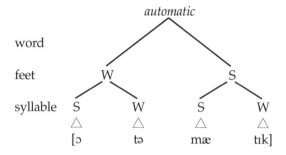

In order to have two feet in the structure, a word does not need to have an even number of syllables, because one foot can have more than one unstressed syllable. Consider the following:

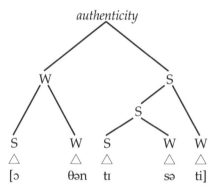

This five-syllable word demonstrates the fact that the phonological structure is hierarchical and the concept of relative prominence applies at various points in this hierarchy. Syllables are grouped to form feet, and the feet are grouped to form the word. This framework is known as Metrical Phonology.

Metrical phonology is based on the principle that relative prominence is crucial in the phonological representation of suprasegmentals. Various parameters of relative prominence operate within phonological units larger than the segment. Because these prominences are relational rather than local, S and W are defined among sister nodes.

To illustrate the hierarchically organized levels of representation that are posited for prosodic units in metrical phonology, the word *automatic* can be revisited:

word   *automatic*

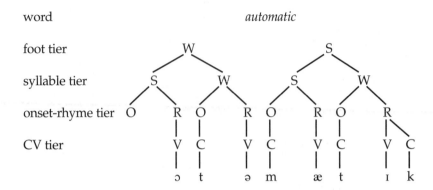

Here, we see that, at the syllable level, first syllables are more prominent than second syllables in both feet. However, at the foot level, these two strong syllables with S belong to feet of different prominence. The third syllable of the word, [mæ], belongs to the foot that is more prominent than the first syllable [ɔ].

The information we have in the tree structures can also be shown by a construction of a metrical grid. A metrical grid is a graphic representation that dispenses with a metrical tree. Instead, a linguistic form is represented as a series of ever-larger constituents. Grids represent the information in the trees by assigning an asterisk to each syllable in the syllable tier; an additional asterisk is assigned to the stronger syllable in each foot. Finally, at the word level, another asterisk is assigned to the strongest foot. This is shown with the word *automatic*:

```
word                    *
foot            *       *
syllable        *   *   *   *
              [ɔ  tə  mæ  tɪk]
```

Because at every grid level, a relation of relative prominence is defined on competing grid marks, it follows that every domain has a single highest column. The difference between the words *hotel* and *urbane* shown via trees earlier can also be shown with the grids:

```
word              *               *
foot          *   *               *
syllable      *   *           *   *
            [ho  tɛl]       [ər  ben]
```

Although this introductory text will not go into the higher structures, the procedures shown for the metrical analysis of words can also be applied to strings of words, which makes it possible to study the rhythmic patterns of phrases and sentences.

DEVELOPMENTAL IMPLICATIONS

The topics discussed in this chapter also have remedial implications. First, the sonority scale seems to be a factor in certain phonological phenomena. Yavas (1994) reported on a Portuguese-speaking subject's syllable-final /r/-deletion rule, which seems to be directly related to the saliency of acoustic changes created by sonority indexing of sounds. The deletions occurred in two different contexts. In the first one, /r/ targets in syllable-final-within-word (SFWW) position (e.g., [barku] "ship") were deleted if the following consonant was a sonorant, and they were correctly realized if the following consonant was an obstruent. In the second, /r/ targets were deleted in syllable-final-word-final (SFWF) position after vowels /i, e/. After /a, o/, however, the targets were correctly realized. The author suggested an explanation based on the sonority changes for the deletions in SFWW. The transition from /r/ to a sonorant creates a less salient acoustic change in comparison to the transition from /r/ to an obstruent. These can be calculated from the sonority indices of the sound types, /r/: 7, sonorant consonants: 5–6, obstruent:1–4. The degree of salient acoustic change also seems to explain the retention or deletion of target /r/ in SFWF position. The transition from /i, e/, which have 20–21 decibels of acoustic power, to /r/, which has 20 dB, does not create a salient acoustic change. On the other hand, /o/ and /a/, with 25–26 dB of power, would establish a more salient change with their transition to /r/, which has 20 dB of acoustic power.

The topic of salient changes in terms of sonority also seems to explain the relative ease or difficulty of segmentation of syllable constituents. Adults seem to have greater difficulty in separating the coda consonant from the nucleus when the coda is a nasal or a liquid (sonorant) than when it is a stop or a fricative (obstruent) (Treiman, 1988). The explanation offered for this fact suggests that liquids cohere with vowels to a greater degree than nasals do, and nasals in turn do so more than obstruents. This continuum is a reflection of the sonority indexing discussed earlier in this chapter.

The significance of sonority sequencing in the speech of children with phonological disorders has also been noted by Chin (1996). One child, referred to as S25, had the following regularity: Target words with labial stops and coronal stridents were realized with initial consonant clusters consisting of a labial stop followed by a coronal fricative. This pattern occurred independently of the order of the targets and of the location of the target within the syllable:

badge	→	[pʃæ]	*push*	→	[pʃʌ]
sharp	→	[pʃar]	*spoon*	→	[psu]

For example, in *push* we have the order of labial + coronal coming from the onset and the coda, respectively, whereas in *spoon* we have the order coronal + labial both occurring in the onset. Analyzing these and similar examples, Chin came to the conclusion that the subject used a metathesis rule to convert the targets into a labial stop + a coronal fricative. The reason offered for this was the sonority sequencing principle that dictates the rise of sonority from the margin to the center of the syllable. If the target word obeys this principle, the rule of metathesis does not apply. If, however, the target does not agree with this principle, it is modified.[9]

Two other subjects with consonant cluster reductions reported by Chin revealed an interesting situation for which explanations were again based on sonority indices of sounds. S6 employed consonant cluster reduction for some targets

stove	→	[sov]
snow	→	[so]
sky	→	[saɪ]

while not reducing the other target clusters

play	→	[ple]
brush	→	[bwʌs]
sleep	→	[slip]
twin	→	[twɪn]

Examining these and similar examples, Chin found that cluster reduction occurred when the difference in sonority index was 3 or greater from C1 to C2. If this condition was not met, the reduction did not apply. In other words, using the principle of minimum distance in sonority, the target clusters were treated differently by the subject. For example, in *stove*, the sonority indexing for the cluster is 3 to 1 = −2; in *snow*, it is 3 to 5 = 2. In the former, the result is −2, indicating a decrease in sonority from C1 to C2; in the latter, although the result in changing sonority is not negative, it still is less than what is demanded by S6. In the second group of words in which the clusters were not reduced, the sonority differences from C1 to C2 are equal to or greater than 3. For example, *brush* shows a transition of 2 to 7 = 5, whereas *play* obtains the same result via 1 to 6. The minimum required, 3, is shown by the target *sleep* , in which the transition is from 3 to 6.

Another of Chin's subjects (S25) had the following patterns:

a. stop + approximant → stop
   twin   → [dɪn],   *drum* → [dʌm],   *play*   → [be],
b. fricative + sonorant → fricative
   few   → [fu] ,   *swim* → [sɪm],   *shrub* → [ʃʌb]
c. fricative + stop → stop
   spoon   → [bun],   *stove* → [dov],   *sky*   → [daɪ]

In (a) and (b) words, the first member of the cluster is maintained and the second member is deleted. In (c) words, however, the reverse is true. The explanation offered by Chin takes into consideration the rise in sonority from the onset consonant to the nucleus. In other words, between the onset and the nucleus the greater sonority difference determines which member of the initial consonant cluster will be dropped. In (a) words, which have the stop (Sonority index: 1–2) + approximant (S.I. 6–7) going to vowels (S.I. 8–10), dropping of the approximant will create a greater rise in sonority from the stop to the vowel (1–2 to 8–10). For, words in (b), the same principle also holds; a fricative to a vowel establishes a greater rise in sonority (3–4 to 8–10) than does sonorant to vowel (5–7 to 8–10). In the last group (c), the words require the deletion of the first member (fricative) of the cluster, as this creates a transition from the second member, stop (S.I. 1–2) to the vowel (S.I. 8–10). The sonority factor in the separation of segments in syllable constituents also has been observed in 4- and 6-year-olds (Yavas & Gogate, in preparation). Children who are given the task of separating onsets (4-year-olds) and codas (6-year-olds) found the task easiest when the consonants in question were stops (maximum degree of difference from the nucleus). This was followed by fricatives, nasals, and liquids, in that order. Taking these cases into consideration, we can say that constraints based on relative sonority play a crucial role in developing phonologies.

More behavioral evidence on sonority as a factor comes from second language studies. As we saw in Chapter 8, the success rate in acquisition of English coda consonants follows the sonority ranking of the syllable-final consonant. Data from Japanese, Cantonese, and Korean learners of English revealed that, independent of their first language patterns, the learners had greater difficulty in acquiring obstruent codas than they did in acquiring sonorant codas (Eckman & Iverson, 1994).

In addition to sonority values of segments, the hierarchical view of prosodic structures also has implications that are relevant to developmental patterns. In this framework, it is believed that the child comes to the language-learning process with a set of universally determined templates (Bernhardt & Stoel-Gammon, 1994). For example, this would include the basic syllabic structure CV or CVV (with a long vowel or a diphthong). Through his or her exposure to the ambient language, the child learns to encode other more complex syllable types. Because the hierarchical view treats levels of representation as independent, the learning of syllable shapes and segments can occur separately. The learner, via the ambient language, is introduced to the principles of the relationship between stress and prosodic structure. This hierarchical view suggests a developmental progression from higher elements to the elements that are lower in the tree. For example, the syllable unit will be acquired earlier than phonemes, and the onset and rhyme will be acquired in between. The difficulties encountered by a child regarding the diphthongs and coda consonants may be handled at different times because of the suggested independence of the nucleus and coda (Bernhardt, 1994).

The role of stress in production accuracy has long been noted; in general, targets in stressed syllables have a greater chance of being realized accurately than ones in unstressed syllables. Stress also seems to explain seemingly irregular incorrect productions. Yavas and Hernandorena (1991) reported that their 7-year-old Portuguese-speaking subject replaced the targets /ʃ/ and /ʒ/ either with [tʃ] and [dʒ], respectively, or with [t]. This variability, however, lent itself to a regularity that was based on the stress. When the target palato-alveolars were in stressed syllables, the realization was [t] (e.g., achei [aʃe] "I found" → [ate], *cachorro* [ka-ʃoxu] "dog" → [tatoxu]). If, however, the target was in an unstressed syllable, the substitute was an affricate (e.g., *relogio* [xelɔʒju] "clock" → [xelɔdʒju], *bicho* [biʃu] "animal" → [bitʃu].)

The relevance of a prosodic unit such as foot to the clinical population has also been cited in the literature. Chiat (1989) reported on a phonologically disordered child, age 4 years 7 months, and found that the subject's stopping of fricatives was dependent on the prosodic and phonotactic structure of the word, which is integrally related to the syllabification of the word. It was observed that the foot was the prosodic domain to which stopping applied; foot-initial fricatives were stopped, whereas other fricatives were correct.

Another case that shows the relevance of the unit foot was given by Yavas (1994). The subject, a 7-year-old Portuguese-speaking girl, regulated her palatal fronting depending on the position of the target in the foot structure. Her realizations were correct when the target sibilants, /ʃ, ʒ/, were in the strong member of a left dominant foot and followed by /i/. Targets that were in other contexts were fronted to [s] and [z].

SUMMARY

In this chapter, we saw that the syllable plays a very important role in phonological description. We looked at the structure of the syllable and its constituents, the onset and the rhyme, which contain the nucleus and the coda. The relationship between sonority and the rules of syllabification was discussed. In the majority of cases, sonority was shown to increase from the syllable margins moving toward the nucleus. Of interest to teachers and parents are the discrepancies between dictionary and spoken rules of syllabification.

It was noted that the syllable is the primary unit for carrying prosodic information such as stress. It was shown that stress rules in languages are sensitive to the syllable weight, which essentially refers to the weight of the rhyme. Sometimes, certain segments or syllables at the word edges do not have any effect on the weight of the syllable and are called extra-metrical. Sequences of syllables consisting of a stressed syllable plus one or more unstressed syllables form a unit of timing called foot. Syllables in a foot, and feet in a word, are in a strength relationship. This hierarchical relative prominence of elements is the trademark of a model of phonology called metrical phonology. All of these units may have implications for developmental phonology. Clinical implications to date have been found in operations applying to feet, preference for sonority sequencing, and importance of stress.

NOTES

1. In more casual speech, the initial vowels of Atlantic and Atlanta (but not of *atlas*) may be reduced to schwa. However, the point we would like to make is that, while the unreduced initial vowels for the words in the right column would sound natural, the same will not be true for the words in the left column; these words will sound quite unnatural if they are uttered with an initial unreduced vowel.

2. Although the nucleus position is commonly occupied by a vowel or a diphthong, the range of segments that can be syllabic nuclei varies from language to language. Some languages, English among them,

allow nasals and liquids to be syllabic. Although rare, some languages also allow fricatives in this position.

3. There are differing views by different scholars on how to handle such
cases which will not be detailed here.

4. This is the problem that was created by the examples of ambisyllabicity. For example, if we divide *Africa* as [æ.frɪ.kə] and start the second
syllable with [fr], following the maximum onset principle, then we
will have [æ] as the only element ofthe first syllable that carries the
stress. Because stressed syllables are heavy and should have a branching rhyme, we have a conflict here. The branching rhyme requirement
of a heavy syllable demands [f] as the coda of the first syllable, whereas the maximum onset principle wants the same segment as the first
consonant of the two member onset of the second syllable. Ambisyllabicity seems to be the solution to this problem.

5. This rule is not exceptionless. Words such as *follow* and *borrow* are
stressed on the first syllable, despite the fact that their second syllables have diphthongized vowels.

6. Disyllabic adjectives are subject to the same rule as verbs.

7. Words such as *committee* and *coffee* are exception to this.

8. There are exceptional cases, however. For example, -ity shifts the
stress in publicity, and possibility, but not in *divinity* and *obesity*. Similarly, -ic in Arabic, Catholic, and lunatic, and -ion in television, and
intersection are exceptions, as the stress does not fall on the syllable
immediately preceding these suffixes.

9. Chin recognizes the strangeness of the consonant cluster production
of the subject when the target has none. He suggests that the target
segments may have been perceived as being unordered.

EXERCISES

1. It is suggested that the number of peaks of sonority in a word should be equal to the number of syllables in that word. Examine the following words and determine which ones do or do not follow this principle:

   a. cardiograph   b. photography
     [   ]   [   ]
   c. economics   d. strawberry
     [   ]   [   ]
   e. fertility   f. reconcilable
     [   ]   [   ]

2. Divide the following words into their syllables according to the principles discussed in this chapter.

   a. stripes   b. obstruction
     [   ]   [   ]
   c. satisfactory   d. hostility
     [   ]   [   ]
   e. Cambridge   e. bibliography
     [   ]   [   ]

3. Which of the following words would have ambisyllabic consonants?
   Draw the tree diagram showing the ambisyllabicity.

   final, medicine, origin, medium, deepen, happen, punish

4. Is stress predictable in the following group of English words ending in *a*? If yes, describe the pattern. Words are given in regular orthography with an acute accent placed on the stressed syllable.

Cánada	Flórida	Nebráska	Albérta
álgebra	vértebra	Atlánta	veránda
Minnesóta	cínema	Ágatha	Matílda
Arizóna	Therésa	Sonóma	bazóoka

5. Consider the following nouns with more than two syllables. First, transcribe the word phonetically and place the stress on the appropriate syllable. Then state why stress is placed on that syllable.

synopsis	[	]
appendix	[	]
gelatin	[	]
pelican	[	]
harmonica	[	]
hypothesis	[	]

6. Consider the following disyllabic verbs. First, transcribe the verb phonetically and place the stress on the appropriate syllable. Then state why stress is placed on that syllable.

consist	[	]
suffer	[	]
rally	[	]
exempt	[	]
contain	[	]

invite   [   ]
shiver   [   ]

7. Is stress predictable in the following list of trisyllabic English verbs? If yes, describe the pattern. Verbs are given in regular orthography with an acute accent placed on the stressed syllables.

díagnose   mánifest   devélop   solícit
éxercise   rídicule   cómplement   abólish
imágine   remémber   súpplement   pérsecute

8. Is stress predictable in the following Arabic data? If yes, describe the pattern. On the basis of what you found, state whether Arabic is a type A or type B language. In the data, syllable boundaries are shown with a $ sign, and C indicates a pharyngealized consonant.

a. [ga $ rí: $ da]   "newspaper"

b. [fu $ ká: $ ha]   "humor"

c. [ká $ ta $ bu]   "they wrote"

d. [má $ ra $ ʔa]   "broth"

e. [bi $ síl $ la]   "green peas"

f. [fa $ súl $ ja]   "green beans"

g. [wá $ la $ di]   "my boy"

h. [ki $ ní: $ sa]   "church"

i. [za $ kít $ ta]   "jacket"

j. [ga $ wán $ ti]   "gloves"

k. [ṭa $ ṛáb $ lus]   "Tripoli"

l. [ʕí $ na $ ba]   "a grape"

m. [ʕá $ ra $ bi]   "Arabic"

n. [ẓá $ ḷa $ ṭa]   "stone"

9. The addition of suffixes has varying effects on word stress in English. Give three words for each of the suffixes in these categories:

a. suffixes that have no effect on the word stress:

-less	*-able*	*-ment*	*-some*	*-ful*
——	——	——	——	——
——	——	——	——	——
——	——	——	——	——

b. suffixes that move the stress to the syllable immediately before them:

-ic	*-ity*	*-ial*	*-ify*	*-tion*
——	——	——	——	——
——	——	——	——	——
——	——	——	——	——

10. Show the relative prominence of feet by drawing binary trees of the following words:

   facility   *satisfactory*

   funeral   *delineate*

Chapter 10

FEATURE GEOMETRY AND UNDER-SPECIFICATION

In the last chapter, separate hierarchically organized levels of representation (tiers) were posited for prosodic units. Accordingly, the representation of a word consisted of word level, foot tier, syllable tier, onset-rhyme tier, and CV tier before it reached the segmental representation. In recent nonlinear phonological models, this hierarchical structure also is extended to the segmental level, and the combination of features in a segment is viewed as hierarchically organized. Because these hierarchical representations are represented as tree structures, we refer to this theory of features as the theory of feature geometry.

This chapter first looks at the problems the earlier feature proposals created and examines how this new proposal of feature geometry may remedy these situations. After establishing the superiority of this new approach, the relevance for the clinical population will be reviewed.

FEATURE GEOMETRY

As we saw earlier in our presentations, the standard feature theory focuses on the segmental properties of the features without reference to their hierarchical organization, and the features composing a sound are represented as an unorganized bundle, allowing each feature to act independently of all others. Although Stevens and Keyser's (1989) model incorporates a hierarchical organization via primary and secondary features, it is not concerned with any dependency relationships among features. This, however, gives the wrong impression that features may freely combine for the phonemes of a language or for the natural classes relevant for the phonological rules.

To start with, as shown by Kenstowicz (1994), certain features do not define any natural class and, thus, play a supplementary role in the subclassification defined by another feature. For example, the features [anterior] and [distributed] only seem relevant for coronal consonants, but these feature values also have appeared for velars or glottals in the formulations we have considered. Although, by default, these consonants will be [–distributed], it will allow the possibility of a contrast [+/–distributed] velars or glottals, which is not correct. There are no examples in languages in which [t] is combined with [h] for a phonological grouping demanded by [–distributed]. Similarly, it does not make much sense to talk about the features [lateral] or [strident] when dealing with vowels. In other words, there is a need to clarify certain combinatory limitations regarding the features.

Another point refers to the fact that certain features form recurrent groupings with regard to phonological rules (Clements, 1985). For example, assimilations dealing with [high], [back], and [low] are common in vowels. However, it would be rather unusual, if not impossible, to witness an assimilatory event among [high], [nasal], and [ATR]. That is, we should have a principled way to show that the features [high], [back], and [low] have a special affinity, whereas the other three, [high], [nasal], and [ATR] do not enjoy such a relationship.

Yet another problem that existed in standard feature theory with respect to the implicit claim was that, if one value of a feature denotes a natural class, then the other value of the same feature should do so also. For example, considering the two features [anterior] and [coronal] that are used to designate the places of articulation, the following combinations are possible:

labial : [+anterior, –coronal]
alveolar: [+anterior, +coronal]
palatal : [–anterior, +coronal]
retroflex: [–anterior, +coronal]
velar : [–anterior, –coronal]
uvular : [–anterior, –coronal]

As a result, the following natural classes result:

[+coronal] : (alveolar, palatal, retroflex)
[–coronal] : (labial, velar, uvular)

The problem with such groupings is that, although the former, [+coronal], is frequently attested in phonological rules of languages, the latter, [–coronal] class, is never found together for a phonological event. That such groupings should be captured and the significant generalizations should be correctly identified led phonologists to the idea that features are organized in hierarchical tree structures with each branch corresponding to what has been called a tier.

The basic idea of feature geometry is that features are organized around six active articulators which reflect the anatomical structures involved in the production of speech. These are the glottis, soft palate, lips, tongue blade, tongue body, and tongue root. Most features are the sole responsibility of a particular articulator. For example, [labial] is uniquely related to the lips, whereas [nasal] is the exclusive responsibility of the soft palate. Such features are called articulator-bound features. On the other hand, other features are not dedicated to a particular articulator and can be executed by several different articulators. These features, called articulator-free, fall into two groups: the major class features [consonantal] and [sonorant], which are placed at the root of the tree, and the stricture (manner) features [continuant], [strident], and [lateral].[1]

Root features [consonantal] and [sonorant] jointly define the major classes of sounds and create the linkage of the segment to the prosodic tiers above. Among the four possible combinations of these two features, one [–consonantal, –sonorant] is excluded, because it is an impossibility. The remaining combinations define the following major classes:

	Obstruents	*Liquids, nasals*	*glides, vowels*
consonantal	+	+	–
sonorant	–	+	+

Manner (stricture) features [continuant], [strident], and [lateral] come directly from the root and thus are classified as articulator-free.

One of the cavity nodes, laryngeal, defines the glottal characteristics of the segment such as voicing and aspiration, while the other cavity node, supralaryngeal, dominates two class nodes, [soft palate] and [oral place]. Here, the first determines the difference between nasal and non-nasal segments, and the second [oral place] dominates the articulator nodes [labial], [coronal], and [dorsal]. Unlike most other features, the articulator features—[labial], [coronal], and [dorsal]—are privative (one-valued), rather than binary. This is because phonological rules operate only on the positive values of these categories. For example, as mentioned above, although there are rules and processes involving labial and coronal segments, no generalization seems to be made on the [–labial] or [–coronal] groups. Finally, articulator class nodes dominate binary valued features. The labial place is related to lip articulations, bilabials and labiodentals /p, b, m, w, f, v/, rounded vowels, and /r/. It dominates the binary value [round]. The coronal place is related to articulations with the tongue tip or blade, which covers interdentals, alveolars, palato-alveolars, and palatals /θ, ð, t, d, s, z, n, r, l, ʃ, z, tʃ, dʒ, j/. It dominates the terminal features [anterior] and [distributed]; the former separates palatals [–anterior] from the rest [+anterior], and the latter isolates the interdentals via [+distributed]. Coronal place is considered the universally unmarked (default) place (Paradis & Prunet, 1991). Dorsal place is related to articulations made with the back of the tongue. It covers velar consonants /k, g, ŋ/ and vowels, and dominates terminal features [high], [low], and [back]. The tree model presented in Figure 10–1 is based on Halle (1992).

The trees for some segments are shown below:

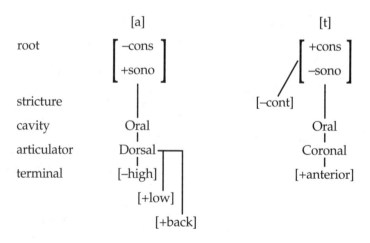

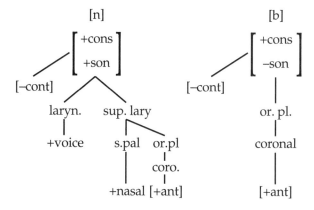

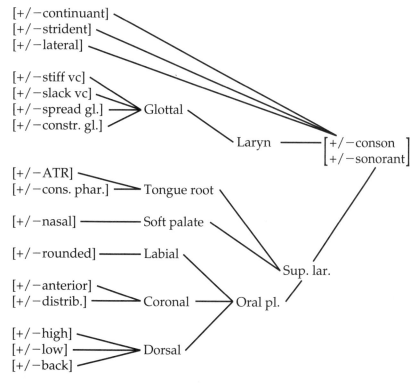

Figure 10–1. Feature tree (Adapted from "Phonological Features;" by M. Halle. In International Encyclopedia of Linguistics [Vol. 3, pp. 207–212]. Oxford: Oxford University Press).

In the tree, any given terminal feature implies the presence of the corresponding articulator and all higher nodes. Thus [anterior] or [distributed] implies the presence of Coronal; [back] implies Dorsal, and so on. This correctly predicts that if one segment assimilates to another in coronality, it necessarily assimilates [anterior] and [distributed] at the same time. This is supported by data from diverse languages. In the tree, the dependency and dominance relationship is crucial; any nonterminal node forms the root of a subtree composed of all the nodes it dominates. Dorsal groups [high], [low], and [back]. Oral place groups Labial, Coronal, and Dorsal and, thus, groups the dependents of Dorsal [high], [low], and [back]. On the other hand, there is no importance of the linear appearance of the branches that appear on the same level. For example, branches emanating from the same node (Labial, Coronal, and Dorsal) can be exchanged freely in their linear representation.

In reviewing the problems that were created by the standard feature theory that were mentioned at the beginning of this chapter, we can see how this new way of looking at the features through the hierarchical feature tree can remedy the situation.

First of all, both [anterior] and [distributed] are ancillary features and subclassify only [+coronal] segments. This is clearly shown in the hierarchical tree structure by making both of these features daughters (emanating from the same node) of Coronal. In other words, both [distributed] and [anterior] only can be accessed through the Coronal articulator.

The tree structure also has a formal means of expressing the features that have certain affinities and co-occur in rules. For example, it was noted earlier that [high], [low], and [back] group together in languages, whereas [high], [nasal], and [ATR] do not. The tree structure reveals this nicely in that features that can co-occur ([high], [low], and [back]) all are dominated by the same node, Dorsal, whereas the ones that do not co-occur ([high], [nasal], and [ATR]) are dominated by different nodes, Dorsal, Soft Palate, and Tongue Root, respectively.

Also mentioned was the situation in which a particular value of a feature defines a natural class successfully, whereas the opposite value of the same feature creates a totally nonfeasible group of sounds. This was exemplified by [+/−coronal]; although the class of [+coronal] sounds (alveolar, palatal, and retroflex) are frequently attested in the phonological rules of languages, the [−coronal] class that will group labials, velars, and uvulars is never found. This problem of the standard feature theory does not exist if these sounds are examined in terms of the articulators of the hierarchical tree.

Articulator	Sounds
LABIAL	labial
CORONAL	alveolar, palatal, retroflex
DORSAL	velar, uvular

This classification groups sounds in accordance with their behavior in phonological rules.

Rules in the nonlinear framework are handled by two operations, called spreading (linking) and deletion (delinking) from one tier to another. The linking and delinking operations may apply to constituents at all levels. This includes features, segments, onset-rhyme, and syllables.

Immediately adjacent tiers in the tree form a plane with nodes that are connected by association lines, indicating a temporal overlap. A node dominated by one root node can be associated with a node dominated by another root node. There are three principles of association between tiers. First, one or more constituents may be linked to a constituent on another tier. This is well exemplified by the feature geometry tree shown earlier in which one or more features is linked to a dominating node. Second, association lines, the links between the nodes in diagrams, must not cross, suggesting that operations may apply to constituents adjacent at some level. Finally, the direction of association follows the specific parameters of a language. For example, place assimilation of nasals to stops (*balance - imbalance*, Spanish *un beso* [um beso]) is regressive (right-to-left). This way, assimilation is represented establishing a new connection or association between two nodes:

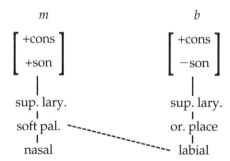

The regressive assimilation exemplified here is represented by the dotted line spreading (linking) of the feature. What this shows is the association of a feature to the corresponding mother node in the adjacent segment; in this particular case, the spreading of the place node. It also shows that /m/ is identical to /b/ in all of its supralaryngeal features except for [nasal].

A progressive assimilation, such as the voicing agreement for the plural formation in English, will be represented as follows:

books [buks]

buk + S

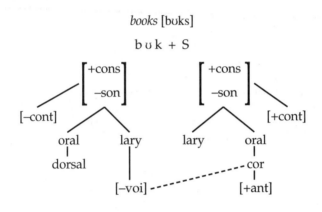

bags [bægz]

b æ g + S

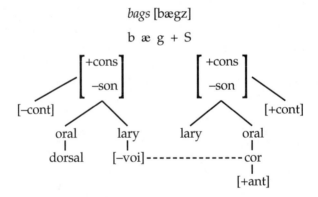

Because the plural allomorphs [s] and [z] are predictable via voicing assimilation, they do not need to be specified for [voice] underlyingly, and the agreement with the final segment of the root is accounted for by spreading of the laryngeal feature [voice]:

laryngeal   laryngeal

[+/−voice]

FEATURE GEOMETRY IN CLINICAL PHONOLOGY

The hierarchical tree structure of feature geometry has remedied many problems that exist in the standard feature theory and it has described phonological events more insightfully than the earlier accounts. The use of feature geometry is not restricted to general phonology, and its applications to phonological development and clinical phonology have been claimed to be quite revealing.

Some phenomena commonly observed in developmental phonology can be dealt with in feature geometry. The following example has an assimilation (consonant harmony) and a deletion (final consonant deletion) in the same word. These two processes will be shown via spreading and delinking, respectively. The word *take* is realized as [ke]. Because this appears alongside *tail* [te], it suggests that the child has underlying dorsal place for *take*, because consonant harmony is responsible for the initial velar in the rendition. The child's rendition of this target as [ke] is explained via spreading (linking) of the dorsal place, and delinking of the second consonant for the final position:

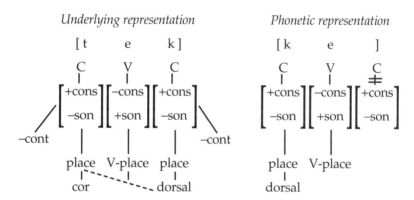

Chin and Dinnsen (1991) demonstrated the applications of feature geometry to phonological disorders using data from 40 children with phonological disorders with regard to certain rule-governed phonological phenomena. One of the authors' examples comes from coalescence, in which a target adult cluster is realized as a single sound, with some features from one of the target cluster elements and some from the other, as exemplified in the following: *swim* → [fɪm], *sweep* → [fɪp]. In all of these coalescence cases, the make-up of the target cluster was [s] + a sonorant, which was usually a labial as in this particular case of [s] and [w]. The traditional systems would have difficulty in deriving a single coalesced sound from two underlying sounds. However, feature geometry efficiently deals with these cases simply by establishing a new connection (reassociating) from the first supralaryngeal node to the second place node in order to derive the coalesced segment. All superfluous structures including the root and all structures beneath it are deleted.

The child's underlying representation for coalesced segment /sw/ will be the following:

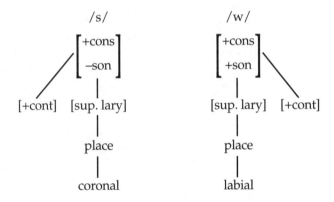

The child's phonetic representation for coalesced segment [f] is given below:

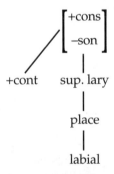

Another interesting example comes from some of the subjects' replacement of the affricates with fricatives, as exemplified in the following: *cage* → [keɪdð], *cagey* → [keɪði]; *witch* → [wɪts], *witchy* → [wɪsi].

In the standard Chomsky and Halle (1968) system, as well as in the Stevens and Keyser (1989) model, this substitution must be shown by changing the feature [continuant] from minus for the affricate to plus for the fricative, and also by changing the plus to minus for [delayed release]. However, a complex segment like an affricate is represented as the simultaneous association of a C slot with two segments in feature geometry, where the stop portion [–continuant]) precedes the fricative portion ([+continuant]), revealing the temporal sequencing.

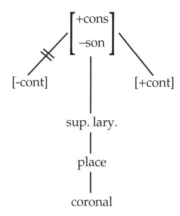

The derivation of the fricative is accomplished simply by delinking the [–continuant] node from the root node. The remaining features account for the fricative. This representation, in addition to avoiding the feature changing rule in traditional systems, also makes the feature [delayed release] superfluous.

Because nonlinear theories emphasize representations rather than rules or processes, this is also reflected in the views on acquisition. Similar to what was said in the previous chapter regarding the prosodic structure, the child is viewed as coming to the language-learning process with a set of universally determined templates with regard to segmental properties. The hierarchical structure suggested for features is one that has certain implications. According to feature geometry, more deeply embedded features in the tree, such as place features, are learned later than features that appear at the higher nodes, especially those at the root node that define major classes (e.g., consonantal, sonorant). As a corollary, common child substitutions involve mismatches in features that are lower in the tree. For example, palatal or velar fronting, which are exemplified in substitutions such as *fish* → [fɪs], (ʃ → s), and *cap* → [tæp], (k → t), involve changes in the place node. On the other hand, an idiosyncratic substitution such as liquid stopping exemplified in *rake* → [dek] (r → d) affects a major class feature, [sonorant], at the root node.

A further implication of feature geometry deals with the independence of the features. For example, because manner (stricture) features such as [continuant] emanate from the root node, there is no dependency of this feature on the place nodes. In other words, [s] may develop independent of [f], as the child's application of [continuant] may not happen in all places of articulation.

One appealing use of feature hierarchy for remediation is that the child's stage of feature acquisition could be established. Once this is determined, remembering that lower features are acquired later, then which features to be added would follow on the basis of the hierarchy. Although this is an attractive idea, it still cannot be considered definitive because dust has not settled yet in the phonological literature about the hierarchy itself. Several different proposals for the hierarchy are currently being debated. Consequently, this makes any application of the hierarchy for remediatiation tentative at best.

It should be pointed out that the segmental realization is contingent the availability of the syllable or word structure. For example, there could be a situation in which all features for a particular segment are established, but the syllable structure is not yet available and the segment does not appear in a particular syllable position. These so-called "word recipes" for certain children have constraints that restrict certain segments to specific word positions.

The relevance of feature geometry to the development and expansion of phonemic inventories in children is an area that has been under investigation. According to the principle of **laryngeal–supralaryngeal cyclicity** advanced by Gierut (Gierut, 1994a, 1994b; Gierut & Morisette, 1995), phonemic inventories are expanded over time by adding a feature distinction from either the laryngeal domain (voicing) or the supralaryngeal domain (place/manner)in alternating fashion. For example, if a child has the following asymmetrical phonemic inventory,

$$p \qquad t$$
$$d$$

we see that the voicing distinction in labials is lacking. This system, then, has a two-way distinction in supralaryngeal dimension as opposed to one in laryngeal. To make this system symmetrical, the expected addition will be /b/, which introduces the second laryngeal (voice, in this case) distinction. The other alternative, namely the introduction of another supralaryngeal distinction by adding /f/ to this system, is disallowed by the laryngeal-supralaryngeal cyclicity principle, as the addition of /f/ would introduce a supralaryngeal distinction (manner, in this case) to an already asymmetrical system.

The principle of laryngeal-supralaryngeal cyclicity does not prohibit the addition of more than one sound to the inventory at the same time. Multiple sounds can be added as long as they all introduce either a laryngeal or a supralarygeal distinction and not both.

The advantage of this new approach via grouping of features into laryngeal and supralaryngeal is seen in its explanatory nature: This principle allows us to account for why certain expansions occur while others do not. The implications of the principle in therapy also have been studied. If we reconsider the asymmetrical system of

$$p \quad t$$
$$d$$

seen earlier, we can entertain the following two possibilities: The first would be an expected distinction in the laryngeal dimension, and the therapy would aim at teaching /b/. The second position might exploit a more advanced situation by skipping the laryngeal addition (/b/), and aiming for another supralaryngeal distinction by teaching /f/. Because it is assumed that establishment of this new target will be done only after acquisition of the untreated laryngeal distinction (/b/), it represents a more advanced achievement. Gierut (1994a) found this alternative to be more efficacious.

Maximal opposition treatment is another contribution of feature geometry (Gierut, 1990, 1991, 1992; Gierut & Neumann, 1992). In traditional minimal pair treatment, the focus is on the minimal difference between the target and the replacement. For example, in a common substitution such as *soup* → [tup], the treatment will focus on the contrast between /s/ and /t/, and the child will be exposed to pairs differing by these sounds. The maximal opposition principle suggests that the erroneously produced target sound be contrasted with another target sound which is maximally different. For example, instead of contrasting with /t/, /s/ is contrasted with a much more different but already-established sound such as /m/. The degree of difference between the two sounds in the pair is determined by the type and number of features that create the difference. Gierut's results suggested that the maximal opposition treatment is more effective than traditional minimal pair treatment in that it introduces more new phonemes to the system. She also found that, when the contrasting pair in question was in opposition in the feature [sonorant], the effectiveness was greater. This is significant because, in feature geometry, [sonorant] is a very important feature and has the highest position in the feature tree. In other words, if the pair differs in [sonorant] (the highest feature) and also in lower features such as voice, place, and manner, the geometry can predict that many new phonemes can be added, because contrasts will be created at all tiers of the tree. This will not happen in conventional minimal pair treatment in which only the terminal (lower level in the geometry) features are involved in the contrast.

UNDERSPECIFICATION

Certain properties of a sound are predictable given its other properties. Such predictable redundancies are part of every language and, instead of being part of the underlying form, they can be given as redundancy rules. For example, in English, all sonorants are voiced. Thus, specification for [voice] for these segments may be dispensed with. The concept of underspecification, which is another trademark of nonlinear phonological models, deals with the question of how much information needs to be specified in the underlying representation.

According to the concept of underspecification, the grammar of a language is simplest when the underlying representations contain the least amount of specification and still maintain the contrasts of the language. English and Sindhi stops made in the same place of articulation provide a familiar example. If we consider the bilabial stops, both English and Sindhi have voiceless unaspirated, voiceless aspirated, and voiced, [p, pʰ, b]. However, there is a fundamental difference in their phonological organization. In Sindhi, these three sounds are used contrastively, as in [pənu] "leaf," [pʰənu] "snake hood," and [bənu] "forest." In English, on the other hand, there is no contrast between the voiceless aspirated and the voiceless unaspirated stops; [p] and [pʰ] are allophones of the same phoneme, and their distribution is predictable. Thus, aspiration is nondistinctive (predictable and redundant) in English and does not need to be shown in the underlying representations. In Sindhi, on the other hand, aspiration must be indicated in the underlying representations.

The example cited above shows that different languages categorize the same phonetic facts differently in phonological terms, and suggests that certain redundancies are language-specific. However, several other redundancies are universal. For example, [+low] implies [–high] universally, as it is impossible for a segment to be made with both low and high tongue positions at the same time. There are also other relationships that show the unmarked (expected) state of affairs. For example, if a segment is [+sonorant], it is more than likely that it will be [+voiced]. Other relationships that result from occurrences in languages of the world include the feature [coronal], which is taken as the universal default place of articulation. This means that coronals are the unmarked, and thus unspecified, consonants for place, whereas the other places (labials and dorsals) are more marked and are specified. Similarly, as far as the manner of articulation is concerned, continuants are treated as marked, thus specified, whereas noncontinuants are unmarked (unspecified). This is derived from the universally observed commonality of stops as opposed to fricatives. Putting all these together, we can say that /t/, a coronal noncontinuant, is the least specified stop and /s/, a coronal continuant, is the least specified fricative. When the two are compared, however, /t/ is less specified than /s/, because it is not specified for continuant.

According to the theory of underspecification, the values that are not present underlyingly are filled by universal and language-specific default rules. There are two different views about the degree of specifications of underlying representations: contrastive specification (Clements, 1985; Steriade, 1987) and radical underspecification (Archangeli, 1988; Kiparsky, 1982). Although both proposals account for redundant feature specification and relations among features, they have different claims on the underspecification of segments. Contrastive specification requires the specification of both values of all and only contrastive features underlyingly; non-contrastive values are left blank. For example, fricatives and stops in the same place of articulation will be specified [+continuant] and [–continuant], respectively. Similarly, in a system that has contrasting voiced and voiceless obstruents, these segments will be specified [+voice] and [–voice], respectively. This point can be illustrated in greater detail by looking at a five vowel system, /i, e, a, o, u/, which is quite common in languages. The fully specified matrix looks like the following:

	i	*e*	*a*	*o*	*u*
high	+	–	–	–	+
low	–	–	+	–	–
back	–	–	+	+	+

From this full specification, the segment pairs that differ by a single feature specification can be extracted. The pairs /i, e/ and /o, u/ can be distinguished in terms of [high]; [low] will be used for the /a/ versus /o/

contrast. Finally, [back] is specified for the contrasts /i/ versus /u/ and /e/ versus /o/. Consequently, once all pairs have been examined and appropriate feature specifications have been marked contrastive, all unmarked feature specifications for each segment are deleted. This way, the following is obtained:

	i	e	a	o	u
high	+	−		−	+
low			+	−	
back	−	−		+	+

The other view, called radical underspecification, requires underlying representations that include the specification of all and only marked (unpredictable) values of features. The predictable values of these features are left blank and are filled in by default rules. Thus, the following will result in the two above-mentioned cases: When there are fricatives and stops in the same place of articulation, only fricatives are specified for [+continuant]; stops will have no specification, because they are the unmarked (expected) segments as opposed to fricatives. As for the other case, in which the system had contrasting voiced and voiceless obstruents, only the [+voice] value would be specified, and the underspecified [−voice] property would be filled in by a rule. The reason for this is that the unmarked voicing condition for an obstruent is the voiceless state. Returning to the five-vowel system, the following values will be inserted by rules and, thus, will be unspecified:

[+low]	→	[−high]
[+low]	→	[+back]
[low]	→	[−low]
[high]	→	[+high]
[back]	→	[−back]

Consequently, the following is obtained:[2]

	i	e	a	o	u
high		−		−	
low			+		
back				+	+

To give an example from consonants, consider the place, manner, and voicing specifications for English stops and fricatives.

	p	b	f	v	θ	ð	t	d	s	z	ʃ	ʒ	k	g
Continuant			+	+	+	+			+	+	+	+		
Voiced		+		+		+		+		+		+		+
Coronal					*	*					**	**		
Labial	+	+	+	+										
Dorsal													+	+

* Coronal : [+distributed]
** Coronal : [–anterior]

Using the model of radical underspecification, the following relationships are seen in the above table: /t/ is completely unspecified, whereas /v/, /ð/, and /ʒ/ are the most specified segments. The explanation for /t/ is that [–continuant] is the unmarked value for manner, [+coronal] is the unmarked value for place, and [–voice] is the unmarked value for obstruents. Thus, for all of these values, /t/ is left unspecified, and the unmarked values are filled in by default rules. The most specified segments in the above table, /v, ð, ʒ/, share [+continuant] and [+voice] (both marked for obstruents). In addition, /v/ is marked for labial because coronal is the unmarked place. Although both /ð/ and /ʒ/ are coronals, they must be specified for [distributed] and [anterior], respectively, because these specifications are necessary to distinguish them from /z/. Interdentals are distinguished from other coronal fricatives in terms of the feature [+distributed], and the palato-alveolars are distinguished from other coronals in terms of [–anterior]. Some other observations from this table are also apparent. Both /p/ and /k/ are specified for the place of articulation because neither one is coronal; they are unspecified for [continuant] because both are stops and unspecified for [voice] because both are voiceless. The similarity ends there, however. /p/ is specified for [labial], whereas /k/ is specified for [dorsal]. Another type of relationship is observed between /v/ and /z/, which are specified for three features and two features, respectively. Although both need to be specified for [continuant] because they are fricatives, and [voice] because they are voiced, only /v/ must be specified for place ([labial]) because /z/ is the unmarked (unspecified) coronal.

To summarize, whereas contrastive underspecification takes the segment as the basic unit, radical underspecification considers the feature as the unit. As such, the latter seems to be a more plausible approach in a feature-based theory of phonology.

With this information, the comparison of English and Sindhi stops can be revisited. Recall that voiceless aspirated, voiceless unaspirated, and voiced stops are in contrast in Sindhi. What this means is that the feature that is used for aspiration, [spread glottis], must be specified in the underlying form, because /pʰ/ is distinct from /p/. In English, however, this is not the case; the stops in [pʰɪt] and [spɪt] are unspecified [spread glottis] at the underlying level. The stop in [pʰɪt] will be converted into [+spread glottis] via the context-sensitive rule of English which states that voiceless stops are aspirated at the beginning of stressed syllables. As for [spɪt], the default rule assigns [–spread glottis].

DEVELOPMENTAL AND CLINICAL IMPLICATIONS

There are several developmental implications of underspecification. One of them concerns the issue of how much featural information must be present in the underlying form and in the changes in the complexity of that featural information during development. As mentioned earlier, underspecification theory claims that the underlying representations should contain only nonredundant properties of segments, and the predictable featural properties should be supplied by universal default rules. Accordingly, the child does not need to learn the default rules. What the child needs to learn is the distinctive features to encode the lexicon and the context-sensitive rules for the marked features of the ambient language. For example, because the unmarked value for the voiceless stops is unaspirated, the English rule that aspirates /p, t, k/ in initial position of stressed syllables must be learned via exposure to English. Likewise, a German child does not need to learn the obstruent devoicing rule in final position because, although it is a context-sensitive language-specific rule, it does follow the unmarked (expected) pattern for obstruents.

As far as phonological development is concerned, there are two competing views regarding how phonological representations change through development. One view holds that the initial representation begins with full specification with all features and feature values present in the underlying form. Through linguistic input from the ambient language, the child discovers the contrastive features for segments and starts eliminating whatever is redundant. The path of development moves from the general to the specific. The contrasting view claims that the child starts out with the universally specified minimal distinctive features [consonantal], [sonorant], and [continuant]. Through exposure to the ambient language, she or he discovers the relevant contrasts and adds whatever is relevant to the representation. Thus, the development is from less to more complexity in feature specification. Several developmental studies have appealed to these perspectives (Beers, 1996; Dinnsen, 1995; Gierut, 1996; Gierut, Simmerman, & Neuman, 1994; Ingram ,1992; Rice & Avery, 1995).

Several issues in developmental and clinical phonology are related to underspecification. Because underspecification is tied to relative markedness of segments, it is not difficult to establish a relationship between underspecified and preferred segments in development.

First, the order of acquisition seems to be correlated with the degrees of specification of segments. All other things being equal, segments with fewer specified features are acquired earlier than others (Bernhardt, 1992).

Another issue that is related to underspecification and unmarked (preferred) segments is the type of substitutions and targets in developing phonologies. For example, context-free substitutions such as stopping (v → b, ð → d, θ → t, s → t) and fronting (k → t, g → d) reveal the fact that the targets are more specified segments than the substitutes:

ð	→	d		k	→	t
+cons		+cons		+cons		+cons
−son		−son		−son		−son
+cont						
+voice		+voice		Dorsal		
Cor:[+dist]						

In terms of the nonlinear developmental view, these substitutions indicate that the child has not acquired the features [continuant] and [dorsal].

On the other hand, idiosyncratic substitutions such as backing ([pæk] for *pat*, t → k) or spirantization of stops ([sɪk] for *tick*, t → s) reveal situations in which the less specified (more unmarked) targets are replaced by more specified (more marked) substitutes:

t	→	k		t	→	s
+cons		+cons		+cons		+cons
−son		−son		−son		−son
						+cont
		Dorsal				

Underspecification also has influenced the views on treatment. In a detailed tutorial, Bernhardt and Stoel-Gammon (1994) showed that the same data analyzed from the view of underspecification would suggest different intervention targets and strategies than an analysis based on phonological processes. For example, if the child has stopping of the fricatives, a phonological process-based intervention would suggest /f, s/ as treatment targets, because these are the least marked and developmentally earlier sounds. An approach with underspecification, however, would choose sounds that are more specified. The reason for this is that, if the child is taught the specified features of the target language, the default features and feature values will become available via redundancies in the system. For example, instead of /s/, later developing and more specified /ʃ/ or /θ / would be selected as the target. /ʃ/, because of [–anterior], and /θ /, because of [+distributed], will be more specified than /s/, which is [+anterior] and [–distributed]. This is similar to the idea advanced by Elbert and Gierut (1986) in which targeting of segments for which the child has the least phonological knowledge was suggested. This is recommended to stimulate maximum change in the system.

So far it has been assumed that certain segments are more or less marked than others without making reference to the particular context in which they occur. It should be pointed out, however, that the unmarked valued of a feature may vary by syllable position. In Chapter 7, it was mentioned that the occurrence of certain sounds is more natural than others in certain environments. Similarly, in underspecification theory, Dinnsen (1996) proposed context-sensitive radical underspecification. According to this proposal, the default values of a feature would be different in different contexts. For example, although voiceless stops are less marked than voiced stops in general, this may not be assumed to be so in all contexts. Thus, while the unmarked value for stops is voice] word finally, it will be [+voice] prevocalically. Consequently, a voiced stop will have 0 specification in prevocalic position and will be [+voice] word-finally. A voiceless stop, on the other hand, will have [–voice] specification prevocalically, and with 0 specification word-finally. This way, we can account for both prevocalic voicing (*pea* → [bi]) and final devoicing (*bag* → [bæk]) in a very natural manner, as the substitutes are less marked than the targets in respective contexts.

Consonant harmony is another process for which underspecification is relevant. As stated in Chapter 6, this common assimilatory pattern between noncontiguous consonants has been reported for numerous languages. Studies of this topic point to some general biases. For example, alveolars are replaced by velars and labials much more commonly than the reverse. Although this tendency has been noted in the phonology literature, no satisfactory explanation has been offered. Stoel-Gammon and Stemberger (1994) suggested that the answer lies in underspecification by stating that assimilatory processes show a bias toward replacing underspecified elements with specified elements. The reason proposed for this is that the addition of a feature to an underspecified segment is seen as a natural event and, conversely, deletion of a feature is not. Because the change from an alveolar /t/ to a labial /p/ or a velar /k/ is an addition, and the opposite direction would be a deletion, the former will be favored. In the display below, in which the place, manner, and voicing specifications for English stops are presented, alveolars have no specification for place, whereas labials and velars are specified for this feature. Stoel-Gammon and Stemberger hypothesized that there is a bias for alveolars, which are not specified for place, to assimilate to velars or labials (both specified for place), and the reverse is not common. This can be shown in the following:

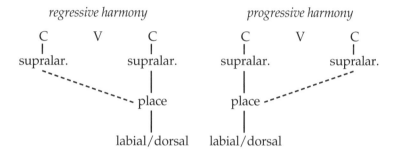

For assimilations that have to do with the manner of articulation, the authors predicted that stops (no specification for manner [continuant]) will assimilate to fricatives (specified for manner, [+continuant]) rather than the reverse. Here again, stops assimilating to fricatives is an operation in which a feature is added, whereas the opposite would entail a deletion of a feature, which is not expected. As far as the assimilations between two segments that are specified for different features are concerned, underspecification does not predict any biases, leaving open the possibility of assimilations in either direction. Thus, for example, the assimilatory events between /p/ and /k/ cannot be determined, because the former is specified for [labial] and the latter for [dorsal].

It is important to note that these predictions that refer to consonant assimilations are the direct opposites of context-free substitutions, fronting, and stopping discussed earlier. In fronting, velars are replaced by alveolars (*key* → [ti], *go* → [do]). Stopping involves the substitutions of fricatives by stops (*van* → [bæn], *sun* → [tʌn]). In these examples, the principle was that the unmarked (unspecified) substitute replaced the more marked (specified) target.

Examining data from 51 children, Stoel-Gammon and Stemberger (1994) found that the context-sensitive consonant harmony conformed to the predictions based on underspecification: place-unspecified alveolars assimilated to more specified labials and velars much more often than the reverse. Similarly, manner-unspecified stops assimilated to specified fricatives much more often than the reverse. Assimilations between two specified groups such as labials and velars, as predicted, did not reveal any significant tendency either way. Thus, underspecification provides a principled account for assimilatory consonant harmony substitutions in developing phonologies, and replaces other inconsistent accounts offered in the literature.

Underspecification is also explanatory for some apparently irregular substitutions that are due to consonant-vowel interactions. Consider the following data from Williams and Dinnsen (1987):

1. tɛi	"catching"		**7.** ko	"comb"		**15.** pɪ	"pinch"	
2. te	"cage"		**8.** kuʔ	"soup"		**16.** puʰ	"push"	
3. tɪkʊ	"chicken"		**9.** kaʰ	"Tom"		**17.** piʔ	"peach"	
4. dɛ	"dress"		**10.** ka	"cough"		**18.** pe	"page"	
5. deʔ	"gate"		**11.** goʔ	"goat"		**19.** bɪ	"big"	
6. dɪ	"swim"		**12.** guʰ	"tooth"		**20.** bɛ	"bed"	
			13. ga	"dog"		**21.** bo	"blow"	
			14. gʊ	"girl"		**22.** buʔ	"boot"	

The subject, N.E. (age 4 years 6 months) revealed that labial consonants are the only ones that are consistently accurate (15–22). Some coronal consonants are replaced by velars (8, 9, 12, 13), but others are accurately produced (4, 6). Similarly, some velar targets are replaced by coronals (1, 2, 5) whereas others are correctly realized (3, 7, 10, 11, 14). Although the situation initially looks chaotic, there is a systematicity in the child's productions. Specifically, coronals appear before front vowels, and velars appear before back vowels. It should be pointed out in passing that, in some of these substitutions, an unmarked sound replaces a marked sound whereas; in others, the reverse is the case. Because labial consonants do appear before any vowel (15–22), the child's system will be judged as having a two-way place contrast between labials and nonlabials. In other words, only labials will be specified for place; other consonants which are regulated by the front/back quality of the following vowel will be left underspecified for spreading. Because labials are specified, they are not prone to spreading. The remaining underspecified consonants (coronals and dorsals) will undergo the assimilatory process via the spread of features from the adjacent specified vowel.[3]

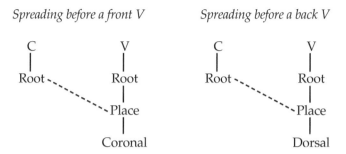

| *Spreading before a front V* | *Spreading before a back V* |

In this way, we can explain that, when coronal targets are before front vowels and velars before back vowels, the child's productions are correct. When the target consonant disagrees with the following vowel in place feature, the production is erroneous.

SHADOW SPECIFICATION

It has been observed that, in the speech of several children with phonological disorders, some target distinctions are merged phonetically. However, some of these phonetic mergers seem to preserve the target distinctions in some nonphonetic way.[4]

Consider the following pretreatment data from a child with phonological disorder age 5 years 5 months (Dinnsen & Chin, 1995, p.138).

[tɪdz]	"kids"	[bæti]	"backy"	[bæt]	"back"
[teɪdz]	"cage"	[dʌti]	"ducky"	[dʌt]	"duck"
[tæts]	"catch"	[buti]	"bookie"	[but]	"book"
[tʌt]	"cut"	[sati]	"sockie"	[sat]	"sock"
[tom]	"comb"	[tad]	"card"		

As we can see, the child neutralizes the target alveolar-velar opposition. A classical process approach to development, given in Chapter 6, represents all of these alveolar substitutes as velars in the child's underlying form. Later, through the process of fronting, these velars are converted to surface alveolars. This account is necessarily abstract because it posits underlying representations with segments that never appear in the child's productions. According to the principles of underspecification, however, the situation is different and the target velars are represented without a specified place feature in the child's system. The substitution of alveolars for velars is done through a default rule that fills in [coronal] as the default place for the unspecified target velars. The claim that is made here is that, because there is no phonetic difference between the surface alveolars used for the ambient alveolars and velars, the two groups are not differentiated by the child. Now, consider the forms that are seen after the therapy (1995, p. 40):

[kɪdz]	"kids"	[bæki]	"backy"	[bæk]	"back"
[keɪdz]	"cage"	[dʌki]	"ducky"	[dʌk]	"duck"
[kɛts]	"catch"	[bʊki]	"bookie"	[bʊk]	"book"
[kʌt]	"cut"	[sɔki]	"sockie"	[sɔk]	"sock"
[kom]	"comb"	[kard]	"card"		

The child who systematically used alveolars for velar targets produced all velars correctly after the therapy without any overgeneralization. In other words, although the velar targets that were previously substituted by alveolars were realized correctly, the alveolar targets that were correct were not converted into velars. This indicates that the child was aware of the target distinctions because, without this awareness, she or he would not have known which alveolars should change to velars. This implies that the distinction between the target alveolars and velars must have been represented and could not have been left unspecified. To account for such cases, a proposal in the form of shadow specification has been made (Dinnsen, 1993; Dinnsen & Chin, 1991, 1993). Shadow specification allows us to make the underlying distinction between two different targets that are realized as phonetically identical. It provides a means for specifying the default value of a feature as opposed to radical underspecification of the same feature for two distinct targets that are merged phonetically. According to this proposal, the alveolar targets that were correctly realized prior to the treatment will be represented as radically underspecified:

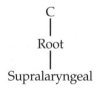

However, the alveolars that were the realizations for the target velars will be shadow-specified for coronal:

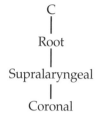

C
|
Root
|
Supralaryngeal
|
Coronal

The concept of shadow specification, advanced to handle cases of target distinctions merged in context-free substitutions, such as fronting of velars and stopping of fricatives, can also be extended to context-sensitive substitutions. A good example is provided by the interaction of consonant harmony with fronting. Here, the central question is whether coronals resulting from fronting of target velars act the same way as other coronals (corresponding to target coronals) with respect to consonant harmony. Dinnsen, Barlow, and Morrisette (1996) analyzed three case studies from normally developing children as well as children with phonological disorders and found individual variation. One child treated coronals that resulted from target velars (the result of fronting) like real coronals; the other children treated the two types of coronals differently. Whereas real coronals were subject to consonant harmony, the coronals that resulted from fronting were not, suggesting a place distinction underlyingly. To account for these differences between children, it was suggested that the ambient coronals and velars that act the same by serving as targets of assimilation are underspecified for place. For children who differentiated the real coronals from the others, the distinction can be shown in terms of underspecification and shadow specification; real coronals will be underspecified whereas the coronals that come from the ambient velars will be shadow specified. This kind of differentiation in the representation also explains the situation in which some children appear to perceive ambient contrasts that they themselves do not produce. The child is capable of handling a phonological difference that does not result in phonetic difference in the production. The authors also addressed the issue of developmental and clinical implications regarding the difference between underspecified and shadow specified forms. The different patterns that are seen in different children suggest two different levels in development. When consonant harmony targets all coronals (corresponding to ambient velars and alveolars), this is an indication that the child does not perceive the ambient distinction.[5] In this case, to make the child aware of the distinction, the recommended path of remediation would be a minimal pair treatment with a focus on both perception and production. If, on the other hand, the child's productions are indicative of different treatment of ambient velars and ambient alveolars evidenced by his or her subjecting only ambient alveolars to consonant harmony, then the child's problem is not one that is related to perception. In this case, what the child needs is to phonetically implement the already existing phonological contrast.

FEATURES, UNDERSPECIFICATION, AND INTERLANGUAGE PHONOLOGY

Feature hierarchy and underspecification also have impacted the field of interlanguage phonology. The explanations of transfer from the first language in the acquisition of second language sounds is an area in which these notions have been utilized. The Feature Competition Model (FCM) advanced by Hancin-Bhatt (1994), similar to the distinctive feature approach given in Chapter 8, assumes that not all features are of the same prominence in a given inventory. Features of greater prominence are claimed to guide what is perceived as L2 sounds and determine the eventual phonological form constructed by the learner. FCM assumes that the underlying representation (UR) is perceptually determined and utilizes feature hierarchy and radical underspecification. It is also assumed that the L2 learner will transfer the feature prominence patterns of his L1 in early L2 learning and, as such, the learning of L2 phonology is constrained by L1 grammar. Because features do not have equal prominence, those with higher prominence will be noticed by the learner before those that are less prominent. As a result, features that are noticed in the input will determine with L1 sound the L2 patterns are associated with.

In deriving feature prominence, two points are of importance. The first is the elimination of redundant features from the UR. This means that, if a feature is not distinctive for a given phoneme, it will not be included in the UR. For example, in English all sonorants are voiced and, consequently, [voiced] is a redundant feature that will not be included in the UR of sonorants. The second point is the elimination of unmarked specification of a distinctive (nonredundant) feature from the UR. For example, [continuant] is a contrastive feature for English obstruents as it separates fricatives [+continuant] from stops and affricates [–continuant]. One of these values is unmarked and will be eliminated from the UR and given by default rules. In the case of the feature [continuant], the [–] value is unmarked and will be absent in the UR.

With these principles, feature prominence can be calculated. This is done by relating the number of phonemic distinctions a particular feature makes in a UR to the total number of phonemes in the language inventory:

$$\text{prominence} = \frac{\text{number of phonemes for which feature is specified}}{\text{total number of phonemes}}$$

To demonstrate how these can be relevant in transfer, Hancin-Bhatt (1994) examined the rendition of English interdental fricatives /θ/ and /ð/ by speakers whose native languages were Japanese, German, and Turkish. In the following, substitutions made by German and Japanese speakers will be looked at. The following table will be used for deriving feature prominences in German obstruents[6]:

	p	b	f	v	t	d	s	z	ʃ	ç	k	g	x
anterior									−				
coronal	−	−	−	−							−	−	
back											+	+	+
continu			+	+			+	+	+	+			+
strident			+	+			+	+	+	+			
voice		+		+		+		+				+	

The following default rules determine the values that are eliminated in the above table:

anterior	→	+anterior	(thus,	only	−anterior is	specified)
coronal	→	+coronal	("	"	−coronal	")
back	→	−back	("	"	+back	")
continu.	→	−cont.	("	"	+cont.	")
strident	→	−strident	("	"	+strident	")
voice	→	−voice	("	"	+voice	")

From the above table, the following feature prominences are derived:

$$\text{continuant} : 7/13 \quad 54\%$$
$$\text{coronal, strident} : 6/13 \quad 46\%$$
$$\text{voice} : 5/13 \quad 38\%$$
$$\text{back} : 3/13 \quad 23\%$$
$$\text{anterior} : 2/13 \quad 15\%$$

On the basis of these, it is suggested that [continuant], because of its high prominence (54%), will be noticed in perception by German speakers who would tend to map the English /θ / and /ð/ with the German anterior, coronal stridents [s] and [z]. This prediction seems to correctly represent what occurs in interlingual transfer.

For Japanese, we have the following table:[7]

	p	b	f	t	d	ts	s	z	ʃ	tʃ	dʒ	k	g
anterior									−	−	−		
coronal	−	−	−									−	−
back												+	+
continu.			+				+	+	+				
strid.						+	+	+	+	+	+		
voice		+			+			+			+		+

Feature prominences derived from the above table show the following:

$$
\begin{aligned}
\text{strident} &: 6/13 \quad 46\% \\
\text{coronal, voice} &: 5/13 \quad 38\% \\
\text{continuant} &: 4/13 \quad 31\% \\
\text{anterior} &: 3/13 \quad 23\% \\
\text{back} &: 2/13 \quad 15\%
\end{aligned}
$$

Because [continuant] is neither very strong nor very weak, it is suggested that it may or may not be noticed, and variations in rendition are possible. However, the English interdental fricative targets are more likely to be misperceived as strident as they are closer to the stronger prominences than the weaker ones.

Although this methodology has considerable success with the above realistic predictions, it does not seem to be free of problems. In the Turkish rendition of the interdental fricatives, we invariably see [t] and [d], and this is problematic. The following table represents Turkish obstruents:

	p	b	f	v	t	d	s	z	ʃ	ʒ	tʃ	dʒ	k	g[8]
anterior									−	−	−	−		
coronal	−	−	−	−									−	−
back													+	+
continu.			+	+			+	+	+	+				
voice		+		+		+		+		+		+		+

This table gives us the following prominences:

$$
\begin{aligned}
\text{voice} &: 7/14 \quad 50\% \\
\text{coronal, continuant} &: 6/14 \quad 43\% \\
\text{anterior} &: 4/14 \quad 29\% \\
\text{back} &: 2/14 \quad 14\%
\end{aligned}
$$

Although it is not the strongest, [continuant], with its relatively high prominence, should create opportunities for variable renditions. However, the fact that Turkish speakers invariably choose [t] and [d] and never utilize [s] and [z] casts doubts on the ability of this methodology to successfully predict transfer in interlanguage substitutions. In conclusion, the idea of the feature competition model is an attractive one but requires further elaborations before it can be considered a solid approach for predictions of transfer.

SUMMARY

This chapter looked at more recent developments regarding the hierarchical arrangement of features. This model, called feature geometry, suggests that in representing a segment, features are organized in such a way so that some of them are grouped together within superordinate nodes, and all features are combined in a single hierarchically arranged structure known as a feature tree.

A related topic that has been dealt with here is underspecification, which suggests that the values of certain distinctive features need not be underlyingly specified, and the values that are not present underlyingly are filled by universal and language-specific default rules. This viewpoint indicates that markedness is intimately related to underspecification. Finally, shadow specification, an extension of underspecification, has also been considered. Developmental and therapeutic implications of these developments were discussed.

NOTES

1. It should be pointed out that the relation between feature trees and articulatory processes is still rather vague with respect to the organization of manner features. Although manner features, [strident], [lateral], and [continuant], are attached to the root node, their applications reveal the involvement of certain specific articulators. For example, [strident] applies only to coronal and labial articulations. In other words, strident is attached to the root of the tree, yet it relates only to a node that is deeply embedded in that tree. Another problem is related to [lateral]; although this, too, is attached to the root (i.e., articulator-free), it is almost always restricted to Coronal consonants. Finally, [continuant] seems to combine freely with the Labial, Coronal, and Dorsal and, consequently, may be attached to the oral cavity node.

2. Other possibilities also exist. For example, taking only one of the two top implicational relationships ([+low] → [–high] or [+low] → [+back]), we can come up with different radically underspecified tables. The one given here is claimed to be the pattern by universal preferences.

3. This assumes, after Clements and Hume, (1995), that a unified set of features can be used for both vowels and consonants.

4. These cases are not the same as others reported in the literature (Forrest, Weismer, Hodge, Dinnsen, & Saxman, 1990; Tyler, Edwards, & Saxman, 1990) in which children maintained ambient distinction phonetically as well as phonemically, but in a nonambient fashion.

5. This can also be interpreted that the child has a simpler production system with greater and more general output constraints.

6. Hancin-Bhatt, based on Benware (1986), included /z/ in the inventory of German. However, because this is a marginal phoneme restricted to certain borrowings, it is excluded here. There are some matters of dispute for German obstruents. The first concerns the status of /ç/ and /x/. A common interpretation is based on the fact that [ç] is found after front vowels, after /n, l, r/, and in word-initial position, and [x] occurs only after central and back vowels, and never in word-initial position. This classic case of complementary distribution has one exception. The diminutive suffix *-chen* [çən] is invariable and gives rise to some contrasts between [ç] and [x] as seen in the following examples: *Tauchen* [tauçən] "little rope" versus *tauchen* [tauxən] "to dive"; *Kuhchen* [ku:çən] "little cow" versus *Kuchen* [ku:xən] "cake". Thus, this table reflects the contrasts supported by only these limited examples. Another problem involves the status of the affricates [pf] and [ts], as to whether they should be treated as unit phonemes or clusters of two phonemes. Hancin-Bhatt did not consider these as unit phonemes and excluded them from the table of obstruents. One can easily see, however, that if these disputed cases are interpreted otherwise, the computation of feature prominences for German obstruents would be different.

7. This is basically what Hancin-Bhatt gives (based on Vance (1987). The only modification made here is the exclusion of /h/. The reason for this is to maintain uniformity, as /h/ is not included in German and Turkish inventories. The Japanese inventory is also controversial. First, most orthodox inventories of Japanese do not include /f/. Second, most analyses do not recognize the phonemic distinction be-

tween /s/, /ts/, /dz/ and /ʃ/ and give the following allophonic distribution: [ʃ] is an allophone of /s/, [dz] is an allophone of /z/, [tʃ] is an allophone of /t/ before /i/, and [ts] is an allophone of /t/ before /u/.

8. I give my own analysis of Turkish, as I find Hancin-Bhatt's version (taken from Lees, 1968) implausible.

EXERCISES

1. Arrange the consonants of English according to feature geometry places of articulation (labial, coronal, dorsal).

2. Draw the trees for the following segments:

Example: /i/

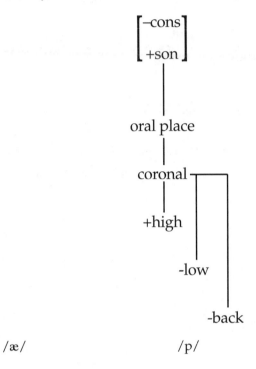

/æ/   /p/   /s/

3. It is suggested that the more deeply embedded features in the tree would be learned later than the features that appear at higher nodes. As a corollary, common child substitutions are expected to create mismatches in features that are lower in the tree and, conversely, unusual substitutions involve the higher features.

Example:

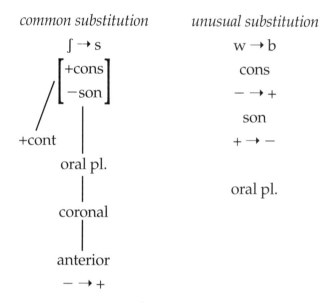

common substitution   unusual substitution

(common substituion   (unusual substitution
involving lower feature)   involving higher features)

Examine the following common and unusual substitutions and state if they support the principle suggested above:

a. f → w   b. ð → d   c. θ → t

d. j → t   e. w → v   f. k → t

4. It is also suggested that, all other things being equal, segments with fewer specified features would be acquired earlier than others. As a corollary, in context-free common child substitutions, the replacements would be less specified/marked than the targets that are more specified/marked, and in unusual substitutions the converse will hold.

Example:

common substitution		*unusual substitution*	
θ → t		d → ð	
+cons	+cons	+cons	+cons
−son	−son	−son	−son
+cont			+cont
		+voice	+voice

Cor: [+dist]

(less specified replacing more specified)	(more specified replacing less specified)

Examine the following common and unusual substitutions and state if they support the above hypotheses.

a. w → v   b. s → t   c. l → ð

d. θ → s   e. b → v   f. ʃ → s

5. Consider the following inventories and determine which
   are permissible expansions and which are not according
   to the laryngeal-supralaryngeal cyclicity:

<table>
<tr><td></td><td>p</td><td>t</td><td></td><td></td><td></td><td>p</td><td>t</td><td>k</td></tr>
<tr><td></td><td>b</td><td>d</td><td></td><td></td><td></td><td>b</td><td>d</td><td>g</td></tr>
<tr><td>a.</td><td>p</td><td>t</td><td>k</td><td></td><td>a.</td><td>p</td><td>t</td><td>k</td></tr>
<tr><td></td><td>b</td><td>d</td><td></td><td></td><td></td><td>b</td><td>d</td><td>g</td></tr>
<tr><td></td><td></td><td></td><td></td><td></td><td></td><td></td><td></td><td></td></tr>
<tr><td>b.</td><td>p</td><td>t</td><td>k</td><td></td><td></td><td></td><td>s</td><td></td></tr>
<tr><td></td><td>b</td><td>d</td><td>g</td><td></td><td>b.</td><td>p</td><td>t</td><td>k</td></tr>
<tr><td></td><td></td><td></td><td></td><td></td><td></td><td>b</td><td>d</td><td>g</td></tr>
<tr><td>c.</td><td>p</td><td>t</td><td>k</td><td></td><td></td><td>f</td><td>s</td><td></td></tr>
<tr><td></td><td>b</td><td>d</td><td></td><td></td><td></td><td></td><td></td><td></td></tr>
<tr><td></td><td></td><td>s</td><td></td><td></td><td>c.</td><td>p</td><td>t</td><td>k</td></tr>
<tr><td></td><td></td><td></td><td></td><td></td><td></td><td>b</td><td>d</td><td>g</td></tr>
<tr><td>d.</td><td>p</td><td>t</td><td>k</td><td></td><td></td><td></td><td>s</td><td></td></tr>
<tr><td></td><td>b</td><td>d</td><td></td><td></td><td></td><td></td><td>z</td><td></td></tr>
<tr><td></td><td>f</td><td></td><td></td><td></td><td></td><td></td><td></td><td></td></tr>
</table>

d. p   t   k
b   d   g
f

6. What would be your suggested pair for a maximal opposition treatment for the following child substitution?
a. k → t
b. ʃ → s
c. v → b

7. Features also are used in the prediction of sound substitutions in second/foreign language learning. The Feature
Competition Model discussed in this chapter tries to predict substitutions with the prominence of each feature by
dividing the number of phonemes for which the feature is
specified by the total number of phonemes. Examine the
obstruents of Spanish given below and state if the Feature
Competition Model is successful in predicting the replacement of [t] for the English target /θ / by speakers of
Spanish.

          p b f t d s tʃ k g x
ANTERIOR
CORONAL
CONTINUANT
STRIDENT
VOICE

Use the following default rules in filling the underspecified inventory:

[anterior]	→	[+anterior]
[coronal]	→	[+coronal]
[continuant]	→	[–continuant]
[strident]	→	[–strident]
[voice]	→	[–voice]

8. The same English target, /θ /, has the replacement [s] by French speakers. Examine the obstruents of French given below and state whether the Feature Competition Model can successfully predict the replacement.

	p	*b*	*f*	*v*	*t*	*d*	*s*	*z*	*ʃ*
ANTERIOR									
CORONAL									
CONTINUANT									
STRIDENT									
VOICE									

REFERENCES

Adams, C. (1979). *English speech rhythm and the foreign learner.* The Hague: Mouton.

Anderson, J. M. (1986). Suprasegmental dependencies. In J. Durand, (Ed.), *Dependency and non-linear phonology.* London: Croom Helm.

Archangeli, D. (1988). Aspects of underspecification theory. *Phonology, 5,* 183–207.

Asher, J., & Garcia, R. (1969). The optimal age to learn a foreign language. *Modern Language Journal, 53,* 334–341.

Bankson, N. W., & Bernthal, J. E. (1990). *Bankson-Bernthal test of phonology.* Chicago: Riverside Press.

Barlow, J. (1996). Variability and phonological knowledge. In T. Powell (Ed.), *Pathologies of speech and language: Contributions of clinical phonetics and linguistics* (pp. 125–133). New Orleans, LA: International Clinical Phonetics and Linguistics Association.

Beatens-Beardsmore, H. (1982). *Bilingualism: Basic principles.* Clevedon, Avon: Tieto Ltd.

Beers, M.(1996). Acquisition of dutch phonological contrasts within the framework of feature geometry theory. In B. Bernhardt, J. Gilbert, & D. Ingram (Eds.), *Proceedings of the UBC International Conference of Phonological Acquisition* (pp. 28–41). Somerville, MA: Cascadilla Press.

Benware, W. (1986). *Phonetics and phonology of modern German.* Washington DC: Georgetown University Press.

Berko, J. (1958). The child's learning of English morphology. *Word, 14,* 150–177.

Bernhardt, B. (1992) The application of nonlinear phonology to intervention with a phonologically disordered child. *Clinical Linguistics and Phonetics, 6,* 283–316.

Bernhardt, B. (1994). The prosodic tier and phonological disorders. In M. Yavas (Ed.), *First and second language phonology* (pp. 149–172). San Diego, CA: Singular Publishing Group.

Bernhardt, B., & Stoel-Gammon, C. (1994). Nonlinear phonology: Introduction and clinical application. *Journal of Speech and Hearing Research, 37,* 123–143.

Bird, J., & Bishop, D. V. M. (1992). Perception and awareness of phonemes in phonologically impaired children. *European Journal of Disorders of Communication, 27,* 289–311.

Bird, J., Bishop, D. V. M., & Freeman, N. H. (1995). Phonological awareness and literacy development in children with expressive phonological impairments. *Journal of Speech and Hearing Research, 38,* 446–462.

Blache, S., Parsons, C., & Humphreys, J. (1981). A minimal word pair model for teaching linguistic significance of distinctive feature properties. *Journal of Speech and Hearing Research, 46,* 291–296.

Bleile, K.M. (1991). *Child phonology: A book of exercises for students.* San Diego, CA: Singular Publishing Group.

Bloomfield, L. (1933). *Language.* New York: John Wiley.

Bodine, A. (1974). A phonological analysis of the speech of two mongoloid (Down's syndrome) boys. *Anthropological Linguistics,16,* 1–24.

Bortolini, U., & Leonard, L. (1991). The speech of phonologically disordered children acquiring Italian. *Clinical Linguistics and Phonetics, 5,* 1–12.

Broselow, E. (1993). Transfer and universals in second language epenthesis. In S. Gass & L. Selinker (Eds.), *Language transfer in language learning* (pp. 71–86). Amsterdam: John Benjamins.

Brown, R. (1958). *Words and things.,* Glencoe, IL: Free Press.

Burling, R. (1959). Language development of a Garo speaking child. *Word, 15,* 45–68.

Cairns, H.S., & Williams, F. (1972). An analysis of the substitution errors of a group of standard English-speaking children. *Journal of Speech and Hearing Research, 15,* 811–820.

Camarata, S., & Gandour, J. (1984). On describing idiosyncratic phonologic systems. *Journal of Speech and Hearing Disorders, 49,* 262–266.

Carlisle, R.S. (1988). The effect of markedness on epenthesis in Spanish/English interlanguage phonology. *Issues and Developments in English and Applied Linguistics, 3,* 15–23.

Carlisle, R. S. (1991a). The influence of environment on vowel epenthesis in Spanish/English interphonology. *Applied Linguistics, 12,* 76–95.

Carlisle, R. S. (1991b). The influence of syllable structure universals on the variability of interlanguage phonology. In A. D. Volpe (Ed.), *The Seventeenth LACUS Forum 1990* (pp. 135–145). Lake Bluff, IL: Linguistic Association of Canada and the United States.

Carlisle, R. S. (1994). Markedness and environment as internal constraints on the variability of inter-language phonology. In M. Yavas (Ed.), *First and second language phonology* (pp. 223–250). San Diego, CA: Singular Publishing Group.

Carr, P. (1993). *Phonology.* New York: St. Martin's Press.

Catford, J. C. (1988). *A practical introduction to phonetics.* New York: Oxford University Press.

Chao, Y. R. (1951). The Cantian idiolect: An analysis of the Chinese spoken by a twenty-eight-month-old-child. *University of California Publications in Semitic Philology, 11,* 27–44. Reprinted in A. Bar-Adon & W. F. Leopold (Eds.), (1971), *Child language: A book of readings.* Englewood Cliffs, NJ: Prentice-Hall.

Cheng, L. R. L. (1987). *Assessing Asian language performance: Guidelines for evaluating limited-English-proficient students.* Rockville, MD: Aspen.

Chiat, S. (1989). The relation between prosodic structure, syllabification and segmental realization: Evidence from a child with fricative stopping. *Clinical Linguistics and Phonetics, 3,* 223–241.

Chiat, S. (1994). From lexical access to lexical output: What is the problem for children with impaired phonology? In M. Yavas (Ed.), *First and second language phonology* (pp. 107–134). San Diego, CA: Singular Publishing Group.

Chin, S. (1996). The role of the sonority hierarchy in delayed phonological systems. In T. W. Powell (Ed.), *Pathologies of speech and language: Contributions of Clinical phonetics and linguistics* (pp. 109–117). New Orleans, LA: A Publication of the International Clinical Phonetics and Linguistic Association.

Chin, S. & Dinnsen, D.A. (1991). Feature geometry in disordered phonologies. *Clinical Linguistics and Phonetics, 5,* 329-337.

Chomsky, N., & Halle, M.(1968) *The sound pattern of English.* New York: Harper and Row.

Clements, G. N. (1985). The geometry of phonological features. *Phonology Yearbook, 2,* 225–252.

Clements, G. N., & Hume, E.V. (1995). The internal organization of speech sounds. In J. A. Goldsmith (Ed.), *Handbook of phonological theory* (pp. 245–306). Cambridge, MA: Plackwell.

Clements, G., & Keyser, S. (1983). *CV phonology: A generative theory of the syllable.* Cambridge, MA: MIT Press.

Compton, A., & Hutton, S. (1978). *Compton-Hutton phonological assessment.* San Francisco: Carousel House.

Costello, J., & Onstine, J.(1976). The modification of multiple articulation errors based on distinctive feature theory. *Journal of Speech and Hearing Disorders, 41,* 199–215.

Crocker, J. R. (1969). A phonological model of children's articulation competence. *Journal of Speech and Hearing Disorders, 34,* 203–213.

Crystal C. (1984). *Linguistics encounters with language handicap.* Oxford: Basil Blackwell.

Dauer, R. M. (1983) Stress-timing and syllable-timing re-analyzed. *Journal of Phonetics, 11,* 51-62.

De Boysson-Bardies, B., & Vihman, M. M. (1991). Adaptation to Language: evidence from babbling and first words in four languages. *Language, 67,* 297–319.

De Boysson-Bardies, B., Vihman, M. M., Roug-Hellichius, L., Durand, C., Landberg, I., & Arao, F. (1992). Material evidence of infant selection from target language: A cross-linguistic phonetic study. In C. A. Ferguson, L. Menn, & C. Stoel-Gammon (Eds.), *Phonological development: Models, research, implications*. Timonium, MD: York Press.

Delattre, P. (1965). *Comparing the phonetic features of English, French, German, and Spanish: An interim report*. Heidelberg: Julius Gross Verlag.

Dickerson, L. B., & Dickerson, W. B. (1977). Interlanguage phonology: Current research and future directions. In S. P. Corder & E. Roulet (Eds.), *The notions of simplification, interlanguages and pidgins and their relation to second language pedagogy* (pp. 18–30). Geneva: Droz.

Dinnsen, D. A. (1993). Underspecification and phonological disorders. In M. Eid & G. Iverson (Eds.), *Principles and prediction: The analysis of natural language*. Philadelphia: Benjamins.

Dinnsen, D. A. (1995). Context-sensitive underspecification and the acquisition of phonemic contrasts. *Journal of Child Language, 23,* 57–79.

Dinnsen, D. A. (1996). Context effects in the acquisition of fricatives. In B. Bernhardt, J. Gilbert, & D. Ingram (Eds.), *Proceedings of the UBC International Conference on Phonological Acquisition* (pp. 136–147). Somerville, MA: Cascadilla Press.

Dinnsen, D., Barlow, J., & Morrisette, M. (1997). Long distance place assimilation with an interacting error pattern in phonological acquisition. *Clinical Linguistics and Phonetics, 11,* 319–338.

Dinnsen, D. A., & Chin, S. (1991). Feature geometry in disordered phonologies. *Clinical Linguistics and Phonetics, 5,* 329–337.

Dinnsen, D. A., & Chin, S. (1993). Individual differences in phonological disorders and implications for a theory of acquisition. In F. Eckman (Ed.), *Confluence: Linguistics, L2 acquisition and speech pathology* (pp. 137–152). Amsterdam: John Benjamins.

Dinnsen, D. A., & Chin, S. (1994). Independent and relational accounts of phonological disorders. In M. Yavas (Ed.), *First and second language phonology* (pp. 135–148). San Diego, CA: Singular Publishing Group.

Dinnsen, D. A., & Chin, S. (1995). On the natural domain of phonological disorders. In J. Archibald (Ed.), *Phonological acquisition and phonological theory* (pp. 135–150). Hillsdale, NJ: Lawrence Erlbaum.

Dinnsen, D. A., Chin, S., Elbert, M., & Powell, T. (1990). Some constraints on functionally disordered phonologies: Phonetic inventories and phonotactics. *Journal of Speech and Hearing Research 33,* 28–37.

Dinnsen, D. A., & Elbert, M. (1984) On the relationship between phonology and learning. In M. Elbert, G. Weismer, & D. A. Dinnsen (Eds.), *Phonological theory and the Misarticulating child. ASHA Monographs, 22,* 59–68.

Dodd, B. (1975). Recognition and reproductions of words by Down's syndrome and non-Down's retarded children. *American Journal of Mental Deficiency, 80,* 45–69.

Dodd, B. (1993) Speech disordered children. In G. Blanken, J. Dittman, H. Grimm, J. Marshall, & C. Wallesh (Eds.), *Linguistic disorders and pathologies* (pp. 825–834). Berlin: De Gruyter.

Dodd, B., & So, L. (1994). The phonological abilities of Cantonese-speaking children with hearing loss. *Journal of Speech and Hearing Research, 37,* 671–679.

Dodd, B., Holm, A., & Wei, L. (1997). Speech disorder in preschool children exposed to Cantonese and English. *Clinical Linguistics and Phonetics, 11,* 229–243.

Donegan, P. J., & Stampe, D. (1979). The study of natural phonology. In D. A. Dinnsen (Ed.), *Current approaches to phonological theory* (pp. 126–173). Bloomington: Indiana University Press.

Drachman, G. (1973). Some strategies in the acquisition of phonology. In M. J. Kenstowicz & C. W. Kisseberth (Eds.), *Issues in phonological theory* (pp. 145–159). The Hague: Mouton.

Dunn, C., & Davis, B. (1983). Phonological process occurrence in phonologically disordered children. *Applied Psycholinguistics, 4,* 187–207.

Durand, J. (1990). *Generative and non-linear phonology.* London: Longman.

Dyson, A. T. (1988). Phonetic inventories of 2- and 3-year old children. *Journal of Speech and Hearing Disorders, 53,* 89–93.

Eckman, F. (1977). Markedness and the contrastive analysis hypothesis. *Language Learning, 27,* 315–330.

Eckman, F. (1985). Some theoretical and pedagogical implications of the markedness differential hypothesis. *Studies in Second Language Acquisition, 13,* 23–41.

Eckman, F., & Iverson, G. (1994). Pronunciation difficulties in ESL: Coda consonants in English Interlanguage. In M. Yavas (Ed.), *First and second language phonology* (pp. 251–265). San Diego, CA: Singular Publishing Group.

Edwards, M. L. (1979). *Patterns and processes in fricative acquisition: Longitudinal evidence from six English-speaking children.* Unpublished doctoral dissertation, Stanford University, Stanford, CA.

Edwards, M. L. (1980). *The use of favorite sounds by children with phonological disorders.* Paper presented at the Fifth Annual Boston University Conference on Language Development, Boston, MA.

Edwards, M. L. (1983). Selection criteria for developing therapy goals. *Journal of Childhood Communication Disorders, 7,* 36–45.

Edwards, M. L. (1992). Clinical forum: Phonological assessment and treatment in support of phonological processes. *Language Speech and Hearing Services in Schools, 23,* 233–240.

Edwards, M. L., & Bernhardt, B. (1983). *Phonological analysis of the speech of four children with language disorders.* Unpublished manuscript.

Ferguson, C. A., & Farwell, C. B. (1975). Words and sounds in early language acquisition: English initial consonants in the first fifty words. *Language, 51,* 419–439.

Fey, M. (1985). Articulation and phonology: Inextricable constructs in speech pathology. *Journal of Speech-Language Pathology and Audiology, 9*, 7–16.

Flege, J. E. (1987). The production of "new" and "similar" phones in a foreign language: Evidence for the effect of equivalence classification. *Journal of Phonetics, 15*, 47–65.

Flege, J. E. (1991). Age of learning affects the authenticity of voice-onset-time (VOT) in stop consonants produced in second language. *Journal of the Acoustical Society of America, 89*, 395–411.

Flege, J. E., & Eefting, W. (1986). Linguistic and developmental effects on the production and perception of stop consonants. *Phonetica, 43*, 155–171.

Flege, J. E., & Eefting, W. (1987). The production and perception of English stops by Spanish speakers of English. *Journal of Phonetics, 15*, 67–83.

Flege, J. E., & Fletcher, K. (1992). Talker and listener effects on degree of perceived accent. *Journal of the Acoustical Society of America, 91*, 370–389.

Flege, J. E., & Port, R. (1981). Cross-language phonetic interference: Arabic to English. *Language and Speech, 24*, 125–146.

Forrest, K., Weismer, G., Hodge, M., Dinnsen, D., & Elbert, M. (1990). Statistical analysis of word-initial /k/ and /t/ produced by normal and phonologically disordered children. *Clinical Linguistics and Phonetics, 4*, 327–340.

French, A. (1989). The systematic acquisition of word forms by a child during his first-fifty-word stage. *Journal of Child Language, 16*, 69–90.

Fries, C. C. (1945). *Teaching and learning English as a foreign language.* Ann Arbor: University of Michigan Press.

Fromkin, V., & Rodman, R. (1993). An introduction to language (5th ed.). New York: Harcourt Brace Jovanovich.

Fry, D. B. (1955). Duration and intensity as physical correlates of linguistic stress. *Journal of the Acoustical Society of America, 27*, 765–768.

Fry, D. B. (1958). Experiments in the perception of stress. *Language and Speech, 1*, 126–152.

Fry, D. B. (1965). The dependence of stress judgements on vowel formant structure. In E. Zwirner & W. Bethge (Eds.), *Proceedings of the Sixth International Congress of Phonetic Sciences* (pp. 306–311). Basel: Karger.

Gamkrelidze, T. V. (1978). On the correlation of stops and fricatives in a phonological system. In J. H. Greenberg et al. (Eds.), *Universals of human language: Vol. 2. Phonology* (pp. 9–46). Stanford, CA: Stanford University Press.

Giegerich, H. (1992). *English phonology.* Boston, MA: Cambridge University Press.

Gierut, J. A. (1985). *On the relationship between phonological knowledge and generalization learning in misarticulating children.* Unpublished doctoral dissertation, Indiana University, Bloomington, IN.

Gierut, J. A. (1990). Differential learning of phonological oppositions. *Journal of Speech and Hearing Research, 33*, 540–549.

Gierut, J. A. (1991). Homonymy in phonological change. *Clinical Linguistics and Phonetics, 5,* 119–137.

Gierut, J. A. (1992). The conditions and course of clinically induced phonological change. *Journal of Speech and Hearing Research, 35,* 1049–1063.

Gierut, J. A. (1994a). Cyclicity in the acquisition of phonemic distinctions. *Lingua, 94,* 1–23.

Gierut, J. A. (1994b). An experiemental test of phonemic cyclicity. *Journal of Child Language, 23,* 291–316.

Gierut, J. A. (1996). Categorization and feature specification in phonological acquisition. *Journal of Child Language, 23*(2), 397–415.

Gierut, J. A., Elbert, M., & Dinnsen, D. A. (1987). A functional analysis of phonological knowledge and generalization learning in misarticulating children. *Journal of Speech and Hearing Research, 30,* 462–479.

Gierut, J. A., & Morisette, M. L. (1995). Triggering a principle of phonemic acquisition. *Clinical Linguistics and Phonetics, 10,* 15–30.

Gierut, J. A., & Neumann, H. J. (1992). Teaching and learning /θ /: A non-confound. *Clinical Linguistics and Phonetics, 6,* 191–200.

Gierut, J. A., Simmerman, C. L., & Neumann, H. J. (1994). Phonemic structures of delayed phonological systems. *Journal of Child Language, 21,* 291–316.

Gildersleeve, C., Davis, B., & Stubbe, E. (1996, November). *When monolingual rules don't apply: Speech development in a bilingual environment.* Paper presented at the annual convention of the American Speech-Language-Hearing Association, Seattle, WA.

Goldstein, B. (1988). *The Evidence of phonological processes of 3 and 4 year old Spanish speakers.* Unpublished master's thesis, Temple University, Philadelphia, PA.

Goldstein, B. (1996). The role of stimulability in the assessment and treatment of Spanish speaking children. *Journal of Communication Disorders, 29,* 299–314.

Goldstein, B., & Iglesias, A. (1996a). Phonological patterns in normally developing Spanish speaking 3 and 4 year olds of Puerto Rican descent. *Language Speech and Hearing Services in the Schools, 27,* 82–90.

Goldstein, B., & Iglesias, A. (1996b). Phonological patterns in Puerto Rican Spanish speaking children with phonological disorders. *Journal of Communication Disorders, 29,* 367–387.

Goldstein, B., & Iglesias, A. (in preparation). The effect of dialect on the analysis of phonological patterns in Spanish-speaking children.

Grunwell, P. (1981). *The nature of phonological disability in children.* New York: Academic Press.

Grunwell, P. (1985). *Phonological assessment of child speech.* London: Nfer-Nelson.

Grunwell, P. (1987). *Clinical phonology* (2nd ed.). London: Croom Helm.

Halle, M. (1959). *The sound pattern of Russian.* The Hague: Mouton.

Halle, M. (1992). Phonological features. In *International Encyclopedia of Linguistics* (Vol. 3, pp. 207–212). Oxford: Oxford University Press.

Halle, M., & Stevens, K. (1979). Some reflections on the theoretical bases of phonetics. In B. Lindblom & S. Ohman (Eds.), *Frontiers of speech communication Research* (pp. 335–349). London: Academic Press.

Hancin-Bhatt, B. (1994). Segment transfer: A consequence of a dynamic system. *Second Language Research, 10*, 241–269.

Hare, G. (1983). Development at 2 years. In J. V. Irwin & S. P. Wong (Eds.), *Phonological development in children: 18–72 months* (pp. 55–88). Carbondale, IL: Southern Illinois University.

Hodson, B. W. (1980). *The assessment of phonological processes*. Danville, IL: Interstate Printers and Publishers.

Hodson, B. W. (1986). *Assessment of phonological processes in Spanish*. San Diego: Los Amigos.

Hodson, B. W., Chin, L., Redmond, B., & Simpson, R. (1983). Phonological evaluation and remediation of speech deviations of a child with a repaired cleft palate: A case study. *Journal of Speech and Hearing Disorders, 48*, 93–98.

Hodson, B. W., & Paden, E. P. (1981). Phonological processes which characterize unintelligible and intelligible speech in early childhood. *Journal of Speech and Hearing Disorders, 46*, 369–373.

Hodson, B. W., & Paden, E. P. (1983). *Targeting intelligible speech*. San Diego, CA: College-Hill Press.

Hodson, B. W., & Paden, E. P. (1991). *Targeting intelligible speech* (2nd ed.). Austin, TX: Pro-Ed.

Hogg, R., & McCully, C. (1987). *Metrical phonology: A coursebook*. New York: Cambridge University Press.

Holden, K. (1972). *Loan-words and phonological systems*. Unpublished doctoral dissertation, University of Texas, Austin, TX.

Holmes, U. T. (1927). The phonology of an English-speaking child. *American Speech, 5*, 219–225.

Householder, F. W. (1971). *Linguistic speculations*. New York: Cambridge University Press.

Hyman, L. M. (1975). *Phonology: Theory and analysis*. New York: Holt, Rinehart and Winston.

Hyman, L. M. (1977). On the nature of linguistic stress. In L. M. Hyman (Ed.), *Studies in stress and accent* (pp. 37–82). Southern California Occasional Papers in Linguistics. Los Angeles: University of Southern California.

Imedadze, N. A. (1967). On the psychological nature of child speech formation under condition of exposure to two languages. *International Journal of Psychology, 2*, 129–132.

Ingram, D. (1976). *Phonological disability in children*. London: Edward Arnold.

Ingram, D. (1978). The production of word-initial fricatives and affricates in normal and linguistically deviant children. In A. Caramazza & E. Zuriff

(Eds.), *Language acquisition and language breakdown* (pp. 63–85). Baltimore, MD: Johns Hopkins University Press.

Ingram, D. (1979). Phonological patterns in the speech of young children. In P. Fletcher & M. Garman (Eds.), *Language acquisition* (pp. 133–149). Cambridge, UK: Cambridge University Press.

Ingram, D. (1981). *Procedures for the phonological analysis of children's language.* Baltimore, MD: University Park Press.

Ingram, D. (1990). Toward a theory of phonological acquisition. In J. Miller, (Ed.), *Research perspectives on language disorders* (pp. 55–72). Boston, MA: College-Hill Press.

Ingram, D. (1992). Early phonological acquisition: A cross-linguistic perspective. In C. A.Ferguson, L. Menn, & C. Stoel-Gammon (Eds.), *Phonological development: Models research, implications* (pp. 17–64). Timonium, MD: York Press.

Ingram, D., & Terselic, N. (1983). Final ingression: A case of deviant child phonology. *Topics in Language Disorders, 3,* 45–50.

Itkonen, T. (1977). Huomita lapsen aanteiston kehitysesta. [Notes on the acquisition of phonology]. *Viritaja, 279–308* [English summary, 304–308].

Jaeger, J. J. (1978). Speech aerodynamics and phonological universals. *Proceedings of the Berkeley Linguistic Society, 4,* 311–329.

Jakobson, R. (1968). *Child language, aphasia, and phonological universals.* The Hague: Mouton.

Jakobson, R., Fant, G., & Halle, M. (1952). *Preliminaries to speech analysis.* (M.I.T. Acoustics Laboratory, Tech. Rep. No. 13.) Boston, MA: M.I.T. Press.

Kahn, D. (1980). *Syllable-based generalizations in English phonology.* New York: Garland.

Katamba, F. (1989). *An introduction to phonology.* London: Longman.

Keating, P. (1990). Coronal places of articulation. In C. Paradis & J. F. Prunet (Eds.), *The special status of coronals* (pp. 29–48). New York: Academic Press.

Kenstowicz, M. (1994). *Phonology in generative grammar.* Cambridge, MA: Blackwell.

Kenstowicz, M., & Kisseberth, C. (1979). *Generative phonology: Description and theory.* New York: Academic Press.

Kent, R. (1984). The psychobiology of speech development: Co-emergence of language and a movement system. *American Journal of Phsiology, 246,* R888–R894.

Khan, L. M.,& Lewis, N. P. (1986). *Khan-Lewis phonological analysis.* Circle Pines, MN: American Guidance Service.

Kiparsky, P. (1982). From cyclic phonology to lexical phonology. In H. van der Hulst & N. Smith (Eds.), *The structure of phonological representation* (pp. 131–175). Dordrecht: Foris.

Kiparsky, P., & Menn, L.(1977). On the acquisition of phonology. In J. MacNamara (Ed.), *Language learning and thought* (pp. 47–78). New York: Academic Press.

Kolaric, R. (1959) Slovenski otroski govor. *Jahrbuch der Philosophischen Fakultat in Novi Sad, 4,* 229–258.

Ladefoged, P. (1993). *A course in phonetics* (3rd ed.). New York: Harcourt Brace Jovanovich.

Lado, R. (1957). *Linguistics across cultures.* Ann Arbor, MI: University of Michigan Press.

Lass, R. (1984). *Phonology.* New York: Cambridge University Press.

Lees, R. (1968). *The phonology of modern standard Turkish.* Bloomington: Indiana University Press.

Leinonen, E. (1991). Functional considerations in phonological assessment of child speech. In M.Yavas (Ed.), *Phonological disorders in children* (pp. 87–120). London: Routledge.

Leonard, L. (1995). Phonological impairment. In P. Fletcher, & B. MacWhinney (Eds.), *The handbook of child language* (pp. 573–602). New York: Blackwell.

Leonard, L., & Brown, B. (1984). The nature and boundaries of phonologic categories: A case study of an unusual phonologic pattern in a language impaired child. *Journal of Speech and Hearing Disorders, 49,* 419–428.

Leonard, L., Schwartz, R., Swanson, L., & Loeb, D. (1987). Some conditions that promote unusual phonological behavior in children. *Clinical Linguistics and Phonetics, 1,* 23–34.

Leopold, W. F. (1947). *Speech development of a bilingual child: A linguist's record: Vol. 1. Vocabulary growth in the first two years.* Evanston, IL: Northwestern University.

Lewis, M. M. (1936). *Infant speech: A study of the beginnings of language.* New York: Harcourt Brace.

Linn , S. C. (1971). Phonetic development of Chinese infants. *Acta Psychologica Taiwanica, 13,* 191–195.

Lisker, L., & Abramson, A. S. (1964). A cross-language study of voicing in initial stops: Acoustical measurements. *Word, 20,* 384–422.

Locke, J. L. (1983). *Phonological acquisition and change.* New York: Academic Press.

Long, M. (1990). Maturational constraints on language development. *Studies in Second Language Acquisition, 12,* 251–285.

Lowe, R. J. (1986). *Assesment link between phonology and articulation.* East Moline, IL: LinguiSystems.

Lowie, W. (1988). *Age and foreign language pronunciation in the classroom.* Unpublished doctoral dissertation, University of Amsterdam, The Netherlands.

Mack, M. (1989). Consonant and vowel perception and production: Early English-French bilinguals and English monolinguals. *Perception and Psychophysics, 46,* 187–200.

Macken, M. A. (1979). Developmental reorganization of phonology: A hierarchy of basic units of acquisition. *Lingua, 49,* 11–49.

Macken, M. A., & Ferguson, C. A. (1983). Cognitive aspects of phonological development: Model, evidence and issue. In K. Nelson (Ed.), *Children's language* (Vol. 4, pp. 256–282). Hillsdale, NJ: Lawrence Erlbaum.

Mackey, W. (1970). Interference, integration and the synchronic fallacy. In J. Alatis (Ed.), *Bilingualism and language contact.* Washinton DC: Georgetown University Press.

Maddieson, I. (1984). *Patterns of sounds.* New York: Cambridge University Press.

Maddieson, I. (1986). The size and structure of phonological inventories. In J. Ohala & J. J. Jaeger (Eds.), *Experimental phonology* (pp. 105–123). Orlando, FL: Academic Press.

Major, R. (1977). Phonological differentiation of a bilingual child. *Ohio State University Working Papers in Linguistics, 22,* 88–122.

Major, R. (1986). Paragoge and degree of foreign accent in Brazilian English. *Second Language Research, 2,* 53–71.

Major, R. (1987). A model for interlanguage phonology. In G. Ioup & S. Weinberger, (Eds.), *Interlanguage phonology: The acquisition of a second language sound system* (pp. 101–124). New York: Newbury House.

Marion, M. J., Sussman, H. M., & Marquardt, T. P. (1993). The perception and production of rhyme in normal and developmentally apraxic children. *Journal of Communication Disorders, 26,* 129–160.

Mason, M., Smith, M., & Hinshaw, M. (1976). *Medida Espanola de articulacion.* San Ysidro, CA: San Ysidro School District.

Maxwell, E. (1979). Competing analyses of a deviant phonology. *Glossa, 13,* 181–213.

Maxwell, E. (1982). *A study of misarticulation from a linguistic perspective.* Unpublished doctoral dissertation, Indiana University, Bloomimgton.

McGregor, K., & Schwartz, R. (1992). Converging evidence for underlying phonological representation in a child who misarticulates. *Journal of Speech and Hearing Research, 35,* 596–603.

McReynolds, L., & Bennett, S. (1972). Distinctive feature generalization in articulation training. *Journal of Speech and Hearing Disorders, 37,* 462–470.

McReynolds, L., & Elbert, M. (1981). Generalization of correct articulation in clusters. *Applied Psycholinguistics, 2,* 119–132.

McReynolds, L., & Engmann, D. (1975). *Distinctive feature analysis of misarticulations.* Baltimore, MD: University Park Press.

Menn, L. (1976). Evidence for an interactionist-discovery theory of child phonology. *Papers and Reports in Child Language Development, 12,* 169–177.

Menn, L. (1978). Phonological units in beginning speech. In A. Bell & J. B. Hooper (Eds.), *Syllables and segments.* Amsterdam: North Holland.

Menn, L. (1983). Development of articulatory, phonetic, and phonological capabilities. In B. Butterworth (Ed.), *Language production* (Vol 2). London: Academic Press.

Menyuk, P. (1968). The role of distinctive features in children's acquisition of phonology. *Journal of Speech and Hearing Research, 11,* 138–146.

Michaels, D. (1973). Sinhalese sound replacements and feature hierarchies. *Linguistics, 170,* 14–22.

Mohring, H. (1938). Lautbildungsschwierigkeit im Deutschen. *Zeitschrift fur Kinderforschung, 47,* 185–235.

Moskowitz, A. I. (1971). *The acquisition of phonology.* Unpublished doctoral dissertation, University of California, Berkeley.

Moskowitz, B. A. (1975). The acquisition of fricatives: A study in phonetics and phonology. *Journal of Phonetics, 3,* 141–150.

Nathan, G. S., Anderson, W., & Budsaba, B. (1987). On the acquisition of aspiration. In G. Ioup & S. Weinberger (Eds.), *Interlanguage phonology: The acquisition of a second language sound system* (pp. 204–212). New York: Newbury House Publishers.

Nettelbladt, U. (1983). *Developmental studies of dysphonology in children.* Lund: CWK Gleerup.

O'Grady, W., Dobrovolsky, M., & Aranoff, M. (1991). *Contemporary linguistics* (2nd ed.). New York: St. Martin's Press.

Oller, D. K. (1980). The emergence of speech sounds in infancy. In G. Yeni-Komshian, J. A. Savanagh, & C. A. Ferguson (Eds.), *Child phonology* (Vol. 1, pp. 93–112). New York: Academic Press.

Olmsted, D. L. (1971). *Out of the mouth of babes: Earliest stages in language learning.* The Hague: Mouton.

Omar, M. K. (1973). *The acquisition of Egyptian Arabic as a native language.* The Hague: Mouton.

Oyama, S. (1976). The sensitive period for the acquisition of a nonnative phonological system. *Journal of Psycho-linguistic Research, 5,* 261–285.

Pacesova, J. (1968). *The development of vocabulary in the child.* Brno: Universita J. E. Purkyne.

Panagos, J., & Prelock, P. (1995). Children's foot capacity for grammatical speech. ASHA Annual Convention Poster. Orlando, FL.

Paolillo, J. (1995). Markedness in the acquisition of English/l/ and /r/. In F. Eckman, D. Highland, P. Lee, J. Milleham, & R. Weber (Eds.), *Second language acquisition theory and pedagogy* (pp. 275–291). Mahwah, NJ: Lawrence Erlbaum.

Paradis, C., & Prunet, J. F. (Eds.). (1992). *Phonetics and phonology: Vol 2: The special status of coronals: internal and external evidence.* San Diego, CA: Academic Press.

Parker, F. (1976). Distinctive features in speech pathology: Phonology or phonemics. *Journal of Speech and Hearing Disorders, 41,* 23–39.

Parucci, R. (1983). *Effects of vowel height on final stops devoicing.* Unpublished master's thesis, University of Maryland, College Park.

Paschall, L. (1983). Development at 18 months. In J. V. Irwin & S. P. Wong (Eds.), *Phonological development in children 18 to 72 months.* Carbondale: Southern Illinois University Press.

Patkowski, M. (1994). The critical age hypothesis in inter-language phonology. In M. Yavas (Ed.), *First and second language phonology* (pp. 205–222). San Diego, CA: Singular Publishing Group.

Penney, G., Fee, E. J., & Dowdle, C. (1994). Vowel assessment and remediation: A case study. *Child Language Teaching and Therapy, 10*, 47–66.

Pike, K. L. (1947). *Phonemics: A technique for reducing language to writing.* Ann Arbor: University of Michigan Publications in Linguistics 3.

Platt, L. J., Andrews, G., Young, M. and Quin, P. (1980). Dysarthria of adult cerebral palsy. II: Phonemic analysis of articulation errors. *Journal of Speech and Hearing Research, 23*, 28–40.

Plevyak, T. (1982). *Vocalic effect on children's final stop devoicing.* Unpublished master's thesis, University of Maryland, College Park.

Pollack, E., & Rees, N. (1972). Disorders of articulation: Some clinical applications of distinctive feature theory. *Journal of Speech and Hearing Disorders, 37*, 451–467.

Pollock, K. E. (1994). Assessment and remediation of vowel misarticulations. *Clinical Communication Disorders, 4*, 23–37.

Pollock, K. E., & Hall, P. K. (1991). An analysis of the vowel misarticulations of five children with developmental apraxia of speech. *Clinical Linguistics and Phonetics, 5*, 207–224.

Poole, I. (1934). Genetic development of articulation of consonant sounds in speech. *Elementary English Review, 11*, 159–161.

Prather, E. M., Hedrick, D. L., & Kern, C. A. (1975). Articulation development in children aged two to four years. *Journal of Speech and Hearing Disorders, 40*, 179–191.

Purschel, H. (1975). *Pause and kadenz: Interferenzerscheinun-gen bei der englischen intonation deutscher sprecher.* Tubingen: Max Niemeyer.

Reynolds, J. (1990). Abnormal vowel patterns: Some data and a hypothesis. *British Journal of Disorders of Communication, 25*, 115–148.

Rice, K., & Avery, P. (1995). Variability in a deterministic model of language acquisition: A theory of segmental elaboration. In J. Archibald (Ed.), *Phonological acquisition and phonological theory* (pp. 23–42). Hillsdale, NJ: Lawrence Erlbaum.

Ritchie, W. (1968) On the explanation of phonic interference. *Language Learning, 18*, 183–197.

Ruder, K., & Bunce, B. (1981). Articulation therapy using distinctive feature analysis to structure the training program: Two case studies. *Journal of Speech and Hearing Disorders, 46*, 59–65.

Ruhlen, M. (1976). *A guide to the languages of the world.* Stanford, CA: Stanford University Press.

Sander, E. (1972). When are speech sounds learned? *Journal of Speech and Hearing Disorders, 37*, 55–63.

Schane, S. A. (1973). *Generative phonology.* Englewood Cliffs, NJ: Prentice-Hall.

Schwartz, R. G., & Leonard, L. B. (1982). Do children pick and choose? An examination of phonological selection and avoidance in early lexical acquisition. *Journal of Child Language, 9*, 319–336.

Schwartz, R., Leonard, L., Loeb, D. F., & Swanson, L. (1987). Attempted sounds are sometimes not: An expanded view of phonological selection and avoidance. *Journal of Child Language, 14*, 411–418.

Scovel, T. (1988). *A time to speak: A psycholinguistic inquiry into critical period for human speech.* New York: Harper and Row.

Selkirk, E. (1982). The syllable. In H. van der Hulst & N. Smith (Eds.), *The structure of phonological representation.* Dordrecht: Foris.

Selkirk, E. (1984). On the major class features and syllable theory. In M. Aranoff & R. Oehrle (Eds.), *Language sound structure: Studies in phonology presented to Morris Halle by his teacher and students.* Cambridge, MA: MIT Press.

Shibomoto, J. S., & Olmsted, D. (1978). Lexical and syllabic patterns in phonological acquisition. *Journal of Child Language, 5,* 417–457.

Shipley, K. G., & McAfee, J. G. (1992). *Assessment in speech-language pathology.* San Diego, CA: Singular Publishing Group.

Shriberg, L., & Kwiatkowski, J. (1980). *Natural process analysis.* New York: John Wiley.

Singh, S., Hayden, M., & Toombs, M. (1981). The role of distinctive features in articulation errors. *Journal of Speech and Hearing Disorders, 46,* 174–183.

Smith, B. L., & Oller, D. K. (1981). A comparative study of premeaningful vocalizations produced by normally developing and Down's syndrome infants. *Journal of Speech and Hearing Disorders, 46,* 46–51.

Smith, B. L., & Stoel-Gammon, C. (1983). A longitudinal study of stop consonant production in normal and Down's syndrome children. *Journal of Speech and Hearing Disorders, 48,* 114–118.

Smith, N. V. (1973). *The acquisition of phonology: A case study.* Cambridge: Cambridge University Press.

Snow, K. (1963). A detailed analysis of articulation responses of "normal" first grade children. *Journal of Speech and Hearing Research, 6,* 277–290.

So, L., & Dodd, B. (1995). The acquisition of phonology by Cantonese-speaking children. *Journal of Child Language, 22,* 473–495.

So, L., & Dodd, B. (1994). Phonologically disordered Contonese-speaking children. *Clinical Linguistics and Phonetics, 8,* 235–255.

Sommerstein, A. (1977). *Modern phonology.* London: Arnold.

Sristava, G. P. (1974). A child's acquisition of Hindi consonants. *Indian Linguistics, 35,* 112–118.

Stampe, D. (1969). The acquisition of phonetic representation. *Papers from the Fifth Regional Meeting of the Chicago Linguistic Society* (pp. 433–444). Chicago, IL: Chicago Linguistic Society.

Stampe, D. (1973). *A dissertation on natural phonology.* Unpublished doctoral dissertation, University of Chicago, Chicago, IL.

Steriade, D. (1987). Redundant values. In A. Bosch, B. Need, & E. Schiller (Eds.), *Papers from the Parasession on Autosegmental and Metrical Phonology* (pp. 339–362). Chicago, IL: Chicago Linguistic Society.

Stevens, K., & Keyser, S. (1989). Primary features and their enhancement in consonants. *Language, 65,* 81–106.

Stevens, K., Keyser, S., & Kawasaki, H. (1986). Toward a phonetic and phonological theory of redundant features. In J. S. Perkell & D. H. Klatt

(Eds.), *Invariance and variability in speech processes* (pp. 426–449). Hillsdale, NJ: Lawrence Erlbaum.

Stockwell, R., & Bowen, D. (1983). *The sounds of English and Spanish.* The Hague: Mouton.

Stoel-Gammon, C. (1984, July). *Phonetic inventories, 15–24 months: A longitudinal study.* Paper presented at the Third International Congress for the Study of Child Language, Austin, TX.

Stoel-Gammon, C. (1985). Phonetic inventories, 15–24 months: A longitudinal study. *Journal of Speech and Hearing Research, 28,* 505–512.

Stoel-Gammon, C. (1990). Issues in phonological development and disorders. In J. Miller (Ed.), *Research on child language disorders: A decade of progress* (pp. 255–265). Austin, TX: Pro-Ed.

Stoel-Gammon, C., & Cooper, J. (1981, August). *Individual differences in early phonological and lexical development.* Paper presented at the Second International Congress for the Study of Child Language, Vancouver, BC.

Stoel-Gammon, C., & Dunn, C. (1985). *Normal and disordered phonology in children.* Austin, TX: Pro-Ed.

Stoel-Gammon, C., & Herrington, P. B. (1990). Vowel systems of normally developing and phonologically disordered children. *Clinical Linguistics and Phonetics, 4,* 145–160.

Stoel-Gammon, C., & Stemberger, J. (1994). Consonant harmony and phonological underspecification in child speech. In M. Yavas (Ed.), *First and second language phonology* (pp. 63–80). San Diego, CA: Singular Publishing Group.

Tahta, S., Wood, M., & Lowenthal, K. (1981). Foreign accents: Factors relating to transfer of accent from the first language to the second language. *Language and Speech, 24,* 265–272.

Templin, M. C. (1957). *Certain language skills in children: Their development and interrelationships.* Institute of Child Welfare Monographs, Vol. 26. Minneapolis: University of Minnesota Press.

Thompson, I. (1991). Foreign accents revisited: The English pronunciation of Russian immigrants. *Language Learning, 41,* 177–204.

Tiffin, B. (1974). *The intelligibility of Nigerian English.* Unpublished doctoral dissertation, University of London.

Toombs, M., Singh, S., & Hayden, M. (1981). Markedness of features in the articulatory substitutions of children. *Journal of Speech and Hearing Disorders, 46,* 184–191.

Treimann, R. (1988). The internal structure of syllable. In G. Carlson & M. Tanenhaus (Eds.), *Linguistic structure in language processing.* Dordrecht, The Netherlands: Kluwer.

Tyler, A., Edwards, M. L., & Saxman, J. (1990). Acoustic validation of phonological knowledge and its relationship to treatment. *Journal of Speech and Hearing Disorders, 55,* 251–261.

Vance, T. (1987). *An introduction to Japanese phonology.* Albany: State University of New York Press.

Van Els, T., & DeBot, K.(1987). The role of intonation in foreign accent. *Modern Language Journal, 71*, 147–155.

Vanvik, A. (1971). The phonetic-phonemic development of a Norwegian child. *Norsk Tidsskrift Sprogvienskap, 24*, 269–325.

Velten, H. V. (1943). The growth of phonemic and lexical patterns in infant language. *Language, 19*, 281–292.

Vihman, M. M. (1971). On the acquisition of Estonian. *Papers and Reports on Child Language Development, 3*, 51–94.

Vihman, M. M. (1976). From pre-speech to speech: On early phonology. *Papers and Reports on Child Language Development, 12*, 230–243.

Vihman, M. M. (1978). Consonant harmony: Its scope and function in child language. In J. H. Greenberg (Ed.), *Universals of human language* (Vol. 2, pp. 281–334). Stanford, CA: Stanford University Press.

Vihman, M. M. (1981). Phonology and the development of the lexicon: Evidence from children's errors. *Journal of Child Language, 8*, 239–264.

Vihman, M. M. (1985). Language differentiation by the bilingual infant. *Journal of Child Language, 12*, 297–324.

Vihman, M. M. (1992). Early syllables and the construction of phonology. In C. A. Ferguson, L. Menn, & C. Stoel-Gammon (Eds.), *Phonological development: Models, research, implications* (pp. 393–422). Timonium, MD: York Press.

Vihman, M. M., Macken, M. A., Miller, R., & Simmons, H. (1981, December). *From babbling to speech: A reassessment of the continuity issue.* Paper presented at the annual meeting of the Linguistic Society of America, New York, NY.

Vincent, N. (1986). Constituency and syllable structure. In J. Durand (Ed.), *Dependency and non-linear phonology*. London: Croom Helm.

Vogel, I. (1975). One system or two: An analysis of a two-year old Romanian-English bilingual's phonology. *Papers and Reports on Child Language Development, 9*, 43–62.

Walsh, H. (1974). On certain practical inadequacies of distinctive feature systems. *Journal of Speech and Hearing Disorders, 39*, 32–43.

Waterson, N. (1971). Child phonology: A prosodic view. *Journal of Linguistics, 7*, 179–211.

Waterson, N. (1978). Growth and complexity in phonological development. In N. Waterson & C. Snow (Eds.), *The development of communication* (pp. 415–442). New York: John Wiley.

Watson, I. (1991). Phonological processing in two languages. In E. Bialystok (Ed.), *Language processing in bilingual children* (pp. 25–48). Cambridge, MA: Cambridge University Press.

Webster, P. E., & Plante, A. S. (1992). Effects of phonological impairment on word, syllable, and phoneme segmentation and reading. *Language, Speech, and Hearing Services in Schools, 23*, 176–182.

Weinberger, S. H. (1994). Functional and phonetic constraints on second language phonology. In M. Yavas (Ed.), *First and second language phonology* (pp. 283–302). San Diego, CA: Singular Publishing Group.

Weiner, F. (1979). *Phonological process analysis.* Baltimore, MD: University Park Press.

Weiner, F. (1981). Treatment of phonological disability using the methods of phonological contrasts: Two case studies. *Journal of Speech and Hearing Disorders, 46,* 97–103.

Weinreich, U. (1953). *Languages in contact.* The Hague: Mouton.

Wellman, B. L., Case, I. M., Mengert, I. B., & Bradbury, D. E. (1931). Speech sounds of young children. *University of Iowa Studies in Child Welfare, 2,* (5).

Williams, A. L., & Dinnsen, D. A. (1987). A problem of allophonic variation in a speech disordered child. *Innovations in Linguistic Education, 5,* 85–90.

Williams, L. (1977). The perception of stop consonant voicing by Spanish-English bilinguals. *Perception and Psychophysics, 21,* 289–297.

Willems, N. (1982). *English intonation from a Dutch point of view.* Dordrecht: Foris Publications.

Wilson, F. (1966). Efficacy of speech therapy with educable mentally retarded children. *Journal of Speech and Hearing Research, 9,* 423–433.

Wode, H. (1981). *Learning a second language: I. An integrated view of language acquisition.* Tubingen, Germany: Narr.

Wolk, L. (1990). *An investigation of young children who stutter and exhibit phonological difficulties.* Unpublished doctoral dissertation. Syracuse University, Syracuse, NY.

Yavas, M. (1988). Padroes na aquisicao da fonologia do portugues. *Letras de Hoje, 74,* 7–30

Yavas, M.(1991). *Phonological disorders in children: Theory, research and practice.* London: Routledge.

Yavas, M. (1994a). Extreme regularity in phonological disorder: A case study. *Clinical Linguistics and Phonetics, 8,* 127–139.

Yavas, M. (1994b). *First and second language phonology.* San Diego, CA: Singular Publishing Group.

Yavas, M. (1995). Phonological selectivity in the first fifty words of a bilingual child. *Language and Speech, 38,* 189–202.

Yavas, M. (1996). Differences in voice onset time in early and later Spanish-English bilinguals. In J. Jensen & A. Roca (Eds.), *Spanish in contact: Issues in bilingualism.* Somerville, MA: Cascadilla Press.

Yavas, M. (1997a). Feature enhancement and phonological acquisition. *Clinical Linguistics and Phonetics, 11,* 153–172.

Yavas, M. (1997b). The effects of vowel height and place of articulation in interlanguage final stop devoicing. *International Review of Applied Linguistics in Language Teaching, 35,* 115–125.

Yavas, M., & Goldstein, B. (in press). Speech sound differences and disorders in first and second language acquisition: Theoretical issues and clinical applications. *American Journal of Speech and Language Pathology.*

Yavas, M., & Hernandorena, C. M. (1991). Systematic sound preference in phonological disorders: A case study. *Journal of Communication Disorders, 4,* 79–87.

Yavas, M., & Lamprecht, R. (1988). Processes and intelligibility in disordered phonology. *Clinical Linguistics and Phonetics, 2,* 329–345.

INDEX

tense/lax, 27–28
cardinal vowels, 28–29
-consonant substitution interaction,
    288–289
English
  distinctive feature matrix, 76
  International Phonetic
    Association (IPA) system, 13,
    28, 29
epenthesis, 107–108, 112
error overview, 157
haplology, 106
loss (phonological processes), 106
naturalness, 177–179
syncope, 106
transcription variation, 34–35

vowel reduction rule, 236

W

Writing, 245–246
  literacy, and phonemic awareness,
    58–59
  phonemics, 54–55

Y

Yoruba language, 200

Z

Zulu language, 21, 22